Signs and Symptoms in
PEDIATRICS
Ready Reckoner

Signs and Symptoms in
PEDIATRICS
Ready Reckoner

Baldev Prajapati MD DPed FIAP MNAMS
Professor and Head
Department of Pediatrics
GCS Medical College
Hospital and Research Centre
Ahmedabad, Gujarat, India

Foreword
Yeshwant K Amdekar

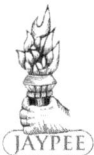

JAYPEE BROTHERS MEDICAL PUBLISHERS
The Health Sciences Publisher
New Delhi | London

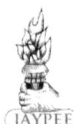 **Jaypee Brothers Medical Publishers (P) Ltd**

Headquarters

Jaypee Brothers Medical Publishers (P) Ltd
EMCA House, 23/23-B
Ansari Road, Daryaganj
New Delhi 110 002, India
Landline: +91-11-23272143, +91-11-23272703
+91-11-23282021, +91-11-23245672
Email: jaypee@jaypeebrothers.com

Corporate Office

Jaypee Brothers Medical Publishers (P) Ltd
4838/24, Ansari Road, Daryaganj
New Delhi 110 002, India
Phone: +91-11-43574357
Fax: +91-11-43574314
Email: jaypee@jaypeebrothers.com

Overseas Office

JP Medical Ltd
83 Victoria Street, London
SW1H 0HW (UK)
Phone: +44 20 3170 8910
Fax: +44 (0)20 3008 6180
Email: info@jpmedpub.com

Website: www.jaypeebrothers.com
Website: www.jaypeedigital.com

© 2023, Jaypee Brothers Medical Publishers

The views and opinions expressed in this book are solely those of the original contributor(s)/author(s) and do not necessarily represent those of editor(s) or publisher of the book.

All rights reserved. No part of this publication may be reproduced, stored or transmitted in any form or by any means, electronic, mechanical, photocopying, recording or otherwise, without the prior permission in writing of the publishers.

All brand names and product names used in this book are trade names, service marks, trademarks or registered trademarks of their respective owners. The publisher is not associated with any product or vendor mentioned in this book.

Medical knowledge and practice change constantly. This book is designed to provide accurate, authoritative information about the subject matter in question. However, readers are advised to check the most current information available on procedures included and check information from the manufacturer of each product to be administered, to verify the recommended dose, formula, method and duration of administration, adverse effects and contraindications. It is the responsibility of the practitioner to take all appropriate safety precautions. Neither the publisher nor the author(s)/editor(s) assume any liability for any injury and/or damage to persons or property arising from or related to use of material in this book.

This book is sold on the understanding that the publisher is not engaged in providing professional medical services. If such advice or services are required, the services of a competent medical professional should be sought.

Every effort has been made where necessary to contact holders of copyright to obtain permission to reproduce copyright material. If any have been inadvertently overlooked, the publisher will be pleased to make the necessary arrangements at the first opportunity.

Inquiries for bulk sales may be solicited at: jaypee@jaypeebrothers.com

Signs and Symptoms in Pediatrics—Ready Reckoner

First Edition: **2023**

ISBN: 978-93-5696-038-1

Dedication

Affectionately dedicated to my Granddaughter, Mishika
And
My beloved teacher, Dr (Mrs) AB Desai
who taught me the art of Pediatrics.

Foreword

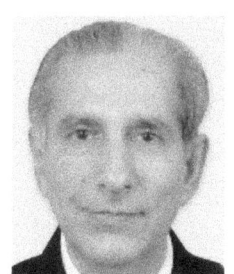

I am happy to write a foreword for the book titled *"Signs and Symptoms in Pediatrics—Ready Reckoner"* authored by Dr Baldev Prajapati – an academician of high standards and teacher par excellence. It is not a textbook or a book on clinical diagnosis. The book presents a discussion of various symptoms and signs in a unique format that includes the basics as well as various causes of each sign/symptom, ranging from common to not-so-uncommon issues met in routine practice. The selection of signs and symptoms included in this book bears the stamp of experience.

Physical signs are often noticed, but not analyzed and interpreted. It is true about not only the obvious signs such as lymphadenopathy or hepatosplenomegaly but also many minor observations. The author has analyzed many minor signs that include gynecomastia, unequal pupils, strabismus or macroglossia and many others. Included are also some pictorial presentations of abnormal facies, the shapes of the chest and umbilical abnormalities.

Each symptom may represent varied causes that demand detailed knowledge which is provided in this book. It is not rare to face symptoms that are difficult to analyze and interpret such as weight loss, oral ulcers, syncope, halitosis, teething issues and many others. Readers will find them useful.

Medicine is a science, full of complexities that are difficult to grasp and remember. This book fills the gap by providing useful material for the reader and a ready-reckoner so as not to miss the probable cause of the presenting signs or symptoms. I am sure this book will enrich our knowledge and it should find a place on our table for instant reference. It will enhance our diagnostic efficiency. I wish the book a great success.

Yeshwant K Amdekar
MD DCH FIAP
Former Professor
Grant Medical College, JJ Hospital, Mumbai
Consultant, SRCC Children's Hospital
Mumbai, Maharashtra, India

Preface

The current modern era of advanced technology has contributed significantly in the field of medicine. But, technology does not absolve the clinician of the need to make a clinical diagnosis, on the contrary, it imposes a great responsibility of using technology judiciously and interpreting it wisely. Therefore, the importance of history and physical examination cannot be overemphasized in the evaluation of sick infants and children. Collecting information in details regarding symptoms and signs and its analysis forms the basis of clinical evaluation. During bed side teaching in my daily round and discussing with students regarding signs and symptoms, I observed the felt need of students for a book exclusively on signs and symptoms in pediatrics. There are several books on clinical examination and voluminous textbooks in pediatrics, but for one or the other reason, they are not able to deal with this important aspect in a reasonably comprehensive way. I started writing a manuscript on particular sign or symptom, discussed in the round and circulating in the groups of students and practicing pediatricians. They felt quite useful in daily practice. At the end of two years, the compilation of these topics was huge. Then, it was decided to arrange them in the format of a book for wide circulation and use.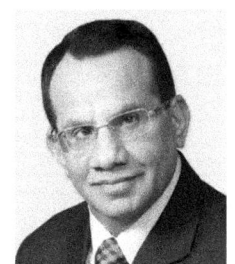

The book has been written in a simplified manner. It covers 102 common pediatric signs and symptoms. Each sign and symptom is elaborated methodologically. It starts with a short introduction which includes the meaning of sign and symptom, prevalence in practice, common points to be covered during collecting information from parents, analysis of data and probable etiology. Common causes for each sign and symptom are enlisted. They are arranged in the sequence of seeing on the practice to highlight their clinical importance and not grouped as system wise. The most common causes are kept first, then less common and rare ones at the last. Very rare causes are not included in the list to maintain the interest of the reader and to avoid undue length of the manuscript. Plenty of tables and clinical photographs are included for easy retrieval of information and good visual impression. Most of clinical photographs are of our own patients.

The book is addressed primarily to undergraduate, MD and DNB students, but it will also be a ready-reckoner for quick and accurate diagnosis for the practicing pediatricians.

I am deeply indebted to living legend, very eminent and most popular pediatric teacher of our country, Dr Yeshwant K Amdekar Sir who taught me the art of clinical pediatrics and teaching skills, for writing the Foreword for this book and his blessings.

My this book is affectionately dedicated to my lovely granddaughter, Mishika. No amount of words can express my gratitude to my wife, Dr (Mrs) Rajal Prajapati, my daughters, Dr Aakanksha and Dr Aalapi and my son-in-laws, Dr Mukund and Mr Sumit who allowed me ample time for completing this book.

Baldev Prajapati

Acknowledgements

I would like to thank the staff of Aakanksha Children Hospital, Ahmedabad, Gujarat, India for their help in preparing this book.

My special thanks to Nisarg Shah who is sincere and dedicated in his work, for type setting and composing.

I also like to thank Shri Jitendar P Vij (Group Chairman), Mr Ankit Vij (Managing Director), Mr MS Mani (Group President), Ms Chetna Malhotra (Senior Director—Professional Publishing, Marketing and Business Development), Ms Pooja Bhandari (Production Head), Ms Rajni D Chauhan (Development Editor), and the staff of M/s Jaypee Brothers Medical Publishers (P) Ltd, New Delhi, India for their generous help in all possible ways to bring out this book.

Contents

1. Abdominal Mass 1
2. Abnormal Shape of Skull 4
3. Altered Sensorium 6
4. Anterior Fontanel 10
5. Ascites 12
6. Ataxia 14
7. Basics of Fever 17
8. Bleeding Manifestations 23
9. Bow Legs 27
10. Bowel Sounds 29
11. Burning Micturition 31
12. Cataracts 32
13. Chest Pain 35
14. Chest Shape 37
15. Clubbing 40
16. Constipation 42
17. Cough 46
18. Crying Child 48
19. Cyanosis 50
20. Delayed Development 52
21. Diarrhea 56
22. Distention of Abdomen 59
23. Dysmorphism 61
24. Dysphagia 65
25. Dyspnea 67

26. Earache (Otalgia) 69
27. Edema 71
28. Encopresis 74
29. Enuresis 76
30. Epistaxis 78
31. Excessive Sweating (Hyperhidrosis) 80
32. Exophthalmos (Proptosis) 82
33. Eye Discharge 84
34. Facial Paralysis/Weakness 85
35. Facies 87
36. Failure to Thrive 92
37. Fatigue 97
38. Feeding Issues 99
39. Fever of Short Duration 101
40. Fever with Skin Rash 105
41. Fever without Focus 119
42. Floppy Infant 124
43. Gait Disorders 127
44. Growth Charts 131
45. Gynecomastia 143
46. Halitosis 145
47. Headache 147
48. Hearing Loss 150
49. Hematuria 152
50. Hemoptysis 154
51. Hepatomegaly 156
52. Hepatosplenomegaly 159

53.	Hoarseness of Voice 161
54.	Hypertension 163
55.	Hypothermia 169
56.	Impairment of Vision and Blindness 170
57.	Inability to Move a Limb 172
58.	Jaundice 174
59.	Lower Gastrointestinal Bleeding 178
60.	Lymphadenopathy 180
61.	Macrocephaly 182
62.	Macroglossia 184
63.	Microcephaly 185
64.	Movement Disorders 187
65.	Neck Masses 190
66.	Nuchal Rigidity 193
67.	Nystagmus 195
68.	Obesity 197
69.	Odynophagia 201
70.	Oral Ulcers 202
71.	Other Clinical Signs 205
72.	Otorrhea (Ear Discharge) 214
73.	Pallor (Anemia) 215
74.	Papilledema 220
75.	Parotid Gland Swelling 222
76.	Pica 223
77.	Pollakiuria (Increased Frequency of Micturition) 224
78.	Polydipsia 226
79.	Polyphagia 227

- 80. Pruritus 228
- 81. Ptosis 229
- 82. Pulse Rate—Abnormality 231
- 83. Pyrexia of Unknown Origin 234
- 84. Recurrent Abdominal Pain 238
- 85. Salivation Disorders 241
- 86. Scrotal Swelling 243
- 87. Seizures 244
- 88. Short Stature 247
- 89. Splenomegaly 251
- 90. Strabismus 253
- 91. Stridor 255
- 92. Syncope 257
- 93. Tall Stature 260
- 94. Teething and Disorders of Teeth 263
- 95. Toeing In 265
- 96. Toeing Out 267
- 97. Umbilicus—Abnormalities 268
- 98. Unequal Pupils 271
- 99. Upper Gastrointestinal Bleeding 273
- 100. Urticaria (Hives) 275
- 101. Vomiting 276
- 102. Weight Loss 279

Index *281*

CHAPTER 1

Abdominal Mass

INTRODUCTION

Abdominal mass, lump, or swelling is a difficult problem in pediatric practice. The adequate clinical work-up is essential before submitting the patient for various investigations to arrive at the precise diagnosis and further management.

Any organ or tissue is capable of developing into a mass. The spectrum of affection includes dilated hollow viscus, inflammatory mass, benign or metastatic, cystic or solid tumors.

Whenever a mass is palpable in the abdomen, one should try to describe the mass with reference to following points:

- Age of appearance of a mass
- Site (may indicate organ of its origin)
- Origin (parietal or intra-abdominal)
- Size
- Shape (round, elongated, irregular)
- Margins (well-defined or ill-defined)
- Surface (smooth or nodular)
- Consistency (cystic, soft, firm, and hard)
- Mobility (with respiration)
- Ballotability
- Presence of signs of inflammation
- Associated signs and symptoms.

AGE-SPECIFIC ABDOMINAL MASSES

Age	Nonmalignant	Malignant
Neonate	• Distended urinary bladder • Unilateral or bilateral hydronephrosis • Multicystic kidney • Horse shoe kidney	• Neuroblastoma • Hepatoblastoma • Wilms tumor • Extragonadal germ cell tumor
1 month–2 years	• Intussusceptions • Choledochal cyst • Appendicular abscess • Hydronephrosis • Multicystic kidney disease	• Neuroblastoma • Wilms tumor • Teratoma
>2 years	• Hepatomegaly and splenomegaly (due to infections, infiltrative, and storage diseases) • Appendicular abscess • Trichobezoar	• Hepatosplenomegaly (leukemia) • Lymphoma • Wilms tumor • Neuroblastoma • Histiocytosis

DIFFERENTIATION ACCORDING TO LOCATION OF MASS

Abdominal Quadrants

- *Right hypochondrium:*
  - Hepatic in origin
  - Enlarged gall bladder
  - Choledochal cyst
  - Subphrenic abscess
- *Epigastrium:*
  - Congenital hypertrophic pyloric stenosis
  - Enlarged left lobe of liver
  - Pseudopancreatic cyst
  - Aortic aneurysm
- *Left hypochondrium:*
  - Enlarged spleen
  - Trichobezoar
- *Right and left lumbar regions:*
  - Hydronephrosis
  - Adrenal mass
- *Umbilical region:*
  - Umbilical hernia
  - Umbilical polyp
  - Umbilical granuloma
  - Congenital omphalocele
  - Gastroschisis
  - Abscess of rectus sheath
  - Mesenteric cyst
- *Right iliac fossa:*
  - Appendicular abscess
  - Intussusception
  - Tuberculous lump
  - Lymphoma of ileocecal region
  - Inguinal hernia
  - Undescended testis (inguinal region)
  - Psoas abscess
- *Left iliac fossa:*
  - Fecal mass
  - Hirschsprung disease
  - Inguinal hernia
  - Undescended testis (inguinal region)
  - Psoas abscess
- *Hypogastirum:* Urinary bladder.

How to Confirm Whether the Mass is Parietal or Intra-abdominal?

- *Straight leg raising test:* The child is asked to raise his extended legs in supine lying-down position and see whether the mass decreases or disappears (intra-abdominal) or becomes prominent (parietal).
- Ask the child to lift his shoulders off the couch while you are pressing firmly against the forehead. You can ask him to raise both extended legs from the couch. If the swelling becomes less prominent or disappears, it indicates intra-abdominal

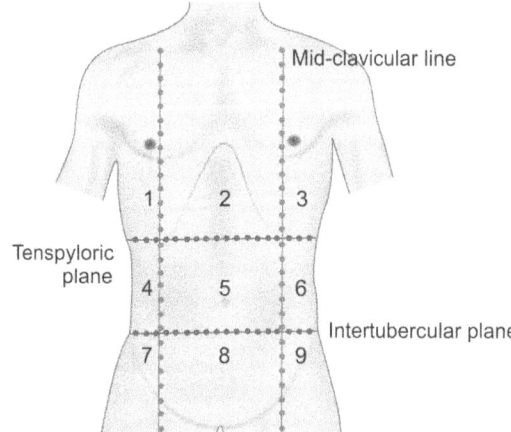

Mid-clavicular line
Tenspyloric plane
Intertubercular plane

1. Right hypochondrium
2. Epigastrium
3. Left hypochondrium
4. Right flank
5. Umbilical
6. Left flank
7. Right groin
8. Pubic
9. Left groin

mass. If it becomes more prominent, it is parietal (in the abdominal wall) mass.

Abdominal Parietal Mass

- Hematoma
- Abscess
- Lipoma
- Hernias
- Seromas
- Metastasis.

ASSOCIATED SYMPTOMS AND SIGNS DIFFERENTIATING ABDOMINAL MASSES

- *Hypertension:* Renal or suprarenal tumor (Wilms tumor, neuroblastoma)
- *Jaundice:* Obstruction to biliary system, choledochal cyst, cholangitis
- *Fever, right lower quadrant mass:* Appendicular abscess, tuberculous mass
- *Nonbilious, projectile vomiting in an infant:* Congenital hypertrophic pyloric stenosis
- *Colicky abdominal pain, bloody diarrhea:* Intussusception
- *Hepatic mass:* Hepatoblastoma, hemangioma
- *Splenomegaly and hematemesis:* Portal hypertension
- *Urinary symptoms:* Hydronephrosis, renal cystic disease
- *Sick appearance, pallor, prolonged fever, cachexia, bleeding tendency:* Leukemia, malignant mass, kala-azar
- A swelling which is firmly adherent to the surrounding structures and is not mobile at all may be a retroperitoneal mass, malignancy, or chronic inflammation.
- Presence of impulse on coughing indicates hernia.
- A renal mass is ballotable.
- Signs of inflammation like redness, induration, warmness, etc. should be noted.
- A strangulated hernia may present as an inflammatory inguinal swelling with severe abdominal pain.

Abnormal Shape of Skull

CHAPTER 2

INTRODUCTION

The shape of the skull is determined by the internal forces, external forces, and at time of closure of the cranial sutures.

CAUSES OF ABNORMAL SHAPE OF SKULL (HEAD) (FIG. 1)

- *Caput succedaneum:* It is the fluid collection in subcutaneous plane over the scalp. It is soft, boggy, and swelling on the presenting part of the head. It is not restricted by structural lines. It is present at birth and usually disappears within 24 hours.
- *Cephalohematoma:* It is the collection of blood under periosteum and is soft and cystic on palpation. It does not cross the suture lines. It appears 24-48 hours after birth and may persist for 4-6 weeks. From soft swelling, it becomes firm and hard in consistency. It may take few months to disappear. It should not be aspirated. It may be responsible for exaggeration of physiological jaundice.
- *Scaphocephaly (dolichocephaly):* Anteroposteriorly skull is elongated due to premature fusion of sagittal suture.
- *Brachycephaly:* Skull is flattened anteroposteriorly (short and square skull) due to premature closure of coronal suture.
- *Plagiocephaly:* Flattening on one side of the skull, usually positional, but it may be due to premature closure of coronal suture on that side.
- *Oxycephaly (towering of skull):* Elongation of the skull like a tower due to premature closure of sagittal and coronal sutures
- *Trigonocephaly:* Positioned skull due to premature closure of metopic suture

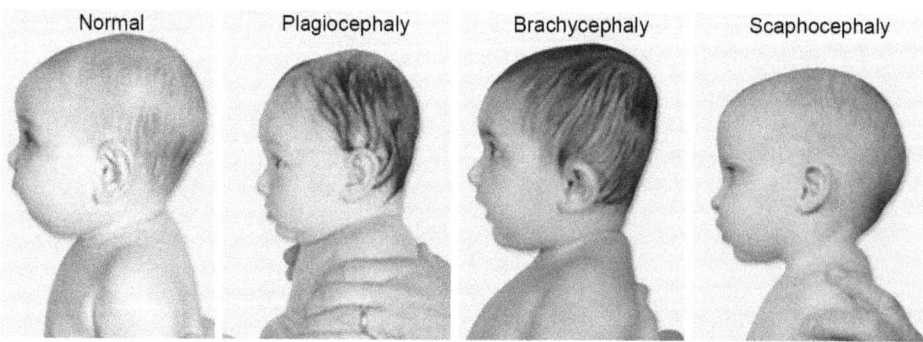

Fig. 1: Normal and abnormal shapes of skull.

- *Macrocephaly:*
  - Neurofibromatosis
  - Achondroplasia
  - Soto's syndrome
- Hydrocephalus
- Microcephaly
- *Craniostenosis:*
  - Apert syndrome
  - Crouzon syndrome
  - Carpenter syndrome
- Mucopolysaccharidosis
- Rickets
- Chronic hemolytic anemia (thalassemia major)
- Forehead bowing (large lateral ventricles)
- Occipital bowing (Dandy–Walker syndrome)
- Bitemporal widening (subdural hematoma)
- Cranial meningocele.

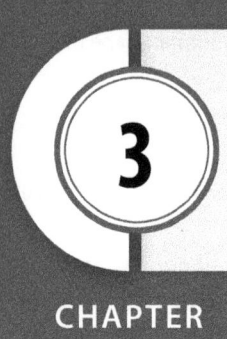

CHAPTER 3

Altered Sensorium

INTRODUCTION

- Altered sensorium is a commonly encountered symptom in pediatric practice. The causes may range from easily reversible (such as hypoglycemia) to relatively permanent (such as stroke) and from benign (such as drug intoxication) to potentially life-threatening (such as meningoencephalitis, hepatic encephalopathy, etc.).
- Consciousness is defined as awareness regarding external as well as internal milieu. It has two components—arousability (wakefulness) and awareness.
- Altered sensorium is described as impairment in arousal and awareness.
- Arousal or wakefulness is a function of ascending reticular activating system, a neuronal network running from the brain stem to thalamus to the cerebral cortex. Arousal is described in terms of whether the sleep-wake cycle is preserved or not. Absence of sleep-wake cycle indicates disruption of ascending reticular activating system. The best example of this disorder is hepatic encephalopathy.
- *Awareness can be assessed differently in different age groups:*
  - Awareness in older children is expressed as interest in surroundings, recognition of parents, indication for bowel or bladder needs, and indication for hunger.
  - Awareness in infants is understood in terms of his behavior. Consolability of child, eye contact with mother, indication for food, interest in toys, etc., are components of behavior of the child to assess his awareness.
- *Cognition* is affected in a child with altered sensorium. Cognitive functions mean the construction of thought process that includes remembering, problem solving, and decision making. It evolves through childhood to adolescence.
- If the levels of arousal are reduced, then awareness is also reduced. One cannot evaluate awareness in an unarousable child.
- Orientation cannot be evaluated properly in children below the age of 5 years. The assessment of orientation should be age-sensitive and questions should be tailored for patient's age:
  - During the first 6 months, the best verbal response is cry.
  - After 1 year, recognizable sounds may be produced.
  - A 3-4 years old alert child should be able to tell his name and gender and identify his parents.

CLINICAL APPROACH IN A CHILD WITH ALTERED SENSORIUM

- Quick evaluation of cerebral cortex and brainstem
- AVPU pediatric response scale
- Glasgow Coma Scale (GCS)

- Body posture
- Doll's eye phenomenon (oculocephalic reflex)
- Pupillary response to light.

Quick Evaluation of Level of Consciousness

- *Consciousness:* Awareness regarding external as well as internal milieu.
- *Drowsy:* Arousable with light stimuli, responding appropriately for some time.
- *Stupor:* Arousable with painful stimuli, remains awake till stimulus is applied, goes to original status as soon as stimulus is removed.
- *Semiconscious:* Nonspecific response to only deep painful stimuli.
- *Unconsciousness:* No response to any stimulus.
- *Coma:* Prolonged stage of unconsciousness. Coma may be followed by vegetative state.
- *Vegetative state:*
  - A vegetative state, or unaware and unresponsive state, is a specific neurological diagnosis in which a person has functioning brainstem but no consciousness or cognitive function. It is also called as post-coma unresponsiveness.
  - It is classified as a permanent (persistent) vegetative state some months (3 months in the US and 6 months in the UK) after a nontraumatic brain injury or 1 year after a traumatic injury.
  - Cerebral cortical functions (e.g., communication, thinking, purposeful movement, etc.) are lost, while brainstem functions (e.g., breathing, maintaining circulation, and hemodynamic stability, etc.) are preserved. Eye opening, occasional vocalization (e.g., crying, laughing), maintaining normal sleep patterns, and spontaneous nonpurposeful movements are often intact.
  - Pain is imparted by a strong pinch, applying pressure over the supratrochlear notch on the medial end of upper margin of orbit, on the sternum, on the finger nail with squeezing big toe, etc.

AVPU Pediatric Response Scale

A *Alert:* Awake, active, appropriately responsive
V *Voice:* Voice responsiveness
P *Pain:* Pain responsiveness
U *Unresponsiveness:* No response to any stimuli.

Glasgow Coma Scale

The name "Glasgow" is derived from the name of a town in Scotland, where this scale was devised.

Parameter	*Glasgow coma scale*
Eye opening	
Spontaneous	4
Response to speech	3
Response to pain	2
Nil	1
Best motor response	
Obeys commands	6
Localized pain	5
Withdrawal of limb	4
Flexion to pain	3
Extension to pain	2
Nil	1
Best verbal response	
Oriented	5
Confused	4
Inappropriate words	3
Incomprehensible sounds	2
Nil	1

Body Posture

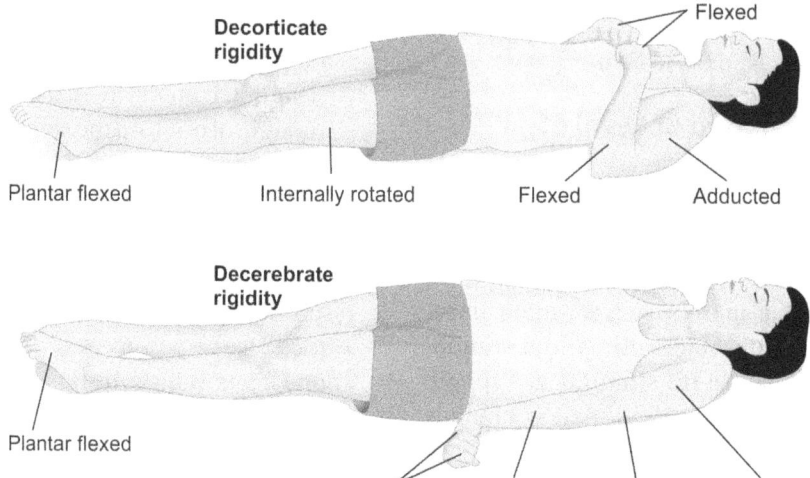

- *Decorticate rigidity:*
  - Abnormal flexor response
  - Indicates lack of cerebral control over brainstem
  - Prognosis is favorable.
- *Decerebrate rigidity:*
  - Abnormal extensor response
  - Lesions in diencephalon, midbrain, or pons
  - Prognosis is not favorable.

Doll's Eye Phenomenon (Oculocephalic reflex)

- The patient is placed in supine and head is suddenly turned toward either side. The patient's eyes lag behind like a doll; there is conjugate deviation of the eyes toward the opposite side.
- Present in normal newborn, in coma, and with impairment of optic fixation
- No importance in a conscious patient
- Absence of doll's eye phenomenon in a comatose child is indicative of damage to brainstem or raised intracranial pressure (ICP).
- Presence of Doll's eye phenomenon in a comatose child is indicative of intact brainstem; lesion is due to cortical lesion.

Pupillary Response to Light

Pupil	Lesion/Dysfunction
Pinpoint (<2 mm)	Pontine, cerebellar
Small (2–3 mm)	Medullary, metabolic (opiates, barbiturates, phenothiazines)
Midsize (5–7 mm)	Midbrain
Dilated, nonreactive	Diffuse damage
Unilateral dilated, nonreactive (unequal pupils)	Uncal herniation

COMMON CAUSES OF ALTERED SENSORIUM

- *Metabolic:*
  - Hypoglycemia
  - Hyponatremia
  - Hypernatremia
  - Diabetic ketoacidosis
  - Inborn errors of metabolism

- Hypoxia
- Hypoperfusion (shock)
■ *Infections:*
  - Bacterial meningitis
  - Tuberculous meningitis (TBM)
  - Encephalitis
■ *Vascular causes:*
  - Cardiovascular (CV) stroke
  - Intracranial hemorrhage
  - Hypertensive encephalopathy
  - Ischemic encephalopathy
■ *Increased intracranial pressure:*
  - Hydrocephalus
  - Space-occupying lesions
■ *Seizures:*
  - Status epilepticus
  - Postictal state
  - Epileptic encephalopathy
■ *Systemic diseases:*
  - Hepatic encephalopathy
  - Uremic encephalopathy
■ *Trauma:*
  - Subdural effusion
  - Intracranial hematomas
  - Diffuse axonal injury
■ *Miscellaneous:*
  - *Toxins (drugs):* Opioids, barbiturates, alcohol, lead poisoning, snake bite, and carbon monoxide poisonous
  - Autoimmune encephalitis
  - Wernicke's encephalopathy
  - *Endocrinal causes:* Myxedema, adrenal insufficiency
  - Hypothermia
  - Heat stroke.

Anterior Fontanel

INTRODUCTION

A neonate has normally six fontanels—anterior, posterior, two mastoid, and two sphenoid, but only anterior and posterior fontanel (PF) are palpable.

- Examination of anterior fontanel (AF) and PF is an integral part of physical examination in infants and young children. One should never miss it.
- Observations should be made whether fontanels are open/close, small/large/normal, bulging/at level/sunken, pulsatile/non pulsatile, etc.
- The AF should be palpated when the infant is quite and sitting or held up right with the head lifted up. A bulging AF in a crying child may mislead.
- AF is about 2.5 × 2.5 cm in size at birth and is diamond shaped. The PF measures <1 cm, allowing only the tip of the little finger at birth.
- The AF closes at 9–18 months of age and PF closes at 2 months of age.
- In a quiet and upright posture of an infant, AF is usually at the level (normal). The bulging AF indicates raised intracranial pressure, while depressed or sunken AF is found with dehydration or marasmic child.
- Mild bulging and pulsatile AF may be found in a normal child.

CAUSES OF DELAYED CLOSURE OF ANTERIOR FONTANEL

- Rickets
- Hydrocephalus
- Congenital hypothyroidism
- Down syndrome
- Edward syndrome
- Patau syndrome
- Malnutrition
- Achondroplasia
- Osteogenesis imperfecta
- Cleidocranial dysostosis
- Mucopolysaccharidosis
- Russell-Silver syndrome
- Hypophosphatasia
- Pyknodysostosis
- Rubinstein-Taybi syndrome
- Delayed closure of PF is commonly found in preterm, rickets, and congenital hypothyroidism.
- Early closure small AF may be seen in microcephaly, craniosynostosis, etc.

CAUSES OF BULGING ANTERIOR FONTANEL

- Crying infant
- *Raised intracranial pressure:*
  - Bacterial meningitis
  - Tuberculous meningitis (TBM)
  - Hydrocephalus
  - Intracranial hemorrhage

- Space-occupying lesion (SOL)
- Pseudotumor cerebri (idiopathic intracranial hypertension)

Causes of Pseudotumor Cerebri (Idiopathic Intracranial Hypertension)

- Nalidixic acid
- Steroids
- Tetracycline
- Fluoroquinolone
- Vitamin A toxicity
- Hypervitaminosis D.

Ascites

CHAPTER 5

INTRODUCTION

- "Ascites" is derived from the Greek word "askites", which means bag or sac.
- Ascites is a condition with pathologic accumulation of fluid (>25 mL in adults) within the peritoneal cavity (normal 1–20 mL).
- The following clinical signs of ascites develop as there is progressive collection of fluid in the peritoneal cavity:
  - *Bulging flanks:* The presence of flank fullness is one of the most sensitive physical signs of ascites. Its absence can rule out ascites with >90% accuracy.
  - *Puddle sign:* To demonstrate puddle sign, the patient lies prone for 5 minutes and is then placed on his hands and knees. The dull note at the central area (umbilical area) denotes ascites. Minimum amount of fluid required to develop puddle sign is 120 mL. Practically, it is cumbersome and is no longer recommended.
  - *Shifting dullness:* It becomes positive if there is >500 mL of fluid. This test has a high sensitivity (85%), but low specificity (50%). Thus, a negative shifting dullness is a useful finding for ruling out ascites.
  - *Horse-shoe dullness:* Tympanic sound is heard on percussion in epigastrium only and rest of the abdomen has dullness. It indicates presence of >750 mL of fluid.
  - *Fluid-thrill:* The presence of fluid thrill means ascitic fluid is >1,000 mL (1,000–1,500 mL).
- In tense ascites, there may be diastasis of the abdominal recti muscles and umbilical hernia.
- Ultrasonography (USG) is extremely sensitive as it can detect as little as 100 mL of fluid.

CLINICAL CLUES TO THE ETIOLOGY OF ASCITES

- *Splenomegaly:* Portal hypertension
- *Starts with puffy face, more in morning and nonprogressive ascites:* Nephrotic syndrome
- *Progressive ascites, but after sometimes it is static (equilibrium is established):* Portal hypertension
- *Progressive ascites:* Exudative inflammation (Tuberculosis)
- *Ascites in Kwashiorkar:* Tuberculosis, unless proved otherwise
- *Starts with edema feet, tender hepatomegaly, and raised jugular venous pressure (JVP):* Congestive heart failure
- Development of ascites, hepatomegaly, and pleural effusion in a case of dengue fever indicates capillary leak stage of the disease

- *Large tender liver and absent hepatojugular reflux (HJR):* Budd–Chiari syndrome
- *Ascites, hepatomegaly, raised JVP, and silent heart:* Constrictive pericarditis
- *History of (H/o) injury to abdomen and abdominal pain radiating to back:* Pancreatic ascites.

SERUM ASCITES ALBUMIN GRADIENT

- The concept of transudative and exudative ascites based on protein level has become obsolete now. It is replaced by high-gradient and low-gradient ascites.
- Serum ascites albumin gradient (SAAG) is measured by subtracting ascitic fluid albumin from serum albumin. Please note that it is not ratio, it is a gradient:
- *High-gradient ascites (SAAG >1.1):*
  - Portal hypertension (accuracy 97%)
  - Budd–Chiari syndrome
  - Portal vein thrombosis
  - Acute liver failure
  - Hypothyroidism
- *Low-gradient ascites (SAAG <1.1):*
  - Tuberculous peritonitis
  - Pancreatic ascites
  - Nephrotic syndrome
  - Biliary ascites
  - Serositis
- Falsely high SAAG in chylous ascites since lipid interferes with albumin estimation
- *Falsely low SAAG:*
  - Hypotension
  - High serum globulin

COMMON CAUSES OF ASCITES

- *Neonatal period:*
  - Urinary ascites (following urinary tract obstruction)
  - Congenital nephrotic syndrome
  - Chylous ascites
  - Acute bacterial peritonitis
  - Meconium peritonitis
  - Hydrops fetalis (hemolytic anemia)
  - Renal vein thrombosis
  - Bile peritonitis
  - Congestive heart failure
- *In children:*
  - Nephrotic syndrome
  - Kwashiorkor
  - Cirrhosis of liver
  - Portal vein obstruction
  - Protein losing enteropathy [tuberculosis, human immunodeficiency virus (HIV), celiac disease, etc.]
  - Peritonitis (bacterial, tuberculous, and bowel perforation)
  - Chronic active hepatitis
  - Budd–Chiari syndrome (hepatic vein obstruction)
  - Constrictive pericarditis
  - Cardiac failure
  - Chylous ascites
  - Inborn errors of metabolism (Wilson disease, tyrosinemia, galactosemia, glycogen storage disease, etc.)
  - Hypothyroidism
  - Systemic lupus erythematosus
  - Pancreatitis
  - Malignancies.

Ataxia

INTRODUCTION

Ataxia is defined as the inability to make smooth, accurate, and coordinated movements.

- Ataxia is usually caused by cerebellar dysfunction or impaired vestibular or proprioceptive afferent inputs to the cerebellum.
- Any of these can be implicated in pathology—cerebellum, spinal cord, brainstem, vestibular nuclei, basal ganglia, frontal lobe, and peripheral sensory nerves.
- Principle cerebellar functions are control and modulation of locomotion, postural control, and voluntary movements.
- Lesions of midline cerebellar vermis produce truncal and gait ataxia, while involvement of lateral cerebellar hemisphere produces a picture dominated by limb ataxia.
- Interruption of afferent and efferent connections within the neocerebellar system results in ataxic gait (swaying in the standing position, staggering while walking with a tendency to fall, and adoption of a compensatory wide base).
- *Romberg sign:* This is the test of proprioception and maintenance of balance is based on vision, vestibular functions, cerebellar functions, and proprioception.
    - The child is asked to stand with his feet close together. The child will sway and tend to fall toward the side of lesion in a case of unilateral cerebellar lesion. In case of bilateral cerebellar lesions, the child will tend to sway backward.
    - If the child can maintain the posture with open eyes, but falls or sways with closed eyes, it indicates lesion of the proprioception (sensory ataxia) (involvement of posterior column of spinal cord). It is called as positive Romberg sign.
- Pure ataxia is rare in acquired ataxia disorders and associated symptoms and signs almost always exist to suggest an underlying cause.
- Ataxia may be acute or chronic, genetic or acquired.

ACUTE CEREBELLAR ATAXIA

- Common age 1–3 years
- It often follows a viral illness such as varicella virus, Coxsackievirus, echo infection, by 2–3 weeks.
- Considered as autoimmune response to viral agent affecting the cerebellum
- Onset is typically sudden.
- Truncal ataxia may be severe that the child is unable to stand or sit.
- Vomiting may occur initially, but fever and nuchal rigidity are absent. Dysarthria may be significant.
- Begins to improve in a few weeks, but may persist for as long as 3 months or longer.
- Prognosis is excellent.

- Acute cerebellitis is a more severe form of cerebellar ataxia with changes on MRI scan. Most common infectious agents causing acute cerebellitis are mumps, Epstein-Barr virus (EBV), mycoplasma, and influenza virus.
- Cerebellar abscess can also occur with bacterial infections.

ACUTE LABYRINTHITIS

- It may be difficult to differentiate from acute cerebellar ataxia in a toddler.
- It is associated with middle ear infection and presents with intense vertigo, vomiting, and abnormalities of labyrinthine functions.

TOXIC CAUSES OF ATAXIA

- Alcohol
- Thallium (used as pesticide)
- Dextromethorphan
- Anticonvulsants (phenytoin, carbamazepine).

BRAIN TUMORS WITH ATAXIA

- Tumors of cerebellum cause ataxia because of direct disruption of cerebellar function or indirectly because of raised intracranial pressure (ICP) from compression of the fourth ventricle.
- Frontal lobe tumor may cause ataxia as a consequence of destruction or interruption of the association fibers connecting the frontal lobe with cerebellum or because of raised ICP.
- Neuroblastoma may be associated with a paraneoplastic encephalopathy characterized by progressive ataxia, myoclonic jerks, and opsoclonus (nonrhythmic conjugate horizontal and vertical oscillations of the eye balls).

METABOLIC DISORDERS CHARACTERIZED BY ATAXIA

- *Abetalipoproteinemia:*
  - Steatorrhea
  - Failure to thrive (FTT)
  - Acanthocytosis [spiculated red blood cells (RBCs)] on peripheral smear (PS) examination.
  - Decreased serum cholesterol and triglycerides
  - Ataxia
  - Retinitis pigmentosa
  - Peripheral neuritis
  - Abnormalities of position and vibration sense
  - Severe vitamin E deficiency
- *Mitochondrial disorders:*
  - Myoclonic epilepsy with ragged red fibers
  - Kearns–Sayre syndrome.

DEGENERATIVE DISEASES WITH ATAXIA

- *Ataxia telangiectasia:*
  - Most common of degenerative ataxia
  - Autosomal recessive
  - Ataxia beginning at age of 2 years and progressive to loss of ambulation by adolescence.
  - Oculomotor apraxia of horizontal gaze, strabismus, and nystagmus are often seen.
  - May present with chorea rather than ataxia.
  - Telangiectasia become evident by mid-childhood and is found on bulbar conjunctiva, over the surfaces of extremities.
  - Skin elasticity is lost.
  - Immunologic functions abnormalities cause frequent sinopulmonary

infections. Decreased serum and secretory immunoglobulin A (IgA).
- Increased chances of development of lymphoma, leukemia, and Hodgkin disease.
- *Friedrich ataxia:*
  - Autosomal recessive disorder
  - Involvement of spinocerebellar tracts, dorsal column in spinal cord, pyramidal tracts, and cerebellum and medulla.
  - Onset is later than ataxia telangiectasia, but usually occurs before the age of 10 years.
  - Ataxia is slowly progressive and involves lower extremities to a greater degree than the upper extremities.
  - Positive Romberg sign, absent deep tendon reflex (DTR), and planter extensor.
  - Dysarthric speech and nystagmus are common. Intelligence is preserved.
  - Skeletal abnormalities such as high-arched feet (pes cavus), hammer toes, and progressive kyphoscoliosis are common.
  - Hypertrophic cardiomyopathy with progressive congestive cardiac failure (CCF) is the cause of death in most patients.
  - There are more than 20 inherited spinocerebellar ataxias.

CONGENITAL ANOMALIES OF POSTERIOR FOSSA PRESENTING WITH ATAXIA

- Dandy-Walker malformation
- Chiari malformation
- Encephalocele
- Agenesis of cerebellar vermis
- *Jobber syndrome and related disorders:*
  - Developmental delay
  - Hypotonia
  - Abnormal eye movements
  - Abnormal respiration
  - MRI of brain is choice of investigation in this group.

COMMON CAUSES OF ATAXIA IN CHILDREN

- *Post infectious:*
  - Varicella
  - Mumps
  - EBV
  - Influenza
  - Coxsackie
- *Toxic—drug induced:*
  - Alcohol
  - Thallium (used in pesticides)
  - Dextromethorphan
  - Phenytoin
  - Carbamazepine
- Posterior fossa tumors (astrocytoma, medulloblastoma)
- Hydrocephalus
- Acute disseminated encephalomyelitis (ADEM)
- Posterior circulation stroke
- Neuroblastoma
- Guillain-Barré syndrome (GBS) and Miller-Fisher syndrome
- Dandy-Walker syndrome
- Arnold-Chiari malformation
- Ataxia-telangiectasia
- Friedrich ataxia.

CHAPTER 7

Basics of Fever

INTRODUCTION

Fever is a very common symptom in our daily pediatric practice. Several studies indicate that >40% of outdoor patients have complaint of fever and daily innumerable phone calls for the practicing pediatrician are for fever.

DEFINITION OF FEVER

- Fever is defined as a rectal temperature ≥38°C (100.4°F).
- Our body temperature fluctuates in a defined normal range [(36.6–37.9°C) (97.9–100.2°F) rectally]. The highest point is reached at early evening and the lowest point is reached in the morning.
- The range of normal temperature is broad, 35.5–37.7°C (96–100°F).

Fever should always be measured by thermometer and documented: Palpation of skin by hands to assess body temperature is widely used by parents. However, it is less accurate and falsely labels children as having fever. To consider fever with warm head and extremities by parents is very common. It should be confirmed by measuring body temperature by thermometer.

MEASUREMENT OF BODY TEMPERATURE

- The measurement of body temperature should reflect the core temperature. The thermometer should be easy, comfortable to use, and give rapid results. It should not cause cross infection. It should not be influenced by environmental temperature. It should be safe and cost-effective. There are several devices available at present.
- *Available different thermometers:*
  - *Mercury clinical thermometer* is not recommended due to possibility of mercury poisoning if it is broken accidentally.
  - *Digital thermometer* is widely used because of its easy use and safety.
  - *Infrared thermometer* is very useful to screen the people for fever without touching the person. It is safe from cross infection point of view, very useful in epidemics like COVID-19.
- *Axillary temperature:*
  - Axilla should be dry.
  - Keep the thermometer in axilla with the bulb of the thermometer toward apex of axilla, the elbow is flexed and the arm is held close to the chest wall.
  - Switch on the thermometer and keep the bulb at the apex of dry axilla till its final beep.
  - The thermometer should be cleaned with 70% isopropyl alcohol after each used, dried and kept in its container.
  - The axillary temperature is 1°C less than the rectal temperature.
- *Oral (sublingual) temperature:*
  - It reflects the temperature of lingual arteries.

- This method can be used in children >5 years.
- The oral temperature is 0.5–1°C higher than axillary temperature.
- *Rectal temperature:*
  - Rectal thermometer is different from clinical thermometer.
  - Having rounded, bulbous tip and low reading (30–40°C).
  - The rectal thermometer should be cleaned with soap and water, wiped dry, and then used.
  - Water-based jelly or lubricant is applied on the tip of the thermometer.
  - Put the baby on his back on a firm surface. Hold the baby's ankles and lift both the legs. Gently, introduce the thermometer in the rectum, directing its tip posteriorly toward the back up to a depth of 2.5 cm. Hold the thermometer till its final beep.
  - Due to accidental perforation of rectum, it is not routinely recommended.
- *Tympanic thermometer:* The degree of temperature of blood supplying to tympanic membrane and that of hypothalamus are very close to each other. Therefore, it is the ideal location for core temperature estimation. They measure the thermal radiation emitted from the tympanic membrane and the ear canal and are called infrared radiation emission detectors (IRED).
- *Temporal artery thermometer:* It reads the infrared heat released by the temporal artery, which runs across the forehead just below the skin. It can be used in 3 months and older children.

MECHANISM OF FEVER

Three different mechanisms can produce fever:
1. Pyrogens
2. Heat production exceeding heat loss
3. Defective heat loss.

Pyrogens

There are two types of pyrogens: Endogenous pyrogens and exogenous pyrogens.

1. *Endogenous pyrogens:*
   a. Endogenous pyrogens include the cytokines interleukin-1 (IL-1) and IL-6, tumor necrosis factor alpha (TNF-α), interferon beta (IFN-β), and IFN-γ. Stimulated leukocytes and other cells produce lipids prostaglandin E2 (PGE2) that also serve as endogenous pyrogens. PGE2 attaches to the prostaglandin receptors in the hypothalamus to produce the new temperature set point.
   b. Besides infectious diseases and drugs, malignancy and inflammatory diseases can produce fever through the production of endogenous pyrogens.
2. *Exogenous pyrogens:*
   a. They come from outside the body and consist of mainly infectious pathogens and drugs. Microbes, microbial toxins, or other products of microbes are the most common exogenous pyrogens, which stimulate macrophages and other cells to produce endogenous pyrogens.
   b. Endotoxin is one of the few substances that directly affect thermoregulation in the hypothalamus as well as stimulate endogenous pyrogens release.

Mechanism of Fever

Invading exogenous pyrogens
↓
Endogenous pyrogens
(Cytokines)
↓
Act on thermosensitive neurons in hypothalamus
↓
Upgrade the set point via prostaglandins
↓
Increase in heat production

(Muscle contractions—rigors)
and decreasing heat loss
(Vasoconstriction—chills)
↓
Rise in body temperature
till a set point
↓
Fever

Many drugs can cause fever and the mechanism for increasing body temperature varies with the class of drugs.

Heat Production Exceeding Heat Loss

The examples include salicylate poisoning and malignant hyperthermia.

Defective Heat Loss

It may occur in children with ectodermal dysplasia and severe heat exposure.

TYPES OF FEVER

The types of fever can provide clues to the underlying etiology. But in this modern time, hardly specific pattern of fever is noted due to self-medication (antipyretics) by the parents, misuse of antipyretics (use of irrational drugs and irrational combinations), overuse of antimalarials and antibiotics, etc. Still, if a specific pattern is observed, it becomes an important clue for the cause of fever.

- *Continuous/persistent/sustained fever:* It is almost same degree of fever through a mild variation of <0.5°C (0.9°F). It is commonly seen in bacterial infections like enteric fever **(Fig. 1)**.
- *Remittent fever:* It is a high grade, persistent fever and variation is >0.5°C (0.9°F) **(Fig. 2)**.
- *Intermittent fever:* Intermittent fever is characterized by febrile periods that are separated by intervals of normal temperature **(Fig. 3)**.

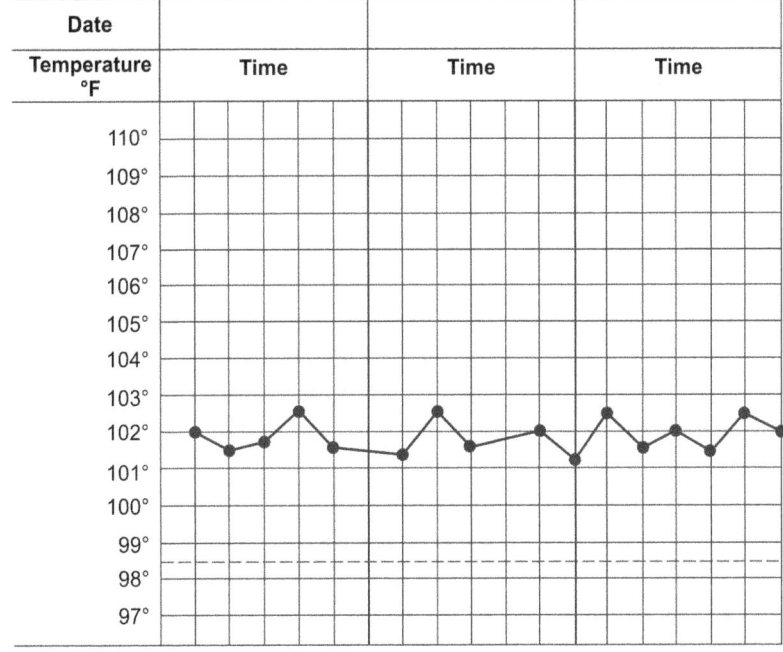

Fig. 1: Continuous fever.

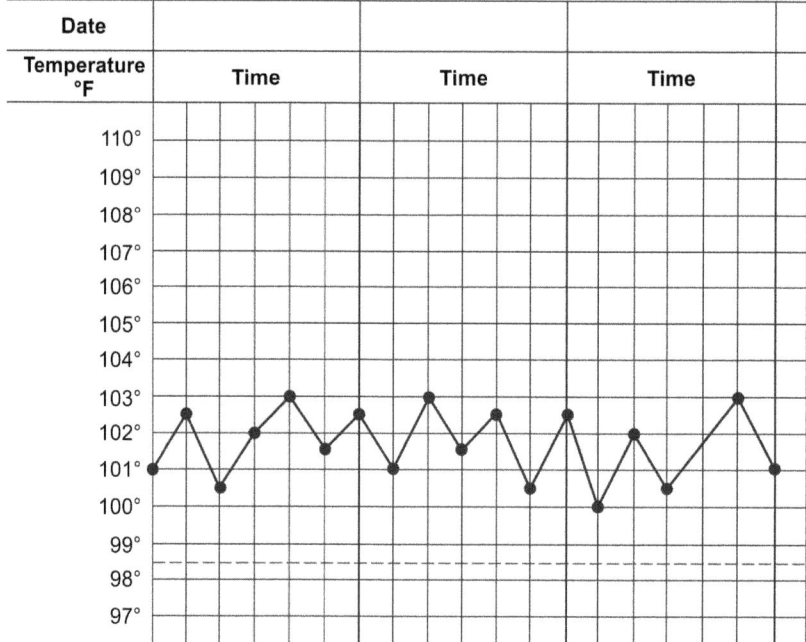

Fig. 2: Remittent fever.

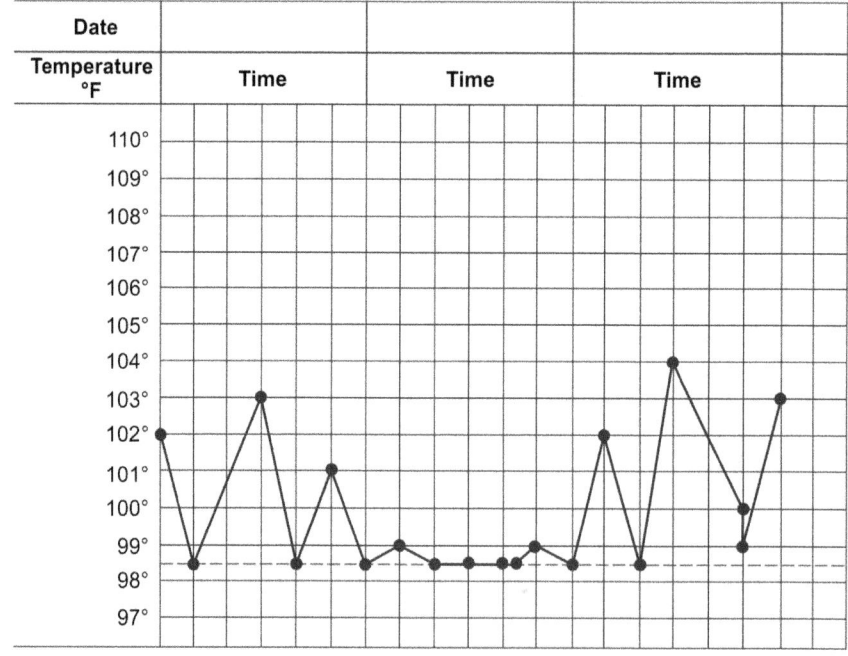

Fig. 3: Intermittent fever.

- Tertian fever is type of relapsing (intermittent fever), it occurs on first and third days. Classical example of tertian fever is malaria by *Plasmodium vivax*.
- Quartan fever occurs on first and fourth day, which is seen in a case of malaria by *Plasmodium malariae*.

- *Hectic fever:* Either an intermittent or remittent fever is considered hectic if the temperature range swings widely throughout the day, with a difference of >1.4°C between the highest and lowest temperatures. It is considered as characteristic of an abscess, collection of pus somewhere in body.
- *Relapsing fever:* This type of intermittent fever spikes up again after days or weeks of normal temperatures.
- *Biphasic fever:* Biphasic fever indicates a single illness with two distinct periods (camel back fever pattern). It has characteristics of viral fevers, dengue fever (DF), leptospirosis, yellow fever, etc **(Fig. 4)**.

Fever is a symptom and not a disease. The presence of fever indicates inflammatory process in body, may be infective or noninfective. Most of the time, fever is harmless, but may be an initiation of some serious condition.

WHY FEVER IS A FRIEND?

- Fever increases white blood cell (WBC) response.
- It decreases endotoxin production or its efficacy.
- Activation of B lymphocytes (humoral immunity)
- Activation of T lymphocytes (cell-mediated immunity)
- It enhances phagocytosis, opsonization, and complement fixation.
- Fever is a beneficial immune response.

RED FLAG CONDITIONS PRESENTING WITH FEVER

- Altered sensorium/drowsiness/irritability/ bulging anterior fontanelle (AF)/signs

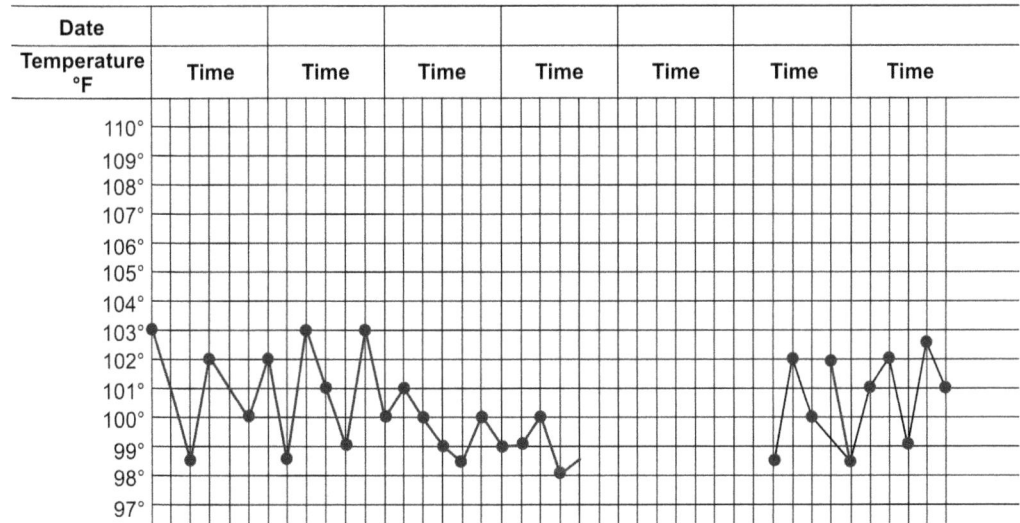

Fig. 4: Biphasic fever.

of meningeal irritation present [central nervous system (CNS) infection].
- Fever in <3 months, particularly neonates
- Poor perfusion (impending shock)
- Increased work of breathing
- Petechial/purpura spots [dengue hemorrhagic fever (DHF)/sepsis/meningococcemia]
- Faucial membrane (diphtheria)
- Immune compromised child
- Severe acute malnutrition
- Abdominal guarding/rigidity (surgical abdomen).

FEVER PATTERN

Try to categorize fever pattern, it will guide for further work up and management.
- *Prolonged fever:* A single illness in which duration of fever exceeds that expected for the clinical diagnosis. For example, >10 days for viral upper respiratory tract infection (URTI), >3 weeks for Epstein-Barr virus (EBV).
- *Recurrent fever:* It is a single illness in which fever and other signs and symptoms wax and wane. It may be due to incomplete antimicrobial therapy of urinary tract infection (UTI) or different conditions developing with fever at different intervals (viral infections, DF, malaria, enteric fever, tuberculosis, etc.).
- *Periodic fever:* The term periodic fever is used narrowly to describe fever syndromes with a regular periodicity, e.g., PFAPA (periodic fever, aphthous stomatitis, pharyngitis, adenitis) syndrome, hyperimmunoglobulin D (IgD) syndrome, cyclical neutropenia, etc.
- *Fever of unknown origin (FUO):*
  - Fever documented by a healthcare provider
  - Fever >38.3°C at several occasions
  - Cause remains unidentified after 3 weeks of evaluation as an outdoor patient or after a week of evaluation in hospital.
- *Factitious fever:* Factitious fever or self-induced fever may be caused by intentional manipulation of the thermometer or injection of pyrogenic material.
- *Double quotidian fever:* Fever that peaks twice in 24 hours is classically associated with inflammatory arthritis.
- *Single isolated fever spike:*
  - Not associated with an infectious disease.
  - Attributed to infusion of blood products, some drugs, some procedures, or manipulation of a catheter on a colonized or infected body surface.

HYPERTHERMIA

- Fever >41.5°C (106.7°F) is hyperthermia.
- Most commonly due to heat exposure, may be due to excessive endogenous heat production, usually not due to infection.
- Setting in thermoregulatory center is unchanged, heat production exceeds to capacity of heat loss.
- Skin is hot and dry.
- Antipyretics do not work. Other measures like to bring down environmental temperature by fan and air condition, tepid sponging, etc.
- *Common causes:*
  - Heat stroke
  - Thyrotoxicosis, pheochromocytoma
  - Cerebral hemorrhage, hypothalamic injury
  - Malignant hyperthermia (succinyl chloride)
  - Drug induced (salicylates, anticholinergics).

8 Bleeding Manifestations

INTRODUCTION

- Blood is a fluid connective tissue.
- Hemostasis is the sum total of specialized functions within the circulating blood and its vessels designed to stop hemorrhage.
- The main three components of hemostasis are:
  1. Intact vascular component
  2. Platelets
  3. Coagulation factors.

INDICATIONS FOR WORKUP FOR BLEEDING DISORDER

- A recent bout of bleeding—spontaneous or after injury or surgery; bleeding is usually prolonged and disproportionate to extent of injury.
- Family history of (H/o) bleeding disorders
- Preparations for surgery or invasive procedures
- Systemic diseases such as liver disorder, renal disorder, and sepsis leading to disseminated intravascular coagulation (DIC).

Whenever a child presents with bleeding manifestations, it is necessary to decide the following:
- Is it significant bleeding?
- Is it due to local cause or generalized hemostasis defect?
- Is it a likely cause of bleeding?
  - Vascular
  - Platelet disorder
  - Coagulation disorder
  - Multiple components.

Whether bleeding manifestations are due to systemic disorder of hemostasis or due to local cause?
- Bleeding from single site and recurs often from the same site, e.g., epistaxis from one nostril, likely local causes such as polyp and foreign body.
- Hematuria, excessive bleeding after tooth extractions, etc., are examples of systemic defect or hemostasis.

CLINICAL APPROACH

- *Features of abnormal bleeding:*
  - Prolonged bleeding after minor trauma
  - Epistaxis for >15 minutes in spite of pressing over it
  - Menstrual periods lasting >7 days with passage of clots
  - Skin bleeding manifestations inconsistent with degree of trauma
- Family H/o bleeding disorder, e.g., hemophilia which is an X-linked disorder
- Mucosal bleeding, bruising, and petechiae are associated with platelet disorders (qualitative or quantitative) and Von Willebrand disease.
- Spontaneous, deep muscle and joint bleeding are commonly seen with coagulation factor deficiency.

- *Neonates:*
  - *Gastrointestinal (GI) tract bleeding:* Swollen maternal blood or hemorrhagic disease of newborn
  - *Bleeding from umbilical stump:* Factor XIII deficiency
  - *Bleeding from circumcision:* Hemophilia.
- Acute onset of bleeding manifestations over a period of days to weeks: Immune thrombocytopenia purpura (ITP), vitamin K deficiency, etc.
- Bleeding following trauma in which there is a good initial hemostasis followed by persistent oozing due to failure to form a firm clot indicates factor XIII deficiency and disorder of fibrinolytic pathway.
- *H/o drug therapy:*
  - Nonsteroidal anti-inflammatory drugs (NSAIDs) (aspirin, ibuprofen, nimesulide, etc.)
  - Steroids
  - Heparin
  - Oral anticoagulants
  - Chloroquine
  - Quinine
  - Valproic acid
- H/o poor wound healing: Factor XIII deficiency.

Bleeding Skin Lesions (Fig. 1)

- *Petechiae:*
  - Pinhead size (<2 mm)
  - Usually due to capillary endothelial damage
  - Pink or brownish in color
  - Blanching on pressure
- *Purpura:*
  - Bleeding into skin (dry purpura) or mucous membrane (wet purpura)

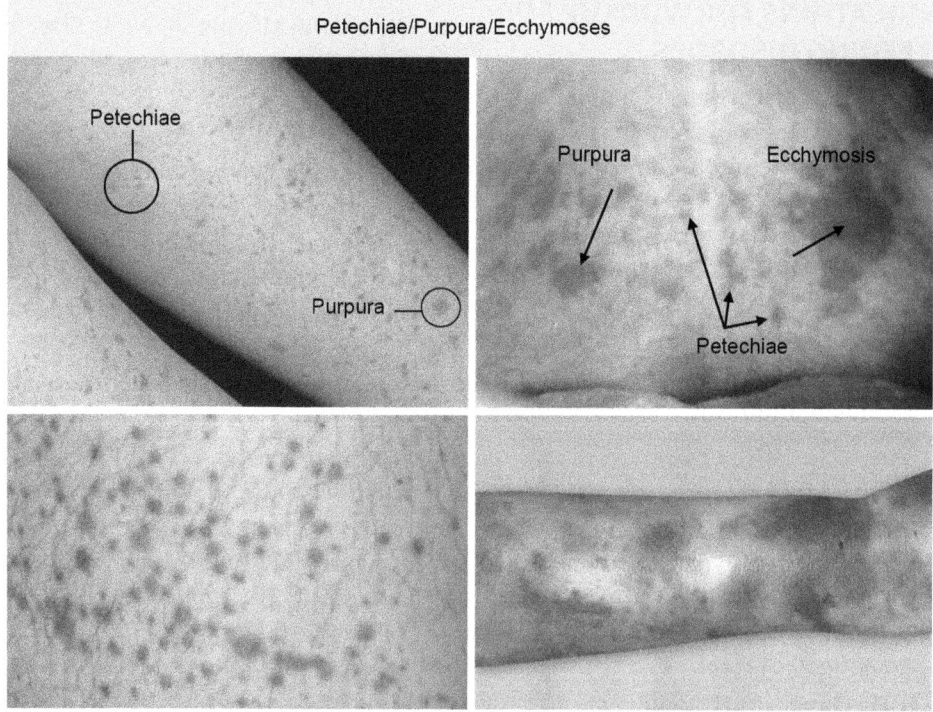

Fig. 1: Bleeding skin lesions.

- 2–5 mm in size
- Bluish in color
- Circumscribed showing clear-cut margin with the surface
- Not blanching on application of pressure
- Wet purpura is more serious
- Due to thrombocytopenia, thrombocytopathy, or vessel damage
■ Ecchymosis:
- Bleeding skin lesion, purplish discoloration due to extravasated blood into skin and mucous membrane
- Bleeding from a large vessel
- >5 mm in size
■ Hematoma:
- Bleeding into muscles and deeper structures
- Large enough to produce an elevation of skin (swelling)
- Mostly due to coagulation disorders
■ Thrombocytopenia with:
- Sick look: Leukemia, dengue fever (DF), and septicemia
- Well-looking: Henoch–Schönlein purpura (HSP)
- Anemia, hepatosplenomegaly and/or lymphadenopathy: Leukemia, and lymphoma
■ Platelet disorders versus coagulation disorders

Clinical signs and symptoms	Platelet disorder or vascular abnormality	Coagulation disorder
Bleeding after minor trauma	Common	No
Bleeding following trauma/surgery	• Immediate • Stops with pressure	• Delayed (1–2 days later) • Does not stop with pressure
Mucosal bleeding	Frequent	Uncommon
Petechiae	Most common	No
Ecchymosis	Small and superficial	Large and deep
Hemarthrosis and muscle bleeding	Uncommon	Very common
Site of bleeding	• Skin • Mucous membrane • Mucosal bleeding: Epistaxis, oral, and GI tract	• Soft tissue • Muscles (hematomas) • Joints
Examples	• ITP • Von Willebrand disease	Hemophilia

(GI: gastrointestinal; ITP: immune thrombocytopenia purpura)

■ Likely inherited disorders:
- Presents usually in infancy and early childhood
- H/o bleeding from umbilical cord without sepsis or slipped ligature
- Cephalhematoma without H/o prolonged or difficult labor
- Bleeding during eruption or fall of deciduous tooth
■ Detailed family H/o bleeding disorder; prepare pedigree covering three generations.
- X-linked recessive pattern:
  ♦ Hemophilia A (factor VIII deficiency)
  ♦ Hemophilia B (factor IX deficiency)
  ♦ Wiscott–Aldrich syndrome

- Autosomal dominant pattern: Von Willebrand disease
- Negative family history does not rule out possibility of inherited bleeding disorder.
- Family history may be negative, if the coagulation defect is mild or there is spontaneous mutation (20% of hemophilia A).
- Milder forms of inherited disorder may present later in life.
■ Previous H/o operations such as circumcision, tooth extraction, tonsillectomy, or major operation practically rule out the possibility of moderate to severe inherited bleeding disorders.

SYNDROMES KNOWN TO BE ASSOCIATED WITH BLEEDING DISORDERS

■ Keloids with afibrinogenemia and factor XIII deficiency
■ Cigarette paper scar and hyperextensible joints: Ehlers–Danlos syndrome
■ Thrombocytopenia, otitis media, eczema, and recurrent infections in Wiscott–Aldrich syndrome
■ Children with albinism may have qualitative functional defects of platelets.
■ Thrombocytopenia with absent (rudimentary) radius in thrombocytopenia-absent radius (TAR) syndrome
■ Giant hemangioma, thrombocytopenia, and DIC in Kasabach–Merritt syndrome.

Common Causes of Thrombocytopenia

■ Immune thrombocytopenia purpura
■ *Infections:*
  - Malaria
  - DF
  - Human immunodeficiency virus (HIV)
  - Kala-azar
  - TORCH (toxoplasmosis, other agents, rubella, cytomegalovirus, and herpes simplex) infections
  - Hepatitis B and C
  - Epstein–Barr virus (EBV)
  - Hemophagocytic lymphohistiocytosis (HLH)
■ *Drugs:*
  - Valproate
  - Penicillins
  - Quinine
  - Digoxin
■ *Thrombotic microangiopathy:* Hemolytic uremic syndrome
■ *Malignancies:* Leukemia and lymphoma
■ *Autoimmune disorders:* Systemic lupus erythematosus (SLE) and Evans syndrome
■ *Bone marrow failure:* TAR syndrome, Fanconi anemia, and Shwachman–Diamond syndrome
■ *Marrow replacement:* Osteopetrosis and Gaucher disease
■ Hypersplenism.

Qualitative Platelet Function Disorders

■ Glanzmann thrombasthenia [glycoprotein 1b (GP1b) deficiency]
■ Bernard–Soulier syndrome
■ Gray platelet syndrome
■ Medications
■ Chronic kidney disease.

Common Coagulation Disorders

■ Hemophilia A
■ Hemophilia B
■ Von Willebrand disease
■ Factors VII, X, and XIII deficiency
■ Afibrinogenemia
■ Liver disorders
■ Vitamin K deficiency
■ DIC.

CHAPTER 9

Bow Legs

INTRODUCTION

- Bow legs (genu varum) is a condition in which a child's legs curve outward at the knees. When a child with bow legs stands with their toes pointing forward, their ankles may touch but their knees remain apart.

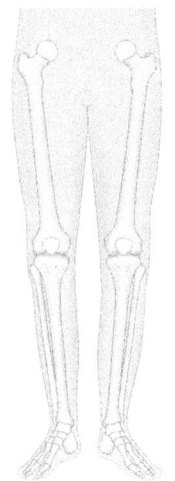
Typical

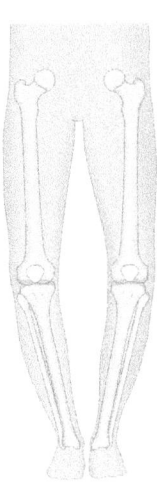
Bow legs

- Bow legs is considered as a normal part of growth in infants and toddlers. In young children, bow legs is not painful or uncomfortable and does not interfere with a child's ability to walk, run, or play.
- Children outgrow bow legs sometime after 18–24 months of age. In rare cases, bow legs may be a sign of growth disorder.

- *Physiological growth of children's legs and knees:*
  - Bow legs is common in children between birth and 24 months.
  - Between 24 and 36 months, toddlers' legs become aligned.
  - Young children, between 3 and 5 years of age, may develop knock knees (genu valgum), a condition in which the knees tilt inward.
  - As children grow, their legs continue to straighten out. By age 7–8 years, they walk normally.

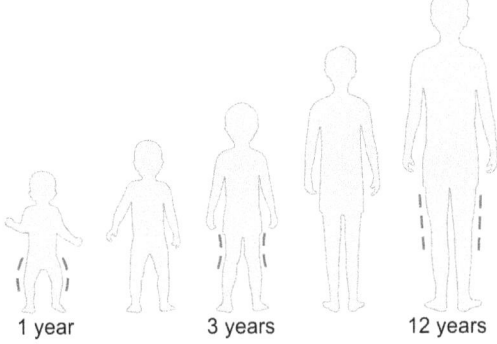
1 year   3 years   12 years

- *Genu varum (bow legs):* The knees are bowed outside and the intercondylar distance is >10 cm. The common conditions are:
  - Physiological in children <2 years of age
  - Rickets
  - Achondroplasia
  - Osteomalacia

- *Genu valgum (knock knees):* The knees are close to each other and the intermalleolar distance is increased. It may be congenital, a normal variant, or in a case of rickets.

SYMPTOMS OF BOW LEGS

1. Knees curve outward
2. Both legs have a similar curve (symmetrical)
3. Awkward walking pattern
4. In toeing (toes point inward)
5. Clumsiness or frequent tripping.

CAUSES OF BOW LEGS

- Physiological up to 2 years of age
- Rickets
- Renal osteodystrophy
- Hypophosphatasia
- Achondroplasia
- Trauma
- Tumors
- Infections
- Blount's disease (tibia vara)
- Congenital
- Neuromuscular disorders.

CHAPTER 10

Bowel Sounds

INTRODUCTION

Bowel sounds are normally best heard near the umbilicus. Normal bowel sounds are intermittent low-to-medium pitched gurgles interspersed with occasional high-pitched, tinkling metallic sounds heard. The frequency of sound is 10–15/min in small intestine whereas 3–5/min in large intestine. However, the sensitivity and specificity of the auscultation of bowel sounds are quite low, differ subjectively by clinician, and will vary from one moment to the next. Before deciding the absence of bowel sounds, one should auscultate for a minimum of 5 minutes.

COMMON CAUSES OF DECREASED/ABSENCE OF BOWEL SOUNDS

- *Normal or benign conditions:*
  - Normal variant: 5–15 bowel sounds/min is normal; however, several minutes may elapse without any sound.
  - Failure to auscultate long enough (minimum 5 minutes)
  - Hunger
- *Paralytic (adynamic) ileus:*
  - Hypokalemia
  - Hyponatremia
  - Hypomagnesemia
  - Uremia
  - Sepsis (toxins)
  - Enteric fever
  - Abdominal surgery
  - Drugs: Loperamide, narcotics, beta (β) blockers, anticholinergic and psychotropic agents
  - Retroperitoneal hemorrhage
  - Vertebral compression fracture
- *Intestinal obstruction:* Partial bowel obstruction often has increased bowel sounds.
- *Peritonitis:*
  - Acute or ruptured appendicitis
  - Intestinal perforation
  - Pancreatitis
  - Pelvic inflammation/infection
  - Solid organ injury following trauma
- *Intestinal ischemia:*
  - Mesenteric artery syndrome
  - Vasculitis (dengue, connective tissue disorders)
- *Miscellaneous (less common):*
  - Diabetic coma
  - Hypoparathyroidism
  - Spinal injury
  - Perforated gall bladder
  - Myocardial infarction
  - Rib fractures.

COMMON CAUSES OF INCREASED BOWEL SOUNDS

High-frequency, loud, low-pitched gurgles (borborygmi) often rising to a high-pitched crescendo that coincides with colicky abdominal pain is pathognomonic of small bowel

obstruction. It is often audible to the unaided ears.
- Hypertrophic pyloric stenosis
- *Mechanical intestinal obstruction:* Small bowel obstruction is the most common. It may be congenital or acquired, partial or complete, and simple or strangulated resulting in bowel ischemia.
  - Congenital small bowel obstruction:
    - Malrotation, with or without volvulus
    - Duodenal atresia or stenosis or annular pancreas (more common in Down syndrome)
    - Jejunal and ileal atresia
    - Annular pancreas
    - Intestinal duplication
    - Intra-abdominal hernia
    - Meconium ileus (common in cystic fibrosis)
  - Acquired small bowel obstruction:
    - Intussusceptions
    - Incarcerated inguinal hernia
    - Postsurgical adhesions
    - Ascariasis (obstructing ball of worms)
    - Crohn's disease (stricture)
  - Colonic obstruction (bowel sounds usually not very increased):
    - Hirschsprung disease
    - Small left colon syndrome (infants of diabetic mothers)
    - Necrotizing enterocolitis
- Acute gastroenteritis
- Early peritonitis
- Intestinal pseudo-obstruction
- Drugs such as prokinetic agents (metoclopramide), antibiotics such as ampicillin, amoxicillin, and macrolides.

11 CHAPTER

Burning Micturition

INTRODUCTION

Burning micturition (painful urination) is also called dysuria. Dysuria can be caused by irritation or inflammation of the urethra. The irritation of the urethra may be due to concentrated urine, application of soap or skin lotion and bubble baths. The inflammation of urethra may be due to pin worm infestation, cystitis, urinary tract infection or infection at other genitourinary sites. Detailed history and physical examination may reveal the cause in most cases, very few patients may require investigations.

Burning micturition is a common complaint by the mother, especially in young children. The causes may vary from simple concentrated urine in summer season, local irritation, and cystitis to urinary tract infection. It may be purely psychogenic in some cases. The clinical evaluation is important to decide the etiology and further management.

- The concentrated urine causing burning micturition is very common. The concentrated urine may be due to less intake of fluids, hot environment, not passing urine for a long time, or febrile status of the child.
- One needs to confirm about water intake of the child and insensible water loss, especially in summer season.
- In neonates, it is quite common to cry before passing the urine and once the baby passes urine, he/she feels comfortable. Baby cries before passing urine due to contraction of bladder muscles which causes discomfort. He/she feels comfortable during the act of micturition and again cries due to soiling of clothes. Continuous crying while passing urine is abnormal, which may be due to irritation, inflammation, or urinary tract infection.
- Local irritation or pain may be due to trauma or inflammation of the external urethral meatus.
- Older child can be asked whether burning micturition is daily with each act or occasionally, whether it is only during start or in later part of act, the latter one is suggesting bladder pathology.
- Child may cry during micturition due to diaper rash.
- *Enterobius vermicularis* (pin worm) infestation may cause urethritis or cystitis and burning micturition, especially in females.
- Color of the urine is an important point. Dark-colored urine indicates concentrated urine. Red-colored urine indicates hematuria, may be due to renal calculus.
- Passing crystals in the urine may be due to calciuria (idiopathic hypercalciuria or renal calculus).
- Associated symptoms such as fever, increased frequency of micturition and abdominal pain suggest urinary tract infection. The loin pain indicates acute pyelonephritis while hypogastric pain suggests cystitis.

Cataracts

INTRODUCTION

A cataract means any opacity of the lens. Cataract is not a common problem in pediatric practice, but it is the most common cause of treatable childhood blindness. Some are detected incidentally on clinical examination, majority are observed by the parents or caretakers, and others may present with visual complaints. Cataracts are more common in low birth weight infants (<2,500 g). The differential diagnosis of cataracts in infants and children includes a wide range of causes such as developmental disorders, congenital infections, inflammatory disorders, metabolic diseases, and toxic and traumatic insults. Cataracts may also develop secondary to intraocular diseases, such as retinopathy of prematurity, retinal detachment, retinitis pigmentosa, and uveitis. Inherited and syndromic conditions also have cataracts, besides other features.

DIFFERENTIAL DIAGNOSIS

Prematurity

A special type of lens changes are seen in preterm babies, called a cataract of prematurity. The cluster of tiny vacuoles in the distribution of the "Y" sutures of the lens is seen in these infants. They can be visualized with an ophthalmic examination, but best seen with the well-dilated pupil. The exact reason is not known, but the opacities disappear within few weeks by their own.

Developmental Variants

Early developmental process may lead to various congenital lens opacities. Discrete dots or white plaque-like opacities of the lens capsule are common and sometimes involve the contiguous subcapsular region.

Congenital Infections

Cataracts in infants and children can be due to congenital infections such as rubella, toxoplasmosis, cytomegalovirus, and herpes simplex virus.

Metabolic Disorders

Cataracts are a prominent manifestations of many metabolic disorders.
- Galactosemia is the most common cause of cataract amongst metabolic disorders. In classic infantile galactosemia, galactose-1-phosphate uridyltransferase deficiency, the cataract is typically of zonular type. Persistent jaundice, hepatomegaly, hypoglycemia, seizures, and cataract in an infant are classical features of galactosemia. With early treatment (galactose-free diet) the lens changes may be reversible.
- In galactokinase deficiency, cataracts are the sole clinical manifestation.

- In children, with juvenile onset diabetes mellitus, lens examination at certain intervals is mandatory. Some develop sunflower-like white opacities and vacuoles of the lens. Others develop cataracts that may progress and mature rapidly, sometimes in a matter of days, especially during adolescence. Congenital lens opacities may be seen in children of diabetic and prediabetic mothers.
- Hypoglycemia in neonates can also be associated with early development of cataracts. Ketotic hypoglycemia is also associated with cataracts.
- An association between cataracts and hypocalcemia is known. Various lens opacities may be seen in patients with hypoparathyroidism.
- Oculocerebrorenal syndrome (Lowe syndrome) is associated with cataracts in infants.
- Sunflower cataract is known to occur in Wilson disease, but is not commonly seen.
- Mucopolysaccharidoses, Niemann–Pick disease, and Fabry disease are other metabolic conditions associated with cataracts.

Inherited Diseases

Many cataracts unassociated with other diseases are hereditary. The most common mode of inheritance is autosomal dominant. Autosomal recessive inheritance occurs less frequently. It is sometimes found in community with high rates of consanguinity. X-linked inheritance of cataracts unassociated with other diseases is relatively rare.

Chromosomal Defects

Lens opacities of different types may occur in association with chromosomal disorders such as Down syndrome (Trisomy 21), Edward syndrome (Trisomy 18), Patau syndrome (Trisomy 13), Turner syndrome (45,X), Noonan syndrome, and various deletion and duplication syndromes.

Trauma

Trauma to the eye is a significant cause of cataracts in children. It may result from blunt or penetrating injuries. Cataracts can be an important manifestation of child abuse.

Radiation

Cataract formation after exposure to therapeutic radiation is dose and duration dependent.

Drugs and Toxins

Of the various drugs and toxic substances that may cause cataracts, steroids are of major importance in children. Steroid-related cataracts are of the posterior capsular type. Steroid-induced cataracts may be reversible in some cases. All children receiving long-term steroid treatment should have periodic eye examination.

Miscellaneous

Several multisystem diseases and eye anomalies are known to manifest with cataracts.

Idiopathic

Many a time, the clinician may not get a cause of cataracts in children in spite of good evaluation.

COMMON CAUSES OF CATARACTS

- *Congenital infections:*
  - Rubella
  - Cytomegalovirus
  - Toxoplasmosis
  - Herpes simplex infection
  - Syphilis

- *Developmental variants:*
  - Prematurity
  - Low birth weight babies
- *Metabolic disorders:*
  - Galactosemia
  - Homocystinuria
  - Wilson disease
  - Fabry disease
  - Abetalipoproteinemia
  - Niemann-Pick disease
  - Refsum disease
  - Mucopolysaccharidosis
- *Chromosomal disorders:*
  - Down syndrome (Trisomy 21)
  - Edward syndrome (Trisomy 18)
  - Patau syndrome (Trisomy 13)
  - Turner syndrome (45,XO)
  - Noonan syndrome
- *Multisystem genetic disorders:*
  - Cockayne disease
  - Marfan syndrome
  - Apert syndrome
  - Crouzon disease
  - Ectodermal dysplasia
  - Lowe syndrome (oculocerebrorenal syndrome)
  - Laurance–Moon–Biedl syndrome
  - Nail-patella syndrome
  - Prader–Willi syndrome
- *Endocrinal disorders:*
  - Diabetes mellitus
  - Hypoparathyroidism
  - Hypoglycemia
- *Ocular anomalies:*
  - Retinitis pigmentosa
  - Coloboma
  - Retinoblastoma
- *Miscellaneous:*
  - Trauma
  - Radiation
  - Juvenile idiopathic arthritis
  - Toxins
  - Drugs (corticosteroids)
- *Idiopathic.*

Chapter 13: Chest Pain

INTRODUCTION

Chest pain is uncommon in children. It is usually not a manifestation of cardiac disease in the pediatric patient; rather noncardiac causes are common. The pediatrician should make every effort to find a specific cause for chest pain before making a referral for cardiac evaluation.

EVALUATION

A three-step diagnostic approach is recommended.

Step 1: The first step should be directed at detecting the three most common causes of chest pain: respiratory diseases, musculoskeletal causes including trauma, and costochondritis. These three account for 45–65% of chest pain in children. A thorough history taking and careful physical examination make the diagnosis of these conditions.

Step 2: The second step is to check for cardiac causes. History, physical examination, especially cardiovascular system in details, chest X-ray, electrocardiogram (ECG), and echocardiogram (echo) study of heart will reveal cardiac condition, if chest pain is due to cardiac cause (5%).

Step 3: If the cardiac cause of chest pain is excluded, then the pain is likely due to a disease of systems such as the gastrointestinal system and is of psychogenic or idiopathic origin (15–45%). Long follow-up may clarify the cause.

CAUSES

The following points may help to locate the cause for chest pain.
- *What seems to bring out the pain:*
  - Increased pain with excessive movement or activity (musculoskeletal); no pain during sleep or while watching television (psychogenic)
- *Site of pain:*
  - Well localized over chest (pleuritic pain)
  - Retrosternal pain [gastroesophageal reflux disease (GERD) and mitral valve prolapse (MVP)]
  - Localized over specific dermatome (herpes zoster)
  - Precordial pain (cardiac causes such as aortic stenosis, pericarditis and arrhythmias)
- *Associated symptoms and signs:*
  - Cough, breathlessness, and fever (respiratory causes such as pneumonia, pleurisy, and pneumothorax)
  - Irritability, arching, and related to food (GERD)
  - Signs of cardiac failure [aberrant left coronary artery originating from pulmonary artery (ALCAPA), aortic stenosis]
  - Syncope (cardiac arrhythmias, aortic stenosis)

- Palpitation (cardiac arrhythmias)
- Skin eruptions (herpes zoster)
- *Aggravating and relieving factors:*
  - Increasing pain with activity or movement: Musculoskeletal, rib fracture
  - Aggravating by breathing and cough: Pleuritic pain
  - Decreases in lateral lying-down position on the same side: Pleuritic pain
  - Sharp, stabbing pain, intensifies during lying down, but sitting up and leaning forward can often ease the pain: Pericardial pain
- History of (H/o) cardiac disease or a cardiac death in family is an important point [ischemic heart diseases and cardiac arrhythmias like Wolff–Parkinson–White (WPW) syndrome].
- Abdominal conditions such as liver abscess, subdiaphragmatic abscess, and pancreatitis can cause chest pain.
- Failure to thrive (FTT), irritability, and arching in an infant may be due to retrosternal pain following reflux esophagitis in a case of GERD.
- An adolescent or a young female presenting with retrosternal chest pain and systolic murmur highly suggests MVP.

COMMON CAUSES OF CHEST PAIN IN CHILDREN

- *Respiratory causes:*
  - Lobar pneumonia
  - Pleurisy
  - Pneumothorax
  - Severe bronchial asthma (may be tightness)
- *Cardiac causes:*
  - Pericarditis
  - ALCAPA
  - Mitral valve prolapse
  - Aortic stenosis
  - Kawasaki disease (due to coronary involvement)
  - Pulmonary valve obstruction
  - Hypertrophic obstructive cardiomyopathy (HOCM)
  - Arrhythmias
- *Miscellaneous:*
  - Trauma
  - Costochondritis
  - Rib fracture
  - Herpes zoster
  - Sickle cell crisis
  - Psychogenic.

Chapter 14: Chest Shape

INTRODUCTION

The shape of the chest can be normal or abnormal. Abnormal shape of chest may cause some respiratory symptoms and signs, which may be benign or manifestations of some serious pulmonary disease. Abnormal shape of chest may be responsible for some cardiac manifestations such as innocent murmur and displacement of apex beat. Cross sections of normal and abnormal forms of chest are shown diagrammatically in **Figures 1A to H**.

NORMAL SHAPES OF CHEST

- Infants have a cylindrical or circular chest, having both transverse and anteroposterior diameters equal.
- Older children and adults have elliptical chest. Elliptical chest has transverse diameter greater than anteroposterior diameter.

ABNORMAL SHAPES OF CHEST

- *Pectus carinatum (pigeon chest)* **(Fig. 2)**:
  - It is also called as keel-shaped chest.
  - Sternum is prominent.
  - It is seen in rickets.
- *Pectus excavatum (funnel-shaped chest)* **(Fig. 3)**:
  - Sternum is depressed and central part of chest is sunken.
  - It reflects excessively compliant chest contents and is often seen in preterm babies.

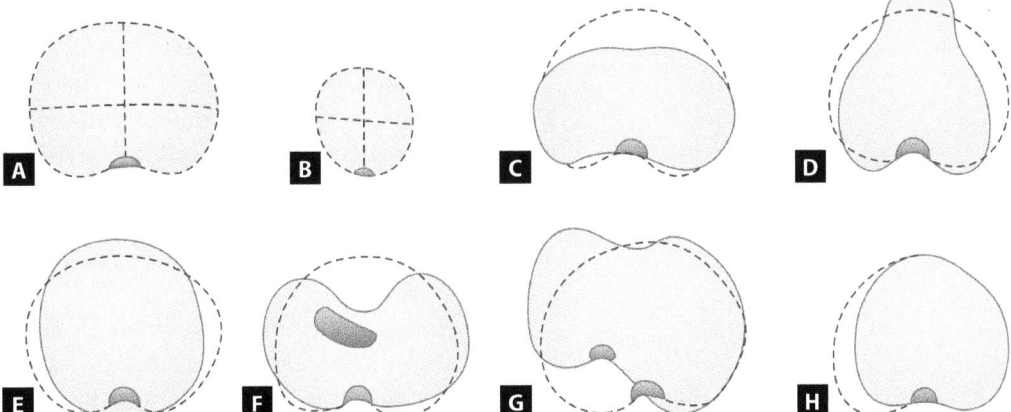

Figs. 1A to H: (A) Adult chest (elliptical); (B) infant chest (cylindrical/circular); (C) flat chest; (D) pigeon chest (rachitic); (E) emphysematous (barrel shaped); (F) funnel chest; (G) kyphoscoliotic chest; and (H) unilateral retraction chest.

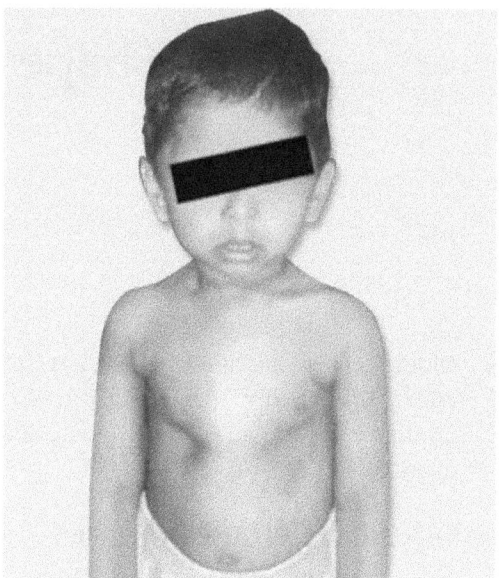

Fig. 2: Pectus carinatum (pigeon chest).

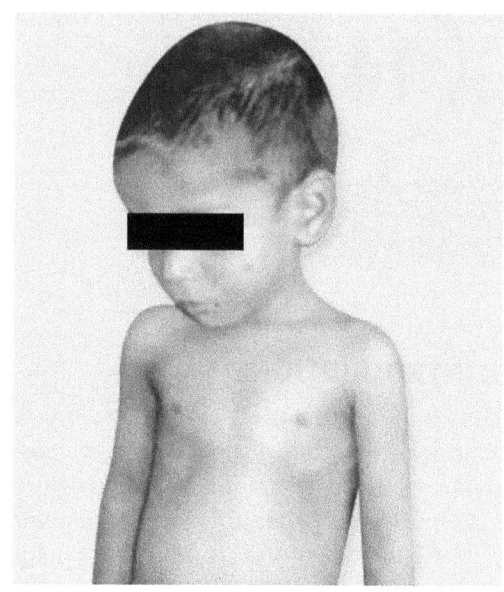

Fig. 4: Harrison's sulcus.

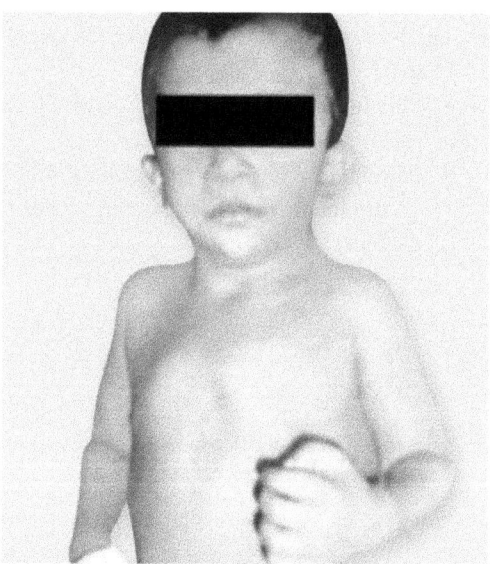

Fig. 3: Pectus excavatum (funnel-shaped chest).

- It can also develop due to bilateral hyperinflated lungs in a child with restrictive lung disease like cystic fibrosis.

- *Barrel-shaped (emphysematous chest):*
  - The chest becomes barrel shaped, appears elongated, and the shoulders are uplifted.
  - Severe hyperinflation in chronic obstructive lung disease such as bronchial asthma results in the chest resembling a barrel.
  - Liver may be pushed down.
- *Harrison's sulcus* (**Fig. 4**):
  - Deep groove along spaces, where the diaphragm is inserted into the inner aspects of ribs, is called Harrison's sulcus.
  - May be a sign of rickets
  - Also seen in children with severe lung diseases
- *Rachitic rosary* (**Fig. 5**): Knob-like swellings at costochondral junctions, seen in rickets.
- *Scorbutic rosary:* There is protrusion of the rib ends because of displacement from the joint. It is seen in a case of scurvy. Scorbutic rosary is sharp and tender.

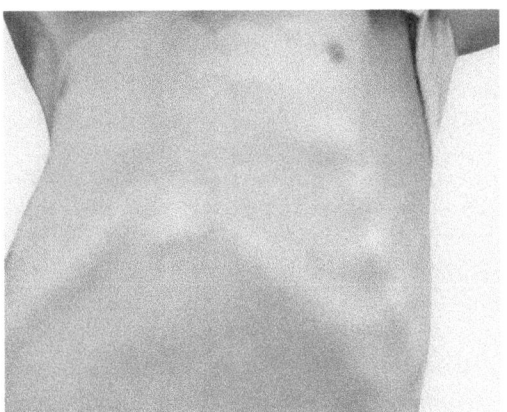

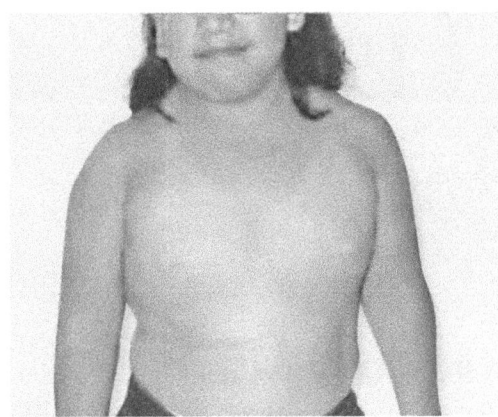

Fig. 5: Rachitic rosary.

Fig. 6: Shield-like chest.

- *Shield-like chest* (**Fig. 6**): Broad chest with widely spaced nipples may be seen in Turner's syndrome.
- Small thoracic cage is seen in Ellis–van Creveld syndrome.
- Kyphosis, lordosis, and kyphoscoliosis like abnormal vertebral column, may give rise to abnormal shape of the chest.

Clubbing

CHAPTER 15

INTRODUCTION

Clubbing is an important clinical sign in medicine. It is thickening of the terminal phalanges and toes due to excessive growth of the connective tissues. Hippocratic nail, watch-glass nails, and drumstick fingers are other names of clubbing.

MECHANISM OF CLUBBING

- The exact mechanism of clubbing is not known. It is believed that endothelial growth factors released during chronic hypoxia and consequent vasodilatation cause the excessive growth of connective tissues, resulting in classical changes of terminal phalanges of fingers and toes, called clubbing.
- Altered prostaglandin metabolism, leading to an increase in the connective tissues, is another probable mechanism.

Methods of Measuring Digital Clubbing (Fig. 1)

- Clubbing may be elicited by rocking the nail on its bed with the examiner's index finger and thumb. It seems to float. It is called fluctuation sign and is an early sign.
- The dorsal surfaces of terminal phalanges of similar fingers are placed together. In a case of clubbing, the normal diamond-shaped window at the base of nail beds disappears. It is called Schamroth sign or Diamond sign. This sign is quite sensitive to pick up even mild clubbing.
- The hyponychial angle is <180° in normal children, but >195° in patients with clubbing.
- The ratio of the distal phalangeal diameter (DPD) to the interphalangeal diameter (IPD) or the phalangeal depth ratio is <1 in normal subjects, but increases to >1 with digital clubbing.

GRADES OF CLUBBING

- *Grade I:* Fluctuation and softening of nail bed
- *Grade II:* Loss of the normal angle between the nail bed and the fold. This is most easily identified by Schamroth sign.
- *Grade III:* Increased convexity of the nails, parrot beak appearance
- *Grade IV:* Drumstick's sign, due to thickening of the whole distal finger
- *Grade V:* Hypertrophic osteoarthropathy (clubbing + thickening of the periosteum). It is less common in children and may be seen in adults.

CAUSES OF CLUBBING

- *Pulmonary causes:*
  - Bronchiectasis
  - Tuberculosis
  - Lung abscess
  - Empyema
  - Cystic fibrosis
  - Interstitial lung disease
  - Sarcoidosis

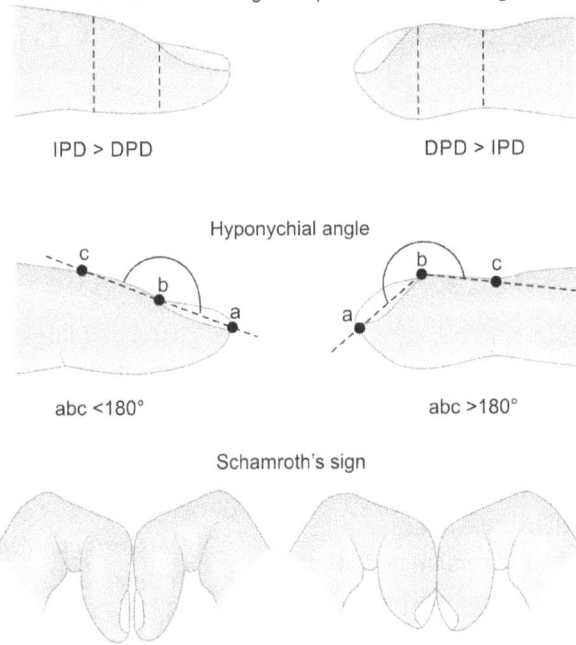

Fig. 1: Methods of measuring digital clubbing.
(DPD: distal phalangeal diameter; IPD: interphalangeal diameter)

- Ciliary dyskinesia
- Mesothelioma of pleura
- *Cardiovascular causes:*
  - Cyanotic congenital heart diseases:
    - Fallot's tetralogy
    - Transposition of great vessels
    - Tricuspid atresia
    - Ebstein anomaly
    - Anomalous pulmonary venous return
  - Bacterial endocarditis
  - Arteriovenous fistula
- *Gastrointestinal causes:*
  - Celiac disease
  - Crohn's disease
  - Ulcerative colitis
  - Cirrhosis of liver
  - Familial polyposis
- *Miscellaneous:*
  - Hereditary (familial)
  - Local trauma to digit
- Scleroderma
- Malignancies such as lymphoma and osteosarcoma
- Pachydermoperiostosis
- Idiopathic
- *Clubbing and anemia:* In a case of anemia, platynychia or koilonychias may be present, but not clubbing. Anemia and clubbing together may be found in the following conditions:
  - Celiac disease
  - Crohn's disease
  - Ulcerative colitis
  - Bacterial endocarditis
  - Arteriovenous fistula
- Clubbing can develop as early as 3 months of age.
- Development of clubbing takes long time, several months. But clubbing may develop in few weeks in a case of lung abscess and bacterial endocarditis.

Constipation

INTRODUCTION

Constipation is a common problem in children. Functional constipation is the most common type of constipation in daily pediatric practice. Functional constipation constituted 30% of pediatric gastroenterology office practice, 4–5% of all referral to pediatric gastroenterology tertiary care centers, and 0.8–1% of all pediatric cases in medical colleges.

DEFINITION

- Constipation may be defined as delay or difficulty in defecation, present for 2 or more weeks and causing significant distress to the child.
- Based on Rome III criteria, Indian Society of Pediatric Gastroenterology, Hepatology and Nutrition and Pediatric Gastroenterology chapter of the Indian Academy of Pediatrics (IAP) has defined criteria of constipation as follows:

  Presence of ≥2 of the following:
  - Defection frequency ≤2 times per week
  - Fecal incontinence ≥1 time per week after the acquisition of toileting skills
  - History of excessive stool retention
  - History of painful or hard bowel movements
  - Presence of large mass in the rectum or on per abdomen examination
  - History of large-diameter stools that may obstruct the toilet
- *Acute constipation:* Less than 4 weeks duration
- *Chronic constipation:* More than 4 weeks duration
- *Stool patterns of normal infants:*
  - The first stool in a neonate is meconium, which is passed in the first 24 hours. Then the child passes six to eight greenish-yellow liquid stools called transitional stools from 2 to 10 days. This is followed by six to eight golden-yellow mature stools per day. However, the normal bowel pattern varies widely. Normal breastfed babies can have as many as seven stools per day or as few as one per 7 days.
  - Infants and toddlers have frequency of stool one to two times per day
  - From the preschool period to adolescence, the bowel frequency is from 3 per day to 3 per week.
- Delayed passage of meconium (>48 hours) in term babies is seen in Hirschsprung disease, intestinal pseudo-obstruction, cystic fibrosis, and hypothyroidism.
- *Constipation may be due to:*
  - Impaired colonic propulsion of luminal contents (fecal retention), e.g., Hirschsprung disease, cerebral palsy, meningomyelocele, and hypothyroidism.

- Increased outlet resistance due to pelvic or anorectal dysfunction (difficulty in defecation), e.g., anorectal malformations such as anal stenosis, anal fissures, and functional constipation.
- Red flags (alarm features) in constipation:
  - Passage of meconium >48 hours in a term newborn
  - Constipation starting in the first month of life or early infancy
  - Family history of Hirschsprung disease
  - Ribbon stools
  - Blood in the stools in the absence of anal fissures
  - Failure to thrive (FTT)
  - Bilious vomiting
  - Severe abdominal distention
  - Abnormal thyroid gland
  - Abnormal position of anus
  - Absent anal or cremasteric reflex
  - Decreased lower extremity strength/tone/reflex
  - Sacral dimple
  - Tuft of hair on spine
  - Gluteal cleft deviation
  - Anal scars
- Age at onset constipation:
  - Delayed passage of meconium (>48 hours) may suggest conditions such as Hirschsprung disease, cystic fibrosis, and hypothyroidism.
  - If onset is in early infancy, organic causes are more likely.
  - Functional constipation often occur at the time of diet changes in infants and at the initiation of toilet training in toddlers.
  - In adolescents, it is due to decreased physical activity, consumption of junk food with *mehnda* (pizza), and irregular lifestyle.
- Pasty stool is seen in Hirschsprung disease and large or hard stool in functional constipation **(Fig. 1)**.

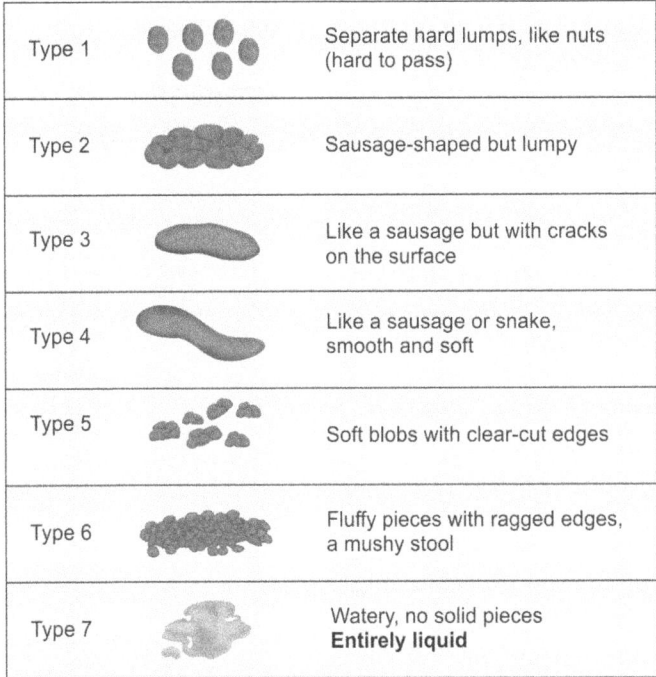

Fig. 1: Bristol stool chart.

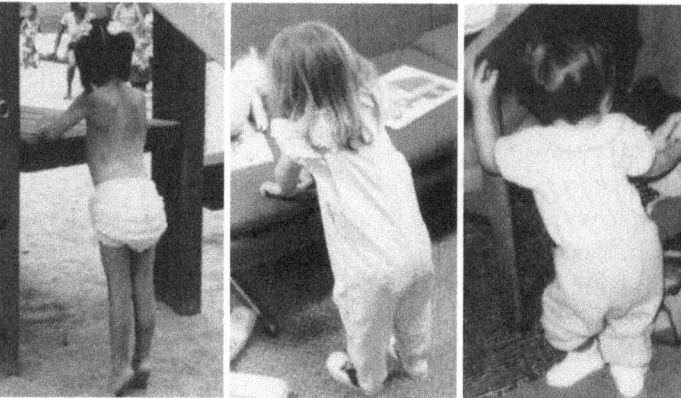

Fig. 2: Retentive Postures.

- Streak of blood with painful defecation suggests anal fissure.
- *Retentive postures:* The child hides behind furniture or goes to a corner, stands on toes with legs crossed and may be red-faced. It is characteristic of functional constipation. Such posturing suggests holding of stool and not straining to pass the stools **(Fig. 2)**.
- Urinary symptoms such as urinary frequency, burning and crying during micturition, urinary retention or incontinence [urinary tract infection (UTI)] with constipation (impacted stool) are known to occur. It is also called a dysfunctional elimination syndrome (DES) or bladder-bowel dysfunction.
- Developmental delay, large, persistent open anterior fontanel, lethargy, dry skin along with constipation are features of hypothyroidism.
- Abdominal distention, enterocolitis (fever, blood in stool, and diarrhea), and FTT are features of Hirschsprung disease.
- Spinal dimple, tuft of hairs, abnormal gait, and other abnormal neurological findings suggest spinal dysraphism, tethered cord, sacral agencies, spinal cord tumor, etc.
- Cerebral palsy, Down syndrome, and neurodegenerative disorders are commonly associated with constipation.
- Meconium ileus, recurrent respiratory tract infections (RTIs), constipation or diarrhea, and FTT are features of cystic fibrosis.
- Abdominal pain, distention of abdomen, constipation, and bilious vomiting are features of mechanical intestinal obstruction, postsurgical intestinal adhesions, etc.
- FTT, refractory iron deficiency anemia, and chronic diarrhea or constipation suggest celiac disease.

PATHOGENESIS OF FUNCTIONAL CONSTIPATION

- Changes in routine
- Changes in diet
- Stressful events
- Postponing defecation (too busy)
- Too early toilet training

↓

Voluntary withholding

↓

Prolonged fecal stasis → Reabsorption of fluid → ↑ in size and consistency

↓

More pain

↓

Painful defecation

↓

Voluntary withholding

COMMON CAUSES OF CONSTIPATION IN CHILDREN

- Functional constipation (95%)
- *Motility-related causes:*
  - Hirschsprung disease
  - Myopathy
- *Congenital anomalies:*
  - Anal stenosis
  - Anteriorly located anus
  - Meningomyelocele
  - Spina bifida
  - Spinal dysraphism
  - Tethered spinal cord
  - Diastematomyelia
  - Sacral agenesis
- *Neurological conditions:*
  - Cerebral palsy
  - Neurodegenerative diseases
- *Endocrinal/metabolic:*
  - Hypothyroidism
  - Diabetes insipidus
  - Renal tubular acidosis
  - Hypercalcemia
- *Drugs:*
  - Codeine
  - Opium
  - Anticonvulsants
  - Antipsychotic
  - Antidiarrheal agents.

Cough

INTRODUCTION

Cough is one of the most common symptoms encountered in daily pediatric practice.
- Cough is a reflex defense mechanism of the respiratory tract. Its main objective is to rid the tracheobronchial tree of foreign particles and mucus.
- *Cough reflex:* The cough reflex involves three main sites:
  1. Cough receptors are located in the nose, sinuses, pharynx, trachea, ear canal, and pleura. Interstitium and lung tissues have "J" receptors for cough. The sensitivity of cough receptors goes on decreasing from upper airway to distal airways.
  2. Cough center is located in the brain stem, to which efferent stimuli arise and are processed.
  3. Effectors like diaphragm and intercostal muscles, actively involved after efferent impulses, are received from the cough center.
- *Mechanism of cough:* The mechanism consists of a short inspiration and inflation of the lungs with air followed by closure of the glottis, compression of the air, and contraction of chest and abdominal muscles. This preparatory stage, during which increased airway pressure is created, is followed by a sudden opening of the glottis and the generation of high-velocity airflow during exhalation.
- *Common etiological principles of cough:*
  - Airway inflammation and production of excessive mucus
  - Spasms of bronchial smooth muscles
  - Direct stimulation of cough receptors
  - Extrinsic pressure: Enlarged lymph nodes (LN), vascular ring, tumors, and retropharyngeal abscess
- Evaluation of cough in a child is always challenging. Only a systemic clinical approach comprising a detailed history and thorough clinical examination is the key to reach the diagnosis. Investigations like complete blood count (CBC) and chest X-ray have their limitations; at most of the occasions, they are normal.

CLINICAL POINTERS SUGGESTING THE CONDITION

- *Onset:*
  - Sudden (hyperacute): Foreign body
  - Acute: viral
  - Recurrent: Bronchial asthma
  - Gradual: Congestive heart failure (L → R shunts)
- *Duration:*
  - Acute: Viral infestations
  - Chronic: Tuberculosis, airway compression by LN or masses (may be progressive as compression increases with enlarging LN or mass)
- *Duration and pattern of cough* (**Fig. 1**):
  - Acute with delayed recovery: Viral

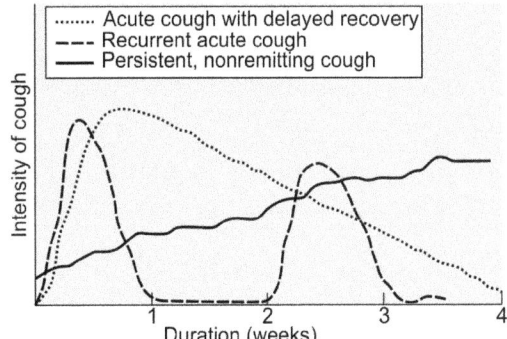

Fig. 1: Pattern of cough and etiology.

- Recurrent: Bronchial asthma.
- Persistent, non-remittent: Tuberculosis.
- *Nature:*
  - Dry: Upper respiratory tract infection (URTI), bronchial asthma
  - Moist (wet): Pneumonia, bronchiectasis, lung abscess, etc.
- *Type:*
  - Barking: Viral croup, laryngitis
  - Spasmodic: Bronchial asthma, allergic
  - Paroxysmal: Pertussis, bronchial asthma
  - Hacking: Tracheitis
  - Staccato cough: Chlamydial infection
- *Whoop:* Pertussis, adenovirus, and chlamydiae
- *Sputum:* Amount, color, odor, and blood
- *Severity:* Disrupts activity, feeding, and sleep
- *Associated symptoms:*
  - Fever (infection)
  - Dyspnea (bronchial asthma, congestive heart failure)
  - Choking (foreign body)
- *Aggravating factors:*
  - Activity (exertional dyspnea)
  - Seasonal: Allergic and bronchial asthma
  - Nocturnal: Bronchial asthma, gastroesophageal reflux disease (GERD), and postnasal drip
  - Posture: More in lying down position (GERD, postnasal drip)
  - Drugs: Angiotensin-converting enzyme (ACE) inhibitors
- *Relieving factors:*
  - Response to bronchodilators (bronchial asthma)
  - Absent cough during sleep: Psychogenic cough (functional).

COUGH IN NEONATES

- Cough in the neonatal period is always abnormal and a cause for concern.
- Although it is common for newborn infants to sneeze, it is abnormal for them to cough.
- The cough reflex is not well developed early in life and is totally absent in preterm babies.
- Causes:
  - Aspirations (GERD, tracheoesophageal fistula)
  - Chlamydial infection
  - Pertussis
- Pleural cough receptors are stimulated by pleurisy, pleural effusion, lobar pneumonia, diaphragmatic hernia, etc.
- Intestinal "J" receptors are stimulated by pulmonary edema, interstitial alveolitis, etc.

Chapter 18: Crying Child

INTRODUCTION

Crying child is a very common symptom, especially in infants and young children, in pediatric outdoor patients. Sometimes, a crying child presents as an emergency and may be difficult for the clinician to decide whether crying in a child is due to a simple cause or a serious condition. Evaluation of the crying child is a challenging situation for a pediatrician.

- Crying is a natural response to any unpleasant stimulus and is the only way of communication for the infants and young children.
- It is said, "Infants do not cry without some legitimate cause".

PHYSIOLOGICAL CONDITIONS

Physiological conditions that make the child cry are:
- Birth cry
- Cry of hunger
- Cry of discomfort
- Cry of emotional deprivation
- Cry of resistance of refusal (do not want)
- Cry of pain
- Cry of habit.

COMMON PATHOLOGICAL CONDITIONS

Common pathological conditions are:
- Infantile colic (2–4 months of age, evening or nocturnal cry)
- Intestinal colic in children
- Earache (otoscopic examination should be routine)
- *Respiratory causes:*
  - Nasal block
  - Nasal foreign body
  - Bronchiolitis (due to hypoxemia)
  - Pleurisy (due to chest pain)
  - Pneumonia (due to respiratory distress)
- *Intracranial pathology:*
  - Central nervous system (CNS) infections (meningitis, encephalitis)
  - Intracranial bleeding (late hemorrhagic disease of newborn).
  - Raised intracranial pressure (ICP) [bulging anterior fontanelle (AF)]
- *Cardiovascular conditions:*
  - Congestive heart failure (CHF) (due to dyspnea)
  - Aberrant left coronary artery originating from pulmonary artery (ALCAPA) (myocardial ischemia) [electrocardiogram (ECG) and echocardiogram (echo) are diagnostic]
- Gastroesophageal reflux disease (GERD) (reflux esophagitis) (crying and arching of body)
- *Crying on handling the child:*
  - Fracture bone
  - Osteomyelitis
  - Septic arthritis
  - Congenital syphilis (hepatosplenomegaly, lymphadenopathy, persistent jaundice, nasal snuffle, perianal excoriation)

- *Surgical conditions:*
  - Acute appendicitis (has been reported in infants and neonates)
  - Intussusception [infants, history of (H/o) upper respiratory tract infections (URTI) or Acute diarrheal disease (ADD), pain in abdomen, mass in abdomen, red currant jelly stool]
  - Torsion of testis (red, edematous scrotum) (never miss to check genitals)
  - Fracture of bones (check for clavicle and limb bones)
  - Septic arthritis
- Night terrors (nightmares) (most common age 18 months to 3 years)
- Drug withdrawal (opium, alcohol)
- Anal fissure (do not miss to examine perianal region for fissure, infection, boil, etc.)
- Constipation
- Urinary retention (urinary bladder is palpable)
- H/o recent vaccination [fever, pain, and excessive crying following diphtheria, tetanus, and pertussis (DPT) vaccination]
- *Drugs:*
  - Anticholinergic drugs (urinary retention)
  - Nalidixic acid, vitamins D and A in excess (benign intracranial hypertension–pseudotumor cerebri)
  - Antihistaminics (excessive crying, seizures, apnea, etc., have been reported, especially in <6 months)
  - Alcohol (withdrawal symptoms)

TYPES OF CRY

- Shrill cry (high-pitched cry) (raised ICP)
- Screaming (intussusception)
- Continuous cry (irritable) (marasmus)
- Intermittent weak cry (kwashiorkor)
- Horse cry (acute laryngitis, croup syndrome, hypothyroidism)
- Cat cry (cri-du-chat syndrome).

Cyanosis

INTRODUCTION

Cyanosis is defined as bluish discoloration of skin, mucous membrane, and nail beds due to deoxygenated (reduced) hemoglobin (Hb) >5 g/dL. In severely anemic children (Hb <5 g/dL), cyanosis may not be apparent in spite of hypoxemia. Apparent clinical presence of cyanosis indicates SPO_2 <85%.

MECHANISM OF CYANOSIS

- When the amount of reduced (deoxygenated) Hb exceeds 5 g/dL in the capillaries, the blood appears dark, giving the tissue a bluish hue. This is seen earliest in the areas with thin skin like palate, tongue, lips, conjunctiva, and nail beds. These structures are also warm due to increased capillary circulation and may be the reason for early detection of cyanosis in these regions. This mechanism is seen in central cyanosis.
- Peripheral cyanosis occurs due to slowing of blood, which allows more time for removal of oxygen (oxygen extraction) by the tissues. It becomes visible on fingers and toes. It is also called as acrocyanosis. It may be seen on the tip of nose and ear lobule. They have a normal systemic arterial saturation. Peripheral cyanosis develops due to vasomotor instability and vasoconstriction following cold, venous obstruction, polycythemia, etc. in neonates. Following rubbing the hands and feet or covering them with clothes, blood circulation improves and cyanosis disappears.
- One should look for cyanosis in the day light. The blue light, blue clothes of the child, and blue curtains in the room may impart bluish hue and may interfere with detection of cyanosis.
- Methemoglobinemia and sulfhemoglobinemia are mimics of cyanosis. In these conditions, cyanosis is due to abnormal pigments. The arterial oxygen tension is normal or elevated despite cyanosis.
- In severe anemia and carbon monoxide poisoning, cyanosis is missed.

TYPES OF CYANOSIS

- Central cyanosis (deoxygenated Hb >5 g/dL)
- Acrocyanosis (peripheral cyanosis) (due to oxygen extraction by the tissues due to cold and stasis of blood)
- Pseudocyanosis (due to abnormal pigments in methemoglobinemia and sulfhemoglobinemia)
- *Differential cyanosis:*
  - Lower limbs are more cyanosed than upper limbs [patent ductus arteriosus (PDA) with reversal of shunt)]
  - Upper limbs are more cyanosed than lower limbs [PDA with reversal of shunt in a child with transposition of the great vessels (TGV)].

- Cyanosis of left upper limb and both lower limbs. (PDA with reversal of shunt in a child with preductal coarctation of aorta).

COMMON CAUSE OF CYANOSIS IN NEWBORNS

- *Respiratory:* Rapid respiration with signs of increased work of breathing, respiratory etiology is likely.
  - Choanal atresia
  - Pierre-Robin syndrome
  - Hyaline membrane disease (HMD)
  - Congenital diaphragmatic hernia (CDH)
  - Meconium aspiration syndrome
  - Airway obstructions
  - Pneumonia, pneumothorax, pleural effusion
- *Cardiovascular:*
  - Tetralogy of Fallot
  - Persistent pulmonary hypertension of the newborn (PPHN)
  - Transposition of the great vessels (TGV)
  - Tricuspid atresia
  - Ebstein anomaly
  - Truncus arteriosus
- *Central nervous system (CNS):*
  - Birth asphyxia
  - Intracranial hemorrhage
  - Seizures
- Methemoglobinemia
- Hypoglycemia
- Polycythemia.

To evaluate the possibility of right to left shunt in the newborns, hyperoxia test should be performed.

COMMON CAUSES OF CYANOSIS IN CHILDREN

- Congenital cyanotic heart diseases like Fallot's tetrad, Eisenmenger's complex, single ventricle, truncus arteriosus, Ebstein anomaly, total/partial anomalous pulmonary venous return, etc.
- Pulmonary causes like pneumothorax, severe bronchial asthma, pulmonary arteriovenous (AV) fistula, severe pneumonia, massive pleural effusion, foreign body, etc.

METHEMOGLOBINEMIA

- Normal hemoglobin has iron in ferrous form. In methemoglobinemia, iron is in the ferric form, designated as methemoglobin (MHb).
- It may be hereditary (absence of reductive pathways) or acquired (due to exposure to toxic substances).
- Nitrates, aniline dyes, dapsone, primaquine, etc. are known to cause methemoglobinemia.
- When MHb levels are >1.5 g/dL, cyanosis is visible.
- In methemoglobinemia, arterial blood is characteristic chocolate-brown colored.
- Arterial oxygen tension is normal or elevated despite cyanosis.
- Ascorbic acid (vitamin C) and intravenous (IV) methylene blue are most effective in this condition. Methylene blue should not be given in a child with glucose-6-phosphate dehydrogenase (G6PD) deficiency.

Delayed Development

INTRODUCTION

A developmental delay referes to a child who has not gained the developmental skills expected of him or her, compared to others of the same age. Delays may occur in the areas of motor function, speech and language, cognitive, play and social skills. There may be deviation or dissociation of development. Delayed development may be restricted to one particular domain or may be global delayed development. It may be simple physiological variation or due to some chronic illness like severe acute malnutrition, autism or serious damage to brain. Methodological evaluation is necessary in each case.

PRINCIPLES OF DEVELOPMENT

- Development is a continuous process from conception to maturity.
- The rate of development may vary in an individual child, but the sequence of development is same in all children.
- The development always proceeds in cephalocaudal direction. A child will learn first to hold his head, followed by sitting, and then walking. This sequence from head to toe will always remain the same, though the age at which each milestone is achieved may differ.
- Development is related to maturation, myelination of the nervous system. The normal development needs an intact anatomical and functionally normal central nervous system (CNS).
  - Anatomical CNS malformations such as anencephaly and meningomyelocele are commonly associated with developmental problems.
  - History of hypoxic ischemic encephalopathy, CNS infection, kernicterus, hypoglycemia, or any other metabolic cause may have delayed development. Such insult during first 5 years of life (while brain is growing) may play an important role in its development.
- Persistent primitive reflexes beyond the age at which they should have disappeared, indicates abnormal development. For example, Moro's reflex disappears by 3 months of age, but presence of Moro's reflex at 7 months of age is suggestive of abnormal development.
- Development in one field may not be parallel to that in other fields and this is termed as developmental dissociation. It helps to decide anatomical localization of the pathology.
- When a child acquires developmental milestones in a nonsequential fashion, it is called as developmental deviation. The child with developmental deviation acquires higher level developmental milestones within a developmental stream before acquiring low-level developmental milestones within that stream. It may be seen in a case of cerebral palsy.

- Developmental delay should be differentiated from developmental regression in which there is loss of milestones which the child has achieved already.

DOMAINS OF DEVELOPMENT
- Gross motor
- Fine motor
- Language (speech and hearing)
- Personal and social milestones.

Important Gross Motor Milestones

Age	Milestone
3 months	Head control (neck holding)
5 months	Rolling over (turning from supine to prone and prone to supine)
6 months	Sitting with support
7 months	Sitting without support
9–10 months	Standing with support
12–13 months	Standing to rise and walking without support
18 months	Running
2 years	Climbing upstair using two feet per step. Kicking a ball
2.5 years	Jumping
3 years	Riding a tricycle, standing on one leg momentarily
4 years	Hopping on one foot. Climbing up and down stairs with one foot per step
5 years	Skipping and jumping

Important Fine Motor Milestones

Age	Milestones
6 weeks	Follows face in midline and turns head toward moving object
4 months	Reaches for toy or red ring or rattle in front with both hands

Contd...

Contd...

Age	Milestones
6 months	Reaches for objects by one hand only (palmar grasp)
7 months	Transfers objects from one hand to another
9 months	Pincer grasp (picks up a pellet with thumb and index finger)
12 months	Throwing the object away
15 months	Able to feed himself with spoon without spilling
18 months	Build tower of three cubes and scribbles
2 years	Vertical and circular strokes
3 years	Copies a circle
4 years	Copies a square and cross
5 years	Draws a triangle

Important Personal and Social Development Milestones

Age	Milestones
4 weeks	Alert to sound
2 months	Social smile
3 months	Recognizes mother
6 months	Smiles at reflection in the mirror
9 months	Waves "bye-bye"
12 months	Plays simple ball games
15–18 months	Holds spoon and feeds without spilling
18–24 months	Copies parents tasks
3 years	Shares toys and knows name and gender. Dry by night
4 years	Attends the toilet alone
5 years	Helps in household works, dresses, and undresses

Important Language Development Milestones

Age	Milestones
4 weeks	Turns head to sound
3 months	Vocalize and cooling sounds
6 months	Speaks monosyllables (ma, ba)
7–8 months	Turns to soft sound out to sight
9 months	Speaks bisyllables (mama, baba)
12 months	Two words with meaning
18 months	10–15 words with meaning. Shows two parts of body
2 years	Uses 2–3 words to make phrases
3 years	Speaks in sentences, tells short stories

RED FLAG SIGNS FOR DEVELOPMENTAL DELAY

- *Gross motor delay:*
  - Tone abnormalities: Hypertonia, hypotonia, dystonia
  - Asymmetry
  - Dysmorphism
  - Persistent primitive reflexes
  - Abnormal deep tendon reflexes (DTR), clonus
  - Hand preferences in <18 months
  - Abnormal gait.
- *Fine motor delay:*
  - Immature grasp till 1 year of age.
  - Poor manipulation of objects till 1 year of age.
  - Excessive clumsiness after 2 years.
  - Assistance in dressing beyond 3 years.
  - Difficulty in buttoning the shirt by 4–5 years.
- *Speech delay:*
  - No babbling: 12 months
  - No single words: 16 months
  - No 2 word phrases: 24 months
  - Regression of language skills at any age
  - Loss of social skills
- *Cognitive delay:*
  - Difficulty in following simple instructions
  - Difficulty in learning new skills
  - Poor expressive language
  - Behavioral problems
  - Poor self-help and increased dependency.

After performing developmental assessment as per standard methods, if there is abnormal development, identify if there is delay, deviation, or dissociation.

- *Global developmental delay* is identified if the developmental quotient (DQ) is <70 in one or more domains.
- *Deviation* is identified if the child develops skill out of the usual sequence, e.g., hand preference by 12 months. This is characteristics of cerebral palsy. Check for other markers of cerebral palsy.
- *Dissociation* is identified if the development is different in different developmental spheres, e.g., autism.

CONDITIONS MIMICKING DEVELOPMENTAL DELAY

- Transient tone abnormalities
- Less environmental stimulation
- Vision and hearing loss
- Epilepsy
- Autism
- Child with chronic illness
- Severe acute malnutrition
- Muscular disorders
- Neurodegenerative disorders
- Spacing-occupying lesion (SOL) of brain
- Hydrocephalus
- Metabolic disorders
- Genetic syndromes.

MARKER FOR CEREBRAL PALSY IN INFANCY

- Acquire handedness before 1 year of age
- Cross midline to pick up a toy
- Persistent fisting after 4 months of age
- Long roll rather than segmental roll

- Leg scissoring when picked up
- Persistent primitive reflexes.

CAUSES OF GLOBAL DEVELOPMENTAL DELAY

- *Prenatal:*
  - *Genetic:* Chromosomal defects
  - *Acquired:* Maternal infections, nutritional deficiencies, fetal alcohol syndrome, maternal substance abuse
- *Perinatal:*
  - Hypoxic ischemic encephalopathy
  - Infections
  - Stroke
  - Hypoglycemia
  - Metabolic disturbances
- *Postnatal:*
  - Infections leading to meningoencephalitis
  - Kernictems
  - Trauma
  - Stroke
  - Severe malnutrition
  - Psychosocial deprivation.

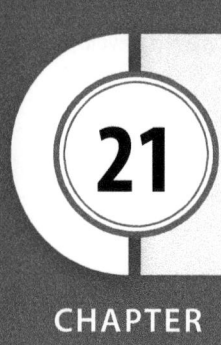

Diarrhea

CHAPTER 21

INTRODUCTION

Diarrhea is defined as a passage of three or more loose or watery stools in a 24-hours period. However, it is the recent change in consistency and character of stool and its water content rather than the number of stools that is important.

What should not be mistaken as diarrhea?
- Frequency of stool several times in a day in breastfed neonates.
- Loose, watery stools in breastfed neonates and young infants (transitional stools or loose, watery stool due to high lactose content of breast milk).
- Gastrocolic reflex in neonates (passage of small stools frequently, just after breastfeeding).
- If the baby remains well hydrated, has no signs of sepsis, feeds well, remains playful, sleeps well, gains weight, and passes urine >5 times in a day, there is no cause of concern. The parents should be reassured accordingly by showing normal growth of the baby, plotted on growth chart.
- *Starvation diarrhea:* In malnourished infants with poor food intake, passage of green colored, frequent stools. It is unused bile due to starvation. With improvement in oral intake, it gets controlled.

MICROANATOMY OF GASTROINTESTINAL SYSTEM IN A CASE OF DIARRHEA

- In adults, about 9 L of fluid (7 L from various body secretions + 2 L from food) reach the proximal small intestine daily. The small intestine absorbs 7.5 L and 1.5 L pass through the ileocecal valve into the colon which in turn absorbs 1.4 L. Hence, large, watery stools resulting in dehydration indicate an acute small intestine disease. Acute rotaviral diarrhea is a classical prototype of small intestinal infection.
- When small intestinal disease is chronic, the children present with infrequent, small stools.
- Since the small intestine is the site for maximal digestion and absorption, incomplete digestion of carbohydrate leads to fermentation of the residue and consequent gas formation and abdominal distention.
- The children with undigested protein and fat present with large quantity, semisolid stools with offensive smell and presence of fat globules. In these children, white stool is due to undigested fat.
- Deficiency of nutrients and failure to thrive are common associated manifestations due to malabsorption syndrome.

- A child with large intestinal diarrhea has small, frequent stools usually associated with blood and mucus. In these children, severe tenesmus and lower abdominal pain are very common complaints. Large bowel problems can also present with constipation, anal fissure, and sentinel tag.

CLINICAL TYPES OF DIARRHEAL DISEASES

- *Acute (watery) diarrheal disease (ADD):*
  - ADD starts suddenly and lasts for few days.
  - Usually, subsides by 1 week, but may go up to 2 weeks.
  - Most common causes of ADD are viral infections, cholera, etc. The classical example of ADD is rotaviral diarrhea.
  - The main dangers are dehydration, electrolytes disturbances, and acute weight loss.
- *Acute bloody diarrhea (dysentery):*
  - Presents with frequency of stool, small quantity with gross blood, and mucus in stool. There may be fever, lower abdominal pain, and tenesmus.
  - Invasive organisms such as *Salmonella*, *Shigella*, enteroinvasive *Escherichia coli* (EIEC), *Campylobacter*, and *Yersinia* are most common for dysentery or colitis. Amoebic dysentery is not common in children.
  - Mucosal ulceration and acute inflammation are responsible for clinical manifestations of disease.
- *Persistent diarrhea:*
  - Starts as acute watery diarrhea and lasts for >14 days.
  - More common in younger children (<18 months). Lack of breast-feeding, bottle-feeding, and antibiotics are other factors.
  - The main causes are persistent infections and malabsorption particularly of carbohydrates (secondary lactose intolerance). Infrequently, dietary protein intolerance is also found.
- *Chronic diarrhea (malabsorption syndrome):*
  - Insidious onset very often, parents do not remember exactly when it started.
  - Malabsorption is the root cause.
  - Common manifestations are persistent or recurrent abnormal stools in form of large quantity (bulky) semi solid, offensive, containing undigested food material (greasy and yellowish).
  - Malnutrition and failure to thrive (FTT) are common results of malabsorption. Dehydration is rare. Multiple nutritional deficiencies are very common associated features.

COMMON CAUSES OF DIARRHEA

- *Acute (watery) diarrheal disease:*
  - *Rotavirus*
  - *Cryptosporidium*
  - Enterotoxigenic *E. coli*
  - *Enterovirus*
  - Cholera
  - *Giardia lamblia*
- *Acute bloody diarrhea (Dysentery):*
  - *Shigella*
  - *Salmonella*
  - Enteroinvasive *E. coli*
  - *Campylobacter jejuni*
  - *Yersinia*
  - *Entamoeba histolytica*
- *Persistent diarrhea:*
  - Age: <18 months
  - Protein-energy malnutrition (PEM) (zinc and vitamin A deficiency)
  - Lack of breast-feeding
  - Bottle-feeding

- Cow's milk
- Inappropriate antibiotics
- Parenteral diarrhea [urinary tract infection (UTI), otitis media]
- *Chronic diarrhea (malabsorption syndrome):*
  - Tuberculosis
  - Human immunodeficiency virus (HIV)
  - Celiac disease
  - Giardiasis
  - Cystic fibrosis
  - Inflammatory bowel diseases (Crohn's disease, ulcerative colitis).
  - Primary immunodeficiency disorders
  - Acrodermatitis enteropathica
  - Intestinal lymphangiectasis
  - Vitamin B-12 malabsorption
  - Lactose deficiency
  - Hyperthyroidism
  - Abetalipoproteinemia
  - Tropical sprue
  - Malignancy (ganglioneuroma).

Distention of Abdomen

INTRODUCTION

Distention of abdomen is a very common complaint by parents in daily pediatric practice. Methodological approach is rewarding.

- The abdomen may be protuberant in infants normally due to lack of tone of abdominal wall muscles.
- It can also be protuberant due to rickets, protein energy malnutrition (PEM), hypothyroidism, mucopolysachharidosis (MPS), Down syndrome, etc.
- Look at the abdomen, whether the abdominal distension is localized or generalized. *If it is localized, it indicates following conditions:*
  - Upper part of abdomen may be full due to organomegaly, commonly hepatomegaly with or without splenomegaly. Hepatomegaly presents as distention of abdomen as it is located anteriorly. Splenomegaly presents as lump in abdomen.
  - In a case of intestinal obstruction, central distention indicates small bowel obstruction.
  - A localized distention may be due to an abdominal lump like Wilms tumor, neuroblastoma, mesenteric cyst, ovarian cyst, etc.
  - A globular suprapubic swelling is usually due to full urinary bladder.
  - Appearance of transient swelling or lump in epigastric region after feeding an infant suggests congenital hypertrophic pyloric stenosis. Many a times, it is noticed by the mother moving on right side and disappearing after vomiting.

GENERALIZED DISTENTION OF ABDOMEN

The traditionally taught five causes of generalized abdominal distention are fluid, flatus, faeces, fat, and fetus.

- Uniform fullness of abdomen along with fullness of flanks indicates ascites. Presence of transversely stretched umbilicus (smiling umbilicus) favors ascites. It can be confirmed with sign of ascites like shifting dullness, horseshoe shape dullness, and presence of fluid thrill.
- Sometimes, large mesenteric cyst or ovarian cyst may mimic ascites.
- Distention of abdomen due to flatus and feces presents as waxing and waning, nonprogressive abdominal distention.
- An excess of adipose visceral fat causes protrusion of abdomen due to central obesity. This body type is also known as "apple-shaped", as opposed to "pear-shaped" in which fat is deposited on the hips and buttocks.

Paralytic ileus also may cause distention of abdomen. *The common causes of paralytic ileus are:*
- Post abdominal surgery
- Hypokalemia
- Bacterial toxins (enteric fever, bacterial sepsis)
- Necrotizing enterocolitis (NEC) in newborns, especially preterm babies
- Antimotility drugs like loperamide.

23 Dysmorphism

INTRODUCTION

Dysmorphology term was coined by Dr David Smith, author of "Smith's Recognizable Patterns of Human Malformation" in 1966, to describe the study of human congenital malformation. It encompasses the variability of normal physical trait as well as pathologic features resulting from abnormal development.

DEFINITION

Dysmorphology is a discipline of clinical genetics which deals with the study of abnormal patterns of human growth, its recognition, and study of congenital human structural anomalies as well as patterns of birth defects.

CONGENITAL MALFORMATIONS (BIRTH DEFECTS)

Congenital malformations (birth defects) can be subclassified as major or minor anomalies:
- *Major anomalies* are those that interfere with the normal functioning of an individual and pose a significant health problem or risk to life, e.g., congenital heart defects, neural tube defects, omphalocele, cleft palate, etc.
- *Minor anomalies* do not interfere with the normal functioning of an individual and usually are only of cosmetic significance, e.g., simian crease, accessory nipple, clinodactyly, preauricular skin tags, etc.
- Major anomalies are present in 2–3% and minor anomalies are present in around 15% of live births.
- Minor anomalies are usually associated with an increased risk of associated major anomalies and therefore presence of minor anomalies should prompt a thorough search for associated major anomalies.

CLASSIFICATION OF CONGENITAL ANOMALIES

Congenital anomalies are classified on the basis of the developmental stage in which the insult occurred, the process that caused the change and the end result into the followings:
- *Malformation:* Primary intrinsic developmental defect usually caused by genetic or environmental or multifactorial causes which occur during the period of organogenesis which is up to 8 weeks post fertilization for most organs, e.g., neural tube defects, ventricular septal defect, polydactyly, etc.
- *Deformation:* Distortion of a normally developed structure caused by mechanical forces usually in the latter half of gestation and most often involving musculoskeletal tissues, e.g., club foot, torticollis, plagiocephaly, etc.
- *Disruption:* Breakdown of an intrinsically normally developing or developed tissue due to some disruptive events such as a mechanical, vascular, or infectious insult, e.g., amniotic band sequence.

- *Dysplasia:* Abnormal cellular organization within a tissue, almost always of genetic origin, e.g., skeletal dysplasia.

SYNDROME

A syndrome is a recognized composite pattern of two or more anomalies with a common specific etiology, e.g., Down syndrome, Turner syndrome, fetal phenytoin syndrome, etc.

ASSOCIATION

An association is a nonrandom occurrence of two or more anomalies that occur together more frequently than expected by chance alone, but without a known specific etiology, e.g., VACTERL association.

VACTERL: **V**ertebral defects, **A**nal atresia, **C**ardiac defects, **t**racheo**e**sophageal (*TE*) fistula, **R**enal anomalies, and **L**imb abnormalities.

APPROACH TO A DYSMORPHIC CHILD

- Gathering information
- Constructing pedigree and analysis of pedigree
- Reviewing past records and prenatal history
- *Clinical assessment:*
  - Visual assessment
  - Measurement
  - Extended family
- Counseling
- Follow-up.

SUSPICION

Genetic etiology is suspected in any child with:
- Congenital anomalies: At least one major and/or two minor anomalies
- Growth deficit [failure to thrive (FTT), short stature, etc.]
- Developmental delay, developmental regression
- Failure to develop secondary sexual characteristics
- Abnormal genitalia
- Unusual or different appearance.

HISTORY

- *Family history:*
  - Three generation family history/pedigree (to define pattern of inheritance)
  - Consanguinity [increased risk of autosomal recessive (AR) disorders]
  - Recurrent abortions, still-births, previously affected babies or relatives (medical record should be checked)
  - Parental age (Advanced maternal age: Trisomy 21, 13, 18). (Advanced paternal age: Achondroplasia, Apert syndrome, Marfan syndrome)
  - Ethnic background
- *Antenatal history:*
  - Drugs (anticonvulsants, methotrexate, retinoic acid, periconceptional folic acid): Fetal phenytoin, valproate syndrome
  - Maternal infections (rubella, toxoplasmosis, etc.)
  - Maternal illness [diabetes mellitus, systemic lupus erythematosus (SLE), phenylketonuria, etc.]
  - Abnormal screening tests [↑ alpha-fetoprotein (AFP), ↓ human chorionic gonadotropin (hCG)]
  - Abnormal ultrasonography (USG) [detection of malformations, intrauterine growth restriction (IUGR)]
- *Perinatal history:*
  - Presentation/mode/complications of delivery
  - Gestational age
  - Apgar score
  - Birth weight, birth length, head circumference, and proportions.

- *Neonatal history:*
  - Feeding history
  - Activity
  - Floppy
  - Complications
- *Postnatal history:*
  - Developmental history
  - Growth pattern (plotted on growth chart)
  - Neurological complications (seizures, vision, hearing, and behavior)
  - Other systemic examination.

PHYSICAL EXAMINATION
General Principles
- Observe the child and his parents to see if the child resembles them or looks different. Also see other available family members for similar or related features.
- Do not make the patient or parents feel conscious or offending during the examination.
- Do not discuss or make any comments about the dysmorphic features in front of the patient and their family. You can do it gently, softly, and indirectly.
- A detailed head-to-toe physical examination with recognition of facial dysmorphism, congenital anomalies, and anthropometric measurements should be taken.
- Abnormalities of growth, body proportions, and asymmetry also should be looked for.
- Knowledge of normal and abnormal phenotypic features and their appropriate description is very important as the first step for diagnosis.
- A keen observation is important to recognize congenital anomalies.
- Recognize variations present in one of the parents and child as these may be normal variants and not of clinical significance.
- Take clinical photographs (with consent of the patient or parents or guardians) for records, syndrome search, referral, and study of evolution of phenotype.

Head-to-Toe Assessment
- *Skull:* Size, fontanelles, shape, sutures, symmetry, etc.
- *Scalp hair:* Color, texture, distribution, hair whorl patterns, position of anterior and posterior hairlines, and sweep of the hair
- *Face:*
  - *Facial appearance:* Coarse facies, Down syndrome facies, myopathic facies, Elfin facies, etc.
  - *Shape, symmetry, and size of face:* Triangular, round, broad, etc.
  - *Face into sections:* Forehead, midface, oral region, etc.
  - View face from front and from sides
  - Lateral profile of face is better for depth or height of structures such as nasal bridge, position of mandible relative to maxilla and midface development.
- *Facial measurements:*
  - Interpupillary distance
  - Inner canthal distance
  - Outer canthal distance
  - Interalar distance
  - Length of philtrum
  - Upper lip thickness
  - Lower lip thickness
  - Intercommissural distance
  - Compare to age and sex norms, < or >2 standard deviation (SD) ≥ abnormal
- *Forehead:*
  - *Size:* Small, tall, and broad
  - *Shape:* Slopping, frontal bossing, bitemporal narrowing, metopic prominence
  - *Supraorbital ridges:* Prominent, underdeveloped

- Maxilla (midface):
  - *Cheek bone:* Prominent, underdeveloped, fullness
  - *Malar region:* Prominent, flat
  - *Midface:* Prominence, retrusion
  - *Nasolabial folds:* Prominent, underdeveloped
- Mandible:
  - *Size and shape:* Micrognathia, retrognathia, prominence
- Eyes:
  - Eyebrows
  - *Palpable fissures:* Length (short/long), slant (up/down)
  - Epicanthal folds
  - *Eye spacing:* Rough guide 1:1:1 for ratio of left palpebral fissure length, inner canthal distance, right palpebral fissure length
  - Palpebral fissure shape, iris color, pupil shape, cornea, sclera, lens, and globe position
- *Nose:* From lateral view, superior, and inferior
  - Nasal root
  - Nasal bridge: Depressed, prominent, broad
  - Nasal tip: Broad, flattened, beak-like
  - Nostrils: Patency and position (anteverted)
  - Alae nasi: Hypoplastic
- Mouth and perioral region:
  - Size and shape of mouth
  - Lip shape, thickness
  - Gum thickness
  - Philtrum: Length
  - Jaw position (micrognathia, retrognathia)
  - Palate
  - Teeth
  - Frenum
  - Tongue: Size, shape, morphology
- Ears:
  - Ear position (low set ears)
  - Ear rotation: Anterior or posterior rotation
  - Ear shape and structure
  - Accessory structures: Skin tags, pits
- Skeleton:
  - Neck: Length, shape, webbing
  - Shape of thorax
  - Sternum: Length, shape (pectus carinatum, excavatum)
  - Spine: Length, straight, curved, (kyphosis, lordosis, scoliosis)
  - Limbs: Length, shape, symmetry
- Joints:
  - Contractures
  - Range of movements
  - Laxity/restriction
  - Soft tissue webbing across joints
- Skin:
  - Texture: Smooth, coarse, dry, ichthyotic
  - Pigmentation: Hypopigmentation, hyperpigmentation, patchy, generalized
  - Naevi/lentigines
  - Redundancy/laxity
- Hands and feet:
  - Shape and size
  - Digit number
  - Digital shape (clinodactyly) and length
  - Webbing between digits
  - Palmar, planter, and digital creases
  - Nail morphology
- Genitals and anus:
  - Phallus size and morphology
  - Development, rugosity, pigmentation of scrotum
  - Size and position of testes
  - Micro- or macropenis
  - Development of labia, clitoris
  - Position of anus and its patency
- Systemic examination in details for malformations, organomegaly, lymphadenopathy, mass, etc.

Dysphagia

INTRODUCTION

The process of swallowing (deglutition) involves the movement of food from the oral cavity to the stomach via pharynx and esophagus. It has three stages: oral, pharyngeal, and esophageal. Anatomical, functional, and iatrogenic causes affecting any of the stages of swallowing can lead to dysphagia.

COMMON CAUSES OF DYSPHAGIA

Disorders Affecting Mouth and Pharynx

- *Mechanical problems:*
  - Cleft palate
  - Macroglossia: It may be due to hemangioma, lymphangioma, cyst, or large tongue with true muscle enlargement.
  - Temporomandibular joint ankylosis: It may be associated with connective tissue disorders.
  - Micrognathia
  - Pharyngeal diverticulum
  - Foreign body
- *Infectious:*
  - Oral infections: Infectious of tongue, gums, tonsils, and buccal mucosa may interfere with swallowing.
  - Retropharyngeal abscess
  - Peritonsillar abscess
  - Cervical lymphadenitis
  - Meningitis
  - Tetanus
  - Diphtheria
  - Poliomyelitis.

Neuromuscular Disorders

- Cerebral palsy
- Guillain-Barré syndrome
- Poliomyelitis
- Palatal paralysis (IX and X cranial nerve palsy)
- Arnold-Chiari malformation
- Cricopharyngeal incoordination
- Werdnig-Hoffman disease
- Myasthenia gravis
- Miscellaneous:
  - Dermatomyositis
  - Dystonia musculorum deformans
  - Prader-Willi syndrome
  - Stevens-Johnson syndrome
  - Juvenile rheumatoid arthritis
  - Familial dysautonomia.

Disorders Affecting Esophagus

- Foreign body
- Esophageal stricture
- Tracheoesophageal fistula
- Vascular anomalies compressing esophagus
- Mediastinal tumor
- Esophageal duplication
- Enlarged left atrium compressing esophagus
- Esophageal tumors such as papillomas, neuromas, lipomas, etc.

- Esophageal web
- Candidiasis
- Crohn disease
- Corrosives
- Gastroesophageal reflux disease (GERD)
- Achalasia
- Esophageal spasm
- Scleroderma
- Dermatomyositis
- Sjögren syndrome
- Guillain-Barré syndrome.

Dyspnea

INTRODUCTION

Looking for following clinical signs and their analysis is rewarding for deriving clinical diagnosis in a child with dyspnea. Occasionally, chest X-ray and ultrasonography (USG) of thorax may not help, but clinical analysis leads for further workup and condition is revealed.

SIGNS OF INCREASED WORK OF BREATHING

- Tachypnea
- Chest retractions (suprasternal, subcostal, and intercostal)
- Use of accessory muscles (sternocleidomastoid muscle)
- Flaring of alae nasi
- Head bobbing
- Abnormal sounds (stridor, wheezing, and grunting)
- Type of breathing
- Altered sensorium and cyanosis.

Tachypnea

The respiratory rate should be counted for complete 60 seconds when the child is quiet (not crying) or sleeping. The cutoff rates for tachypnea at different ages are as follows:

Age	Respiratory rate/min
0–2 months	≥60
2 months to 1 year	≥50
1–5 years	≥40
>5 years	≥30

Chest Retractions

The presence of chest retractions and site of retractions indicate the site of pathology and severity of disease.

- *Subcostal indrawing (SCI):* Increased work of diaphragm (bronchiolitis)
- *Intercostal indrawing (ICI):* Decreased lung parenchymal compliance (pneumonia, congestive heart failure)
- *Suprasternal indrawing (SSI):* Involvement of upper airway [(vascular ring, diphtheria, and acute laryngotracheobronchitis (ALTB)]
- With increased severity of disease, chest retractions may develop at multiple sites, but site of retractions at onset of disease indicates pathology.

Abnormal Chest Sounds

- *Nasal snuffle:* Excessive nasal secretion causing noisy nasal breathing. It is common in infants in the first 3 months of life. If it is since birth with hepatosplenomegaly, lymphadenopathy, and perianal excoriation, congenital syphilis should be considered in differential diagnosis.
- *Snoring:* It is noisy breathing during sleep. It indicates upper airway obstruction in a case of hypertrophy of adenoids or obesity.
- *Rattling sounds:* Throaty, gurgling sounds, commonly heard in a case of laryngomalacia
- *Stridor:* Extrathoracic airway obstruction (vascular ring)

- *Wheeze:* Intrathoracic airway obstruction (bronchiolitis, bronchial asthma)
- *Rales:* Small clicking, bubbling sounds heard in the lungs during inspiration, common in a case of bronchiolitis
- *Grunt:* Lung parenchymal disease (hyaline membrane disease in newborn, severe pneumonia).

Abnormal Breathing

- *Prolonged inspiration:* Upper airway obstruction
- *Prolonged expiration:* Bronchial asthma
- *Rapid breathing without retractions and sounds:* Metabolic acidosis
- *Rapid breathing with minimal retractions:* Congestive heart failure
- *Rapid shallow breathing:* Pleurisy
- *Apneustic breathing:* Central nervous system (CNS) lesion
- Presence of flaring of alae nasi and head bobbing indicates severe respiratory distress.

RESPIRATORY SIGNS AND SITE OF LESION

	Extrathoracic	Intrathoracic	Pulmonary
Tachypnea	+	++	+++
Retractions	++++	++	++
Stridor	+++	+	–
Wheeze	–	++	+++
Grunt	–	–	+

- Altered sensorium and cyanosis are signs of severe hypoxemia.

Earache (Otalgia)

INTRODUCTION

Earache (otalgia) is a common symptom in pediatric practice. The ears have rich sensory innervation from multiple nerves. Therefore, not all ear pain is otologic; it may be secondary too. Earache in most children is the result of acute middle ear infections or chronic accumulation of fluid in the middle ear. Otitis externa is also common in the summer season. Self-induced trauma to the ear canal or tympanic membrane occurs more frequently than generally thought of. They stick all sorts of matter into their ear canals.

The causes of otalgia can be divided into two groups: disorders involving the ear primarily and those in which ear pain is referred from disease in another area, particularly those innervated by cranial nerves with ties to the ear.

PRIMARY OTALGIA

External Ear

- Otitis externa (pinnae and tragus are painful)
- Impacted cerumen (causes occlusion of ear canal leading to ear pain and hearing loss)
- Ear trauma: The ear canal or auricle may be injured by self-induced trauma with sticks, paper clips, and similar objects used to scratch the ears or remove cerumen. Trauma may result from falls, blows, and other forms of trauma.
- Furuncle or abscess
- Foreign body (beads, toys, pins, etc.)
- Cellulitis (red, swollen, and tender auricle)
- Chronic eczema
- Herpes simplex
- Herpes zoster
- Perichondritis.

Middle and Inner Ear

- Acute otitis: This is the most common cause of earache. The tympanic membrane is dull, bulging, and erythematous on otoscopic examination.
- Otitis media with effusion
- Eustachian tube obstruction: Swelling of the lining tissues of the Eustachian tube by infection or allergies may prevent equalization of air pressure between the middle ear and the environment. Serous otitis media may follow long-standing obstruction.
- Barotrauma (sudden changes in air pressure cause acute earache)
- Bullous myringitis (vesicles and hemorrhage may be noted on tympanic membrane).
- Mastoiditis: Untreated middle ear infection may extend to the mastoid cells. The mastoid area becomes erythematous, swollen, and tender on touch. The pinna may be pushed out and forward away from the head.
- Bell palsy

Earache (Otalgia)

- Tumors such as angiomas and rhabdomyosarcoma may result in Eustachian tube dysfunction.
- Temporal bone neoplasma (rare).

SECONDARY OTALGIA

Pain is referred from other sites of the disease:

- Acute pharyngitis
- Tonsillitis
- Retropharyngeal abscess
- Dental problems
- Esophageal foreign body
- Gastroesophageal reflux disease
- Temporomandibular joint dysfunction
- Postauricular lymphadenopathy
- Sinusitis
- Mumps
- Herpes zoster (Ramsay Hunt syndrome).

27 Edema

INTRODUCTION

Edema is defined as excessive accumulation of fluid in the interstitial space or serous cavities. It can be either localized or generalized.
- Apparent puffy face, swelling over feet, or ascites are obvious presentations of edema.
- Excessive weight gain (especially in neonates), tight fitting of clothes or shoes, and feeling discomfort by the child are other indicators of development of edema.

PITTING OR NONPITTING EDEMA

- Pressing over skin of tibia or above the medial malleolus for 30 seconds and development of a pit or depression indicate pitting as edema. Pitting edema is due to fluid collection in subcutaneous plane **(Figs. 1A and B)**.
- Nonpitting edema is commonly due to lymphatic cause like filariasis, lymphangiectasia, and lymphatic obstruction. Turner syndrome, Noonan syndrome, and hypothyroidism are other causes of nonpitting edema **(Fig. 2)**.
  Swelling of the hands and feet (pretibial nonpitting edema) in a short, female infant highly suggests Turner syndrome.

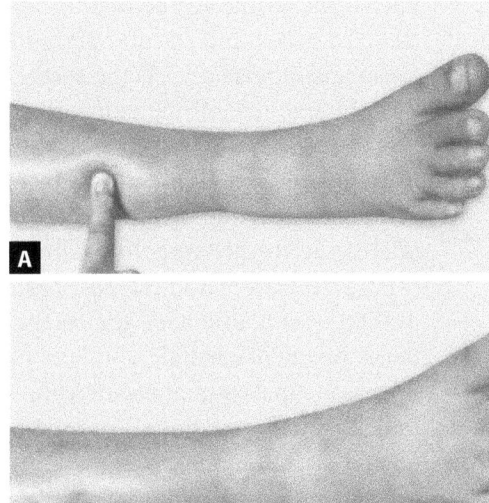

Figs. 1A and B: Dermonstration of pedal edema. It should be pressed over shin of tibia or malleolus for 30 seconds and see for pitting impression.

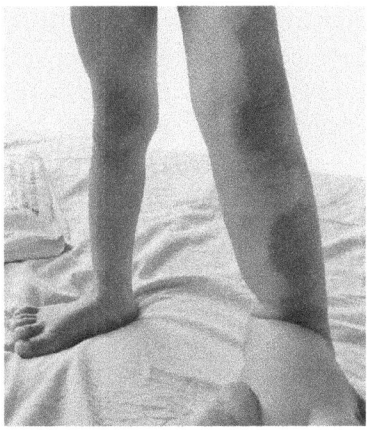

Fig. 2: Nonpitting edema.

LOCALIZED OR GENERALIZED EDEMA

- *Localized edema:* Localized edema (swelling) may be due to insect bite and some pressure effect like tourniquet or tight bandage. Urticaria, cellulitis, and angioneurotic edema are other causes of localized edema.
- *Generalized edema:*
  - Physiologically, balance between hydrostatic pressure and oncotic pressure maintains intravascular compartment fluid volume. Any imbalance in this can lead to edema.
  - Increased hydrostatic pressure in conditions like congestive heart failure (CHF), acute glomerulonephritis (AGN), and hypertension causes oozing of fluid in subcutaneous tissues and development of edema.
  - Increased capillary permeability causes leak of fluid and development of edema as in a case of dengue fever, drug allergies, etc. Henoch–Schonlein purpura, systemic lupus erythematosus (SLE), and Kawasaki disease are other examples.
  - Decreased oncotic pressure (low protein, mainly low albumin) cannot retain the fluid in the intravascular compartment and gets collected in subcutaneous tissues (leading to edema) or serous cavities (resulting in development of ascites, pleural effusion, etc.).
  - Decreased oncotic pressure indicates low serum albumin. It may be due to several reasons like:
    - Decreased intake (nutritional), e.g., Kwashiorkor
    - Decreased synthesis of protein (albumin): Albumin is synthesized by rough endoplasmic reticulum of hepatocytes in the liver. Therefore, decreased synthesis of protein indicates liver disease of hepatocyte origin, e.g., cirrhosis of liver.
    - Loss of protein (albumin) from the body: Loss of protein from the gastrointestinal (GI) tract is due to malabsorption in conditions like celiac disease and human immunodeficiency virus (HIV). Renal loss is known in a case of nephrotic syndrome.

BILATERAL OR UNILATERAL

- *Bilateral:*
  - Cardiac: CHF, pericarditis
  - Renal: Nephrotic syndrome, acute glomerulonephritis
  - Hepatic: Cirrhosis of liver, portal hypertension
  - Endocrinal: Myxedema
  - Allergic: Angioneurotic edema
  - Nutritional: Kwashiorkor
  - Toxic: Epidemic dropsy
- *Unilateral:*
  - Filariasis
  - Cellulitis
  - Deep vein thrombosis
  - Fracture of bones.

ONSET, SITE, AND PROGRESSION

- *Acute onset:* Insect bite, angioneurotic edema (**Fig. 3**), allergic, acute glomerulonephritis (AGN).
- *Insidious onset:* Nephrotic syndrome, hepatic causes (half-life of serum albumin is 21 days).
- *Periorbital edema* (fluid collection starts in periorbital region due to lax subcutaneous tissues and fat): Renal origin, acute conditions like angioneurotic edema and

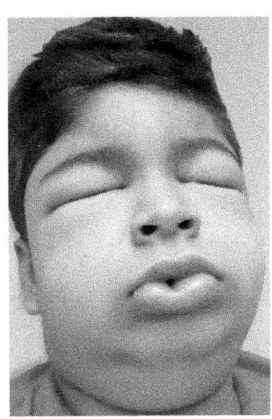

Fig. 3: Angioneurotic edema.

iatrogenic excessive intravenous (IV) fluid therapy.
- *Morning edema:* Renal origin. It develops due to gravitational factor during sleep.
- *Bilateral pedal:* Sacral (dependent) edema, Congestive heart failure due to venous stasis
- *Ascites:* Hypoalbuminemia due to liver disorders.

In any condition with progression of diseases, gradually it becomes generalized anasarca. But site of edema at the onset of disease gives an important clue.

28 Encopresis

INTRODUCTION

- The course of rectum is aligned at an approximate angle of 90° to the anal canal. This sharp bend favors the rectal continence. The contraction of levator ani muscle which causes the straightening of the anorectal canal results in defecation. The sympathetic nervous system causes rectal filling by relaxing the sigmoid and rectum and by contracting the internal anal sphincter. The parasympathetic system causes contraction of sigmoid and rectum while relaxing internal anal sphincter, resulting in emptying of the bowel.
- Defecation is the process of consciously emptying the bowel and continence is the ability to control the act. It is a complex mechanism and is regulated by coordinated actions of sympathetic and parasympathetic nervous systems on the sigmoid, rectum, anus, levator ani muscles, and anal sphincter.
- Incontinence occurs when the pressure induced by peristaltic movement in the distal rectum overcomes the anorectal pressure.
- The bowel control is attained by the age of 2.5 years on an average.

Definition

Encopresis is defined as the involuntary or voluntary passage of formed feces, at inappropriate places, usually in the underwear in the absence of any physical illness, after the age of 4 years. It should occur at least once a month for 3 consecutive months.

Encopresis is more common in boys with the peak age of 5–6 years.

Categories of Fecal Incontinence

True incontinence:
- Impaired neuromuscular function
- Deficient anorectal muscles as in imperforate anus.

Partial incontinence: Insufficient anorectal pressure or impaired sensations of peristaltic movement and bowel distention prevents complete evacuation of the bowel, resulting in continuing passage of a small amount of feces.

Overflow incontinence: Chronic fecal impaction and leakage of liquid feces through the dilated anorectal ring.

CLASSIFICATION OF ENCOPRESIS

- *Primary encopresis:* Children who were never continent since infancy
- *Secondary encopresis:* Children with a typical history of clean periods, followed by relapse of symptoms
- *Retentive encopresis:* Retention of feces for a prolonged time, two-thirds of cases are retentive type, associated with chronic constipation
- *Nonretentive encopresis:* No retention of feces. It is mainly due to behavioral or psychological problem.

CAUSES OF ENCOPRESIS

- *Multifactorial:* Psychological, anatomical, genetic, physiological, and dietary elements
- Chronic constipation (retentive encopresis)
- Two-thirds of cases are retentive type and mainly due to chronic constipation and impaction of fecal matter.
- *Psychological (mainly secondary encopresis):*
  - Stressful family situation such as divorce, birth of a sibling, and transition such as starting school
  - Traumatic or frightening experience such as sexual or physical molestation
- Corrective toilet training
- *Anatomical conditions (primary incontinence):*
  - Spina bifida
  - Meningomyelocele
  - Spinal cord injury
  - Tethered spinal cord
  - Ultrashort-segment Hirschsprung disease
  - Imperforate anus with fistula.

Enuresis

INTRODUCTION

- Micturition is a complex function resulting from coordinated activity of the muscles of urinary bladder (detrusor muscles and internal urethral sphincter muscles) involving integration of both volitional and autonomic nervous system. In infants, it is under control of the autonomic system and as the child grows this act becomes volitional. It is uninhibited for the first 18 months of life and as the child grows, he becomes aware of the sense of bladder fullness and urinary frequency decreases. By 3 years of age, diurnal control is established and by 4 years most children develop nocturnal control also.
- By 5 years of age, 90–95% of children are nearly completely continent during the day and 80–85% are continent at night.

ENURESIS (BED WETTING)

- *Definition:* Voluntary or involuntary repeated passing of urine into clothes or bed, after a developmental age when bladder control should be established (usually 5 years), is called enuresis.
  Bed wetting or urinary incontinence is labeled as enuresis only if urine is being voided twice a week for at least 3 consecutive months, or if it is causing clinically significant distress to the child.
- Nocturnal enuresis refers to voiding during sleep, whereas diurnal enuresis refers to daytime urination; these may or may not exist together.
- 10% of the children with nocturnal enuresis will have diurnal enuresis whereas 50% of children with diurnal enuresis have nocturnal enuresis.
- 10% of the 5-year-old, 5% of the 10-year-old, and 1% of the 18-year-old children will have nocturnal enuresis.
- *Primary enuresis:* It is defined as repeated, at least twice a week for at least 3 consecutive months, passage of urine into clothes or bed wetting during night in a child of more than 5 years in night, who has never been dry in night. Primary enuresis is three times more common in boys. It is mostly idiopathic or behavioral in origin.
- *Secondary enuresis:* The child has been dry for at least 6 months before wetting begins again during sleep. In most of these children, an underlying organic pathology is detected.

TOILET TRAINING

- Physiological readiness for toilet training generally occurs at around 18 months of age; child can delay defecation or urination sufficiently to get to an appropriate place.
- However, cognitive maturity, to use the potty, to remember to use it, and to resist distraction long enough to complete the process, is usually achieved around 24 months.

- The motor skills needed to get in the bathroom, manage clothes, and sit still on the potty are also important, though parents may assist in some of these.

Readiness Criteria (When to Start Toilet Training) for a Developmentally Normal Child

- Child stays dry at least 2 hours at a time during the day or is dry after naps.
- Bowel movements are regular and predictable.
- Facial expressions/posture/words show that your child is about to urinate/defecate.
- Child can follow simple instructions and imitate parental behavior.
- Child can walk to and from the bathroom and help undress.
- Child seems uncomfortable with soiled diapers and wants a clean diaper.
- Child asks to use the toilet or potty chair.
- The child can put on/take off clothes.
- The child follows the parent into the bathroom and expresses interest in the toilet.

CAUSES OF PRIMARY ENURESIS

- Multifactorial
- Could be related to sleep disorders and poor arousability in response to acoustic stimuli.
- Small functional bladder capacity and detrusor overactivity may be important factors.
- *Genetic factors:*
  - Positive family history in most cases
  - 43% risk, if one parent had nocturnal enuresis
  - 77% risk, if both parents were affected
  - 75% of children with nocturnal enuresis have a first-degree relative who had enuresis.
- Stress at school or home may be a psychological cause.
- Delay in neurological maturation to control bladder sphincter in children with mental retardation or spinal cord abnormalities.
- 5% of 10-year-olds and 1% of adolescents may remain enuretic.
- Hyposecretion of arginine vasopressin, decreased responsiveness to low urine osmolarity, and loss of circadian rhythm of antidiuretic hormone secretion are other factors.
- Less than 3% cases have organic causes like obstructive uropathy or urinary tract infections (UTIs).

CAUSES OF SECONDARY ENURESIS

- Too enthusiastic and immature toilet training can result in secondary enuresis.
- Emotional stress
- Parent–child maladjustment
- UTIs
- Diabetes mellitus
- Diabetes insipidus.

Causes of Diurnal Enuresis

- More common in preschool girls, due to micturition deferral, waiting till the last moment to pass urine and then being unable to hold any longer. Usually, settles by the age of 9 years.
- Stress incontinence
- UTI
- Urinary bladder outlet obstruction
- Ectopic ureter
- Diabetes mellitus
- Diabetes insipidus
- Psychological causes such as anxiety, loss of a parent, parental discord, and abusive home environment.
- Some children fail to appreciate the sense of bladder fullness or ignore it while playing.

When both diurnal enuresis and nocturnal enuresis are present, urinary tract anomalies or voiding disorders are likely. Chronic constipation is an important risk factor for enuresis.

Epistaxis

INTRODUCTION

Epistaxis (bleeding from nostril) is common in children usually after the age of 2 years. Most nose bleeds are primary (without any obvious etiology) while others are secondary to a systemic disease like hematological disorder or a local pathology such as nose picking. Children with recurrent epistaxis need to be diagnosed accurately and managed appropriately. Most children with recurrent idiopathic epistaxis tend to get better in adolescence.

CLASSIFICATION

- *Anterior bleeds:* Easily visible and originate from Little's area; this area is copiously supplied by Kiesselbach plexus (superficial capillaries). It is one of the most common areas of bleeds.
- *Posterior bleeds:* These bleeds originate from the posterior part of the nose from the distribution of the sphenopalatine artery. This site of bleeding is characteristic of angiofibroma, seen in adolescent boys.
- *Recurrent epistaxis:* Children with bleeding tendencies or nasal pathology present with recurrent epistaxis.

CLINICAL EVALUATION

- *Initial evaluation:*
  - Aim is to rule out signs of serious disease or hemodynamic alterations.
  - Protecting the airway is vital in posterior nasal bleeds.
  - Concomitant presence of skin and/or retinal bleed should raise the possibility of a serious underlying disease with hematological abnormality due to thrombocytopenia or coagulation disorder.
  - Epistaxis in a febrile child may be due to dengue fever, leukemia, meningococcemia, falciparum malaria, leptospirosis, septicemia, etc.
  - Check for bleeding from other sites; may suggest generalized serious disorder.
- *Systemic evaluation:*
  - Look for pallor, telangiectasia, purpura, mucosal bleeds, lymphadenopathy, hepatosplenomegaly, etc. Examination for retinal bleeding is very vital.
  - Look for manifestations of thrombocytopenia and coagulation disorders.
  - Epistaxis in infancy is most often due to secondary causes such as congenital syphilis, diphtheria, trauma, and nasal foreign body.
- *Nasal examination:*
  - Asymmetry, swelling, and discoloration of external nares may suggest a hematoma ethmoidal disease.
  - Little's area (anterior nares) should be examined for active bleeding and crusting.

- Unilateral, blood-stained nasal discharge is highly suggestive of foreign body or nasal diphtheria.
- The presence of telangiectasia suggests systemic disease.
- Blockage of the nares may be associated with choanal stenosis, deviated nasal septum, angiofibroma, adenoidal, and hypertrophy.
- Most bleeds are single, unilateral, and mild and usually have a benign course.
- Recurrent and mild bleeding from the anterior part of the nose is usually due to excessive drying, trauma from nose picking, and allergic rhinitis.
- History of (H/o) drug such as aspirin, nonsteroidal anti-inflammatory drugs (NSAIDs), and anticoagulants should be confirmed.
- Improper use of nasal sprays used for allergic rhinitis can predispose to nasal bleed.

COMMON CAUSES OF EPISTAXIS

- Idiopathic (from Little's area)
- Nasal picking
- Trauma
- Allergic rhinitis
- Nasal foreign body
- Nasal diphtheria
- Thrombocytopenia
- Coagulation disorders
- Infections such as dengue fever, falciparum malaria, meningococcemia, and septicemia
- Systemic disorders such as sarcoidosis, angiofibroma, Wegener granulomatosis, and hypertension.

Excessive Sweating (Hyperhidrosis)

CHAPTER 31

INTRODUCTION

Sweat glands are appendages of the skin. There are two types of sweat glands, eccrine and apocrine. Eccrine sweat glands are simple, coiled, tubular glands present throughout the body, most numerously on the palms, soles, and face. Apocrine sweat glands, also called odoriferous sweat glands, are known for producing malodorous perspiration. They are mostly confined to the axillary and perineal regions, including the perianal region, labia majora in women, and scrotum in men. Apocrine sweat glands are also present in the nipples and areola.

- Eccrine sweat glands serve thermoregulatory functions via evaporative heat loss. When the internal temperature of the body rises, sweat glands release the water to the skin surface, which quickly evaporates, subsequently cooling the skin and blood beneath. This is the most effective mechanism of thermoregulation in humans.
- Hyperhidrosis is the excessive excretion of the sweat above the quantity needed for thermoregulation.
- Hyperhidrosis can be due to endocrine, neurologic, cardiovascular, neoplastic, and infectious disorders, or secondary to some medication. It is idiopathic in many cases.
- *Physiologic causes:*
  - Exercise
  - Increased environmental temperature
  - Emotional stimuli
  - Anxiety
  - Gustatory stimuli (spicy and hot food)
  - Fever
  - Excessive clothing
  - Obesity
- Familial hyperhidrosis
- *Sweating with infections:*
  - During defervescence
  - Tuberculosis
  - Brucellosis
  - Malaria
- *Endocrinal causes:*
  - Hypoglycemia
  - Hyperthyroidism
  - Pheochromocytoma
  - Pituitary gigantism or acromegaly
  - Phenylketonuria
- *Cardiovascular disorders:*
  - Congestive heart failure: In infants, sweating is common over head, forehead, and neck.
  - Syncope: Pallor, sweating, and restlessness are classical features of syncope.
  - Reynaud phenomenon: Common over hand and feet accompanied by color change.
- *Neurologic disorders:*
  - Benign paroxysmal vertigo
  - Diencephalic syndrome
  - Subacute sclerosing panencephalitis (SSPE)
  - Spinal cord lesions
  - Hydrocephalus
  - Cluster headache

- *Drugs and toxins:*
  - Salicylate intoxication
  - Organophosphorus poisoning
  - Acrodynia (mercury poisoning)
  - Insulin overdose
  - Narcotic withdrawal
- *Miscellaneous:*
  - Familial dysautonomia
  - Rickets
  - Lymphoma
  - Carcinoid syndrome
  - Chediak–Higashi syndrome
  - Thrombocytopenia-absent radius (TAR) syndrome.

HYPOHIDROSIS (DIMINISHED SWEATING)

Hypohidrosis is a rare disorder in which there is diminished sweating in response to appropriate stimuli. The consequences of untreated hypohidrosis are hyperthermia and heat stroke. In an extreme case of hypohidrosis, there is a complete absence of sweating and it is termed anhidrosis.

Common Causes of Hypohidrosis/Anhidrosis

- Ectodermal dysplasia
- Diabetes insipidus
- Fabry disease
- Sjögren syndrome
- Familial dysautonomia
- Drugs:
  - Anticholinergic agents (atropine)
  - Opioids
  - Antihistaminics.

Exophthalmos (Proptosis)

INTRODUCTION

The anterior protrusion of an eye or both the eyes is called exophthalmos (exophthalmus) or proptosis. It is a relatively uncommon finding in the pediatric practice. Unilateral proptosis of an acute onset is often due to orbital cellulitis secondary to ethmoidal sinusitis. If it is bilateral and gradually developing, orbital masses should be considered in its differentials. Neuroblastoma and leukemia are most common in children. Besides history and physical examination, neuroimaging is an important tool in the evaluation of slowly progressive, bilateral proptosis.

COMMON CAUSES OF PROPTOSIS

Infections

- Orbital cellulitis: Acute ethmoiditis is the most common cause of proptosis or periorbital cellulitis. It may develop following trauma or the spread of local infection. Periorbital cellulitis is far more common which may not cause trauma proptosis. Extraocular movements are lost in orbital cellulitis, but not in periorbital cellulitis.
- Osteomyelitis of orbit
- Orbital tuberculosis.

Endocrinal Causes

Hyperthyroidism is a relatively common cause of bilateral exophthalmos, usually slowly progressive in nature. It is more common in adolescent girls. Weight loss, in spite of good appetite, fever, tachycardia, excessive sweating, irritability, and tremors are other features of hyperthyroidism.

Neoplasia

- *Primary orbital tumors*
  - Dermoid tumor
  - Optic nerve glioma
  - Teratoma
  - Retinoblastoma
  - Lacrimal gland tumors
  - Rhabdomyosarcoma
- *Metastatic and secondary tumors*
  - Neuroblastoma: In any child presenting with spontaneous development of purpura of the eyelids and proptosis, consider neuroblastoma unless proved otherwise.
  - Neurofibromatosis: Optic glioma is more common.
  - Leukemia
  - Langerhans cell histiocytosis
  - Lymphoma
  - Metastatic sarcoma
  - Juvenile angiofibroma of the nasopharynx.

Vascular Disorders

- Vascular tumors: Hemangioma and vascular malformations
- Sturge-Weber syndrome

- Lymphangioma
- Cavernous sinus thrombosis
- Carotid-cavernous sinus fistula.

Bone-related Diseases
- Craniosynostosis
- Apert syndrome
- Crouzon syndrome
- Encephalocele
- Osteopetrosis
- Rickets
- Caffey disease.

Hemorrhage
- Scurvy
- Hemophilia
- Trauma: Fracture of the orbital fossa.

Syndromes with Proptosis or Prominent Eyes
- Pycnodysostosis
- Leopard syndrome
- Turner syndrome
- Progeria.

Miscellaneous Causes
- Sarcoidosis
- Congenital hydrocephalus
- Myasthenia gravis.

Eye Discharge

INTRODUCTION

Any discharge from the eyes of a child requires due attention. In newborns, it may be due to conjunctivitis or congenital dacryocystitis. In older children, it may be due to infective or allergic conjunctivitis, trauma, or chronic dacryocystitis.

CONJUNCTIVITIS IN NEONATES

- The sticky eyes without purulent discharge are common during the first 2–3 days after birth. They should be washed with sterile cotton swabs soaked in saline.
- Unilateral conjunctivitis having onset after 5 days of life is often due to *Chlamydia trachomatis*.
- Purulent conjunctivitis is usually due to gram-positive cocci.
- Gonococcal ophthalmia should be suspected, if profuse purulent discharge occurs in one or both the eyes within 48 hours of age.
- Congenital nasolacrimal duct obstruction occurs in approximately 6% of newborns and is the most common cause of persistent tearing and ocular discharge in infants and young children **(Fig. 1)**.

EYE DISCHARGE IN INFANTS AND CHILDREN

- *Viral conjunctivitis:*
  - Adenovirus (fever, pharyngitis, conjunctivitis, cystitis, and lymphadenopathy)

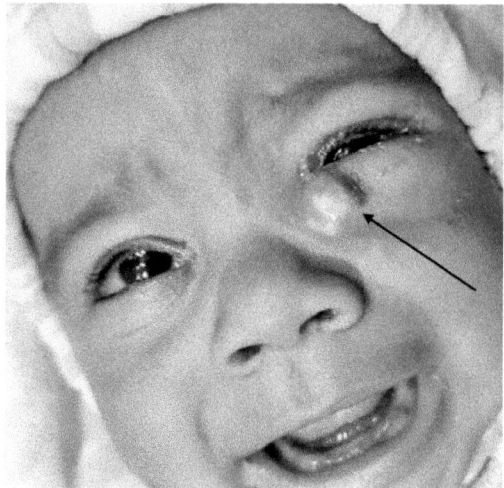

Fig. 1: Dacryocystitis.

  - Human herpes virus
- *Bacterial conjunctivitis:*
  - *Staphylococcus aureus*
  - *Haemophilus influenzae*
  - *C. trachomatis*
  - Gonorrhea
- *Allergic conjunctivitis:*
  - Mucoid discharge and pruritus are common symptoms
  - Symptoms may be seasonal
  - History of atopic disorder to parents
  - Phlyctenular conjunctivitis due to tuberculosis
- Foreign body
- Corneal abrasion
- Glaucoma.

34 Facial Paralysis/Weakness

INTRODUCTION

Facial paralysis or weakness is a relatively uncommon condition in general pediatric practice. Bell's palsy is the most common cause of acquired facial palsy. The causes of facial nerve paralysis or weakness may be divided into some groups like postnatal acquired, birth trauma, and congenital. The causes of upper motor neuron (UMN) type of facial nerve palsy are not included in this.

POSTNATAL ACQUIRED FACIAL NERVE PARALYSIS

- *Bell's palsy:* This is an acute onset lower motor type facial palsy. The exact pathogenesis is not known, but it is thought to follow vasospasm of the blood vessels supplying the facial nerve, leading to edema and resultant loss of function. It may develop following swelling or compression of facial nerve. Onset is usually sudden and often triggered by viral infection. Paralysis is usually unilateral and may be complete or partial and usually transient. Ear pain may be an early symptom. Vertigo, loss of taste, and hyperacusis may also occur.
- *Infectious disorders:*
  - Herpes simplex
  - Herpes zoster
  - Epstein–Barr virus
  - Mumps
  - Human immunodeficiency virus (HIV)
  - Sarcoidosis
  - Lyme disease (bacterial infection caused by infected tics)
  - Acute otitis media
  - Guillain–Barré syndrome (GBS) (in one-third patients of GBS, may be bilateral)
  - Meningitis (bacterial meningitis, tuberculous meningitis)
  - Encephalitis
  - Mastoiditis
  - Brain abscess
- *Traumatic:*
  - Facial trauma
  - Parotid gland or neck surgery
  - Skull fracture
- Osteopetrosis (compression of nerve due to narrowing of foramen)
- *Tumors and neoplasia:*
  - Acoustic neuroma
  - Metastatic tumors
  - Leukemia
  - Eosinophilic granuloma
  - Hemangioma
  - Neurofibromatosis
  - Parotid gland tumors
  - Facial nerve tumors.

PRENATAL/PERINATAL ACQUIRED FACIAL NERVE PARALYSIS

- *Traumatic:*
  - Forceps delivery

- Compression by maternal sacral promontory
- Skull fracture
- Congenital rubella syndrome.

CONGENITAL FACIAL NERVE PARALYSIS

- *Hypoplasia of the depressor anguli oris muscle* (**Fig. 1**): Facial nerve paralysis should be differentiated from hypoplasia of the depressor anguli oris muscle. Asymmetric movements of the face is noted especially on crying in both the conditions—facial nerve palsy and congenital absence or hypoplasia of depressor anguli oris muscle. But in congenital absence or hypoplasia of depressor anguli oris muscle, forehead wrinkles are present, eyes can be closed, and nasolabial folds appear equal. A high incidence of congenital anomalies may be associated with this syndrome, including cardiac, renal, and musculoskeletal.
- *Mobius syndrome:*
    - Absence of seventh nerve nuclei

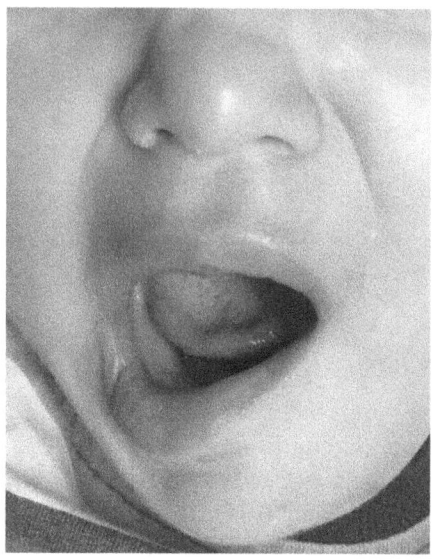

Fig. 1: Hypoplasia of left depressor angularis oris muscle.

- Usually evident at birth
- Bilateral
- Associated bilateral involvement of sixth nerve
- Constant drooling
- Mental retardation.

35 Facies

INTRODUCTION

Reading a face is an art. This art has significance in medical context. The facies are distinctive facial expressions and appearances associated with specific medical conditions, which may be syndromic, endocrinal, metabolic disorder, genetical disorder, or specific disease related.

- *Mongoloid facies* (**Fig. 1**):
  - Seen in trisomy 21 (Down syndrome)
  - Flat facial profile
  - Hypertelorism
  - Upward slant of eyes (Mongoloid slant)
  - Epicanthic folds
  - Low set ears
  - Saddle nose
  - Scrotal tongue
  - Brushfield spots on the iris
- *Coarse facies* (**Figs. 2A and B**):
  - Flat face
  - Short nose
  - Large head (bulging forehead)
  - Dry skin
  - Thick tongue
  - Thickened facial outlines
  - Seen in mucopolysaccharidosis, hypothyroidism, gangliosidosis, Sotos syndrome
- *Hemolytic facies* (**Fig. 3**):
  - Frontal bossing (prominence of frontal and parietal eminences)
  - Depressed nasal bridge
  - Maxillary prominence
  - Prominent malar eminences
  - Malaligned, protruding teeth
  - Typically seen in thalassemia, sometimes may be seen in chronic severe iron deficiency anemia

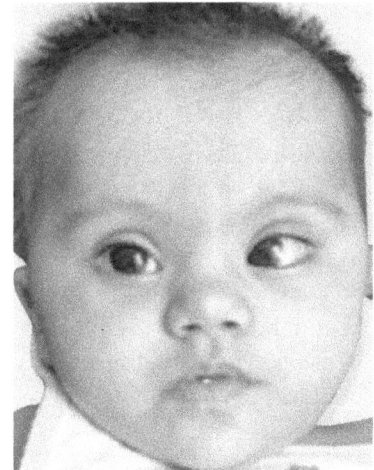

Fig. 1: Mongoloid facies.

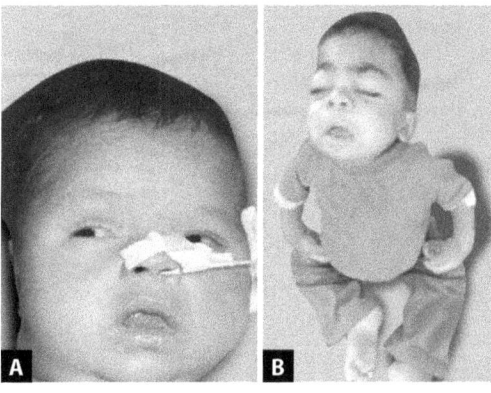

Figs. 2A and B: (A) Hypothyroidism with coarse facial features; (B) mucopolysaccharidosis.

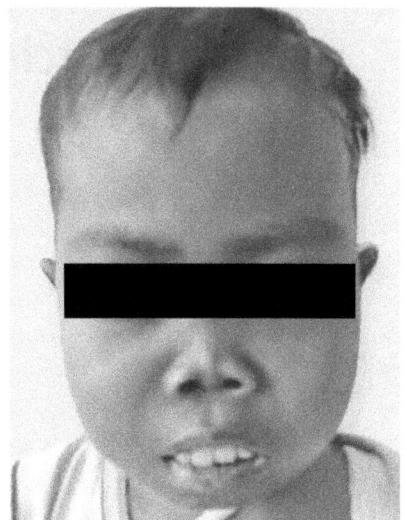

Fig. 3: Hemolytic facies.

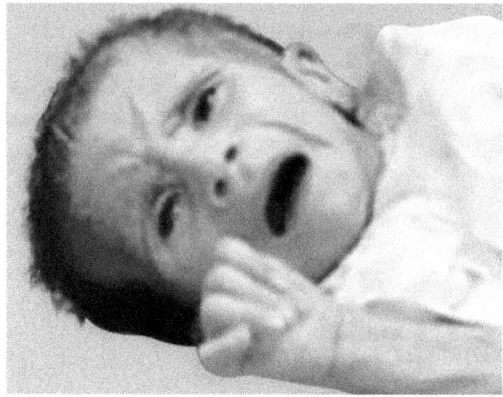

Fig. 5: Monkey facies.

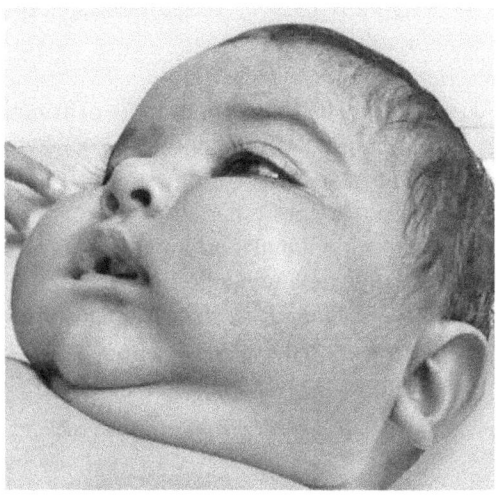

Fig. 4: Moon face (steroid face).

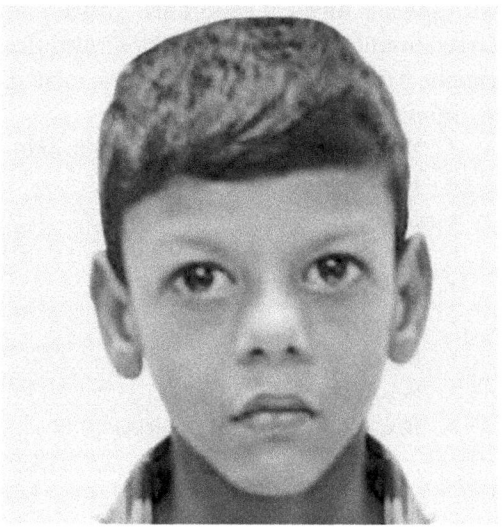

Fig. 6: Elfin facies.

- *Moon face (steroid face, Cushingoid face)* **(Fig. 4)**:
  - Rounded face
  - Prominent cheeks
  - Double chin
  - Puffy chin
  - Puffy appearance
  - Hirsutism
  - Seen in Cushing syndrome and prolonged steroid therapy
- *Monkey facies* **(Fig. 5)**:
  - Marasmic child has typical face
  - Wrinkled, loose, and dry skin
  - Loss of buccal pad of fat results in pits in cheeks, appearing as monkey facies or old-aged appearance.
- *Elfin facies* **(Fig. 6)**:
  - Upturned nose
  - Broad upper lip

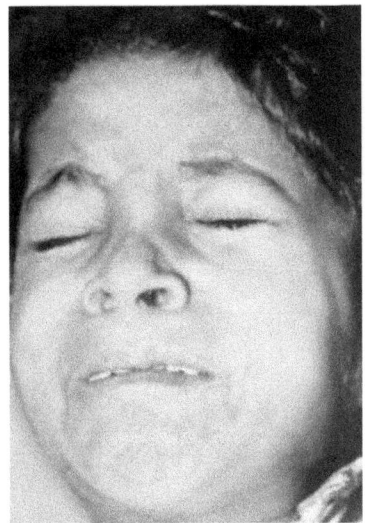

Fig. 7: Risus sardonicus.

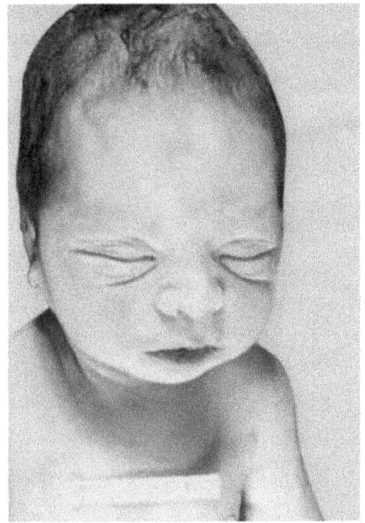

Fig. 8: Potter facies.

- Small mandible
- Prominent maxilla
- Short stature
- Small chin
- *Risus sardonicus* (**Fig. 7**):
  - Fixed, sarcastic grimace
  - Anxious expression
  - Caused by abnormal and sustained spasms of the masseter and other facial muscles that appear to produce grinning.
  - Characteristic clinical feature of tetanus; may be seen in strychnine poisoning
- *Triangular face:*
  - Lower half of the face becomes thin, appearing of a triangle with a tip facing downwards.
  - Common in individuals with osteogenesis imperfect, Russell–Silver Syndrome, Turner syndrome, and Ehlers–Danlos syndrome
- *Potter facies* (**Fig. 8**):
  - Suborbital creases
  - Depressed nasal tip
- Low set ears
- Retrognathia
- Associated with positional deformities of limbs like club feet
- Most common in bilateral renal agenesis
- *Acromegaloid facies* (**Fig. 9**):
  - Forehead and overlying skin is oily and thickened
  - Bulging of forehead
  - Cheek bones are obvious
  - Nose is widened and thickened
  - Prominent jaw
  - Thick lips
  - Seen in acromegaly
- *Adenoid facies* (**Fig. 10**):
  - Open-mouthed
  - Dumb expression
  - Underdeveloped thin nostrils
  - Short upper lip
  - Prominent upper teeth
  - Crowded teeth
  - Narrow upper alveolus
  - High-arched palate
  - Hypoplastic maxilla

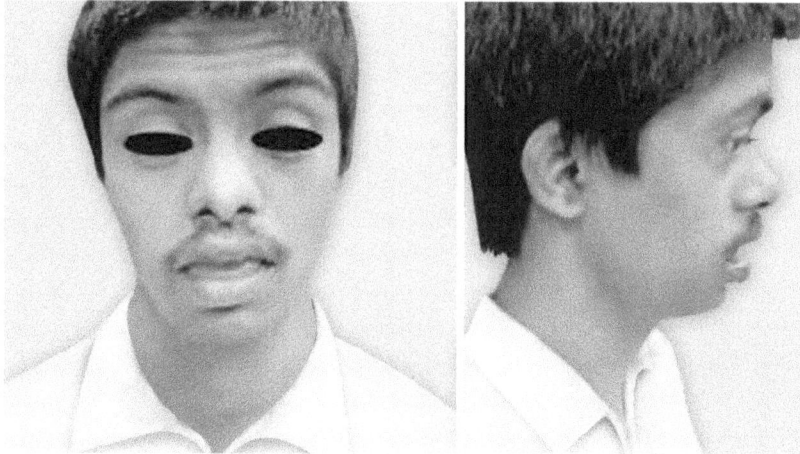

Fig. 9: Acromegaloid facies.

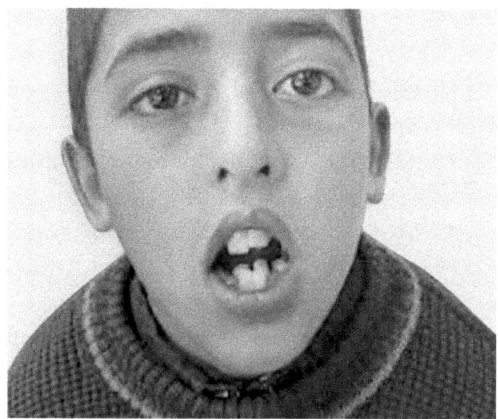

Fig. 10: Adenoid facies.

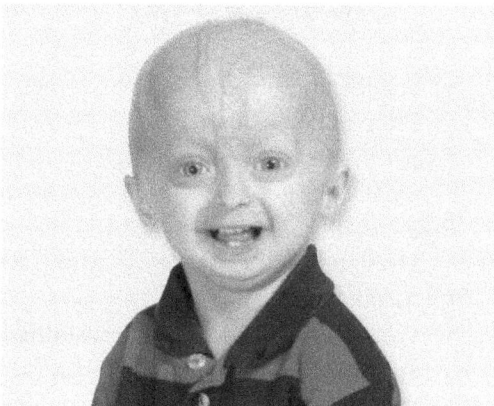

Fig. 11: Progeroid face.

- *Atopic facies:*
  - Cheeks are pale.
  - Perioricular darkening with dry, scaly skin
- *Hippocratic facies:*
  - Pinched expression of face
  - Sunken eyes
  - Relaxed lips
  - Hollow cheeks and temples
  - Observed in one dying after an exhausting illness
- *Leonine facies:*
  - Lion-like face
  - Diffuse infiltration of the skin of forehead, chin, nose, and ears
  - Seen in leprosy, leishmaniasis, sarcoidosis, etc.
- *Mask-like face:*
  - An immobile expressionless face
  - Staring eye
  - Slightly open mouth
  - Seen in parkinsonism and scleroderma
- *Progeroid face* **(Fig. 11):**
  - Triangular, old-looking face
  - Beak-shaped or pinched nose
  - Pseudohydrocephalus

- Wide fontanelle
- Prominent veins
- Sparse scalp hairs
- Lipodystrophy—subcutaneous fat loss from face, extremities, and paravertebral and gluteal region
- Seen in progeria

- *Alagille syndrome* **(Fig. 12)**:
  - Triangular face
  - Hypertelorism
  - Broad forehead
  - Deeply set eyes
  - Pointed chin
  - Straight nose with bulbous tip
  - Cholestasis is common.

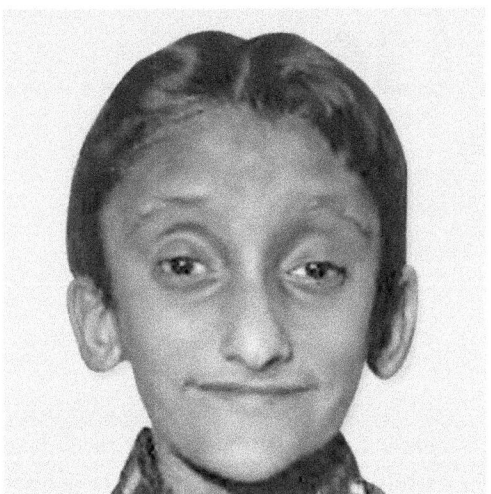

Fig. 12: Alagille syndrome.

Failure to Thrive

CHAPTER 36

INTRODUCTION

- Failure to thrive (FTT) is a condition associated with inadequate growth or inability to maintain adequate growth especially in young children. Most often, it is applied to infants and toddlers <3 years of age. It may be extended up to age of 5 years in developing countries.
- FTT is neither a disease nor a diagnosis. It is a sign indicating that growth of the child is below expected.

CRITERIA TO CONSIDER FAILURE TO THRIVE

- A child <3 years of age whose weight is <80% of the ideal weight for age (**Fig. 1**).
- A child <3 years of age whose weight is <3rd percentile for age, on more than one occasions (**Fig. 2**).
- A child <3 years of age whose weight cross two major percentiles downwards on a standard growth chart (**Fig. 3**).

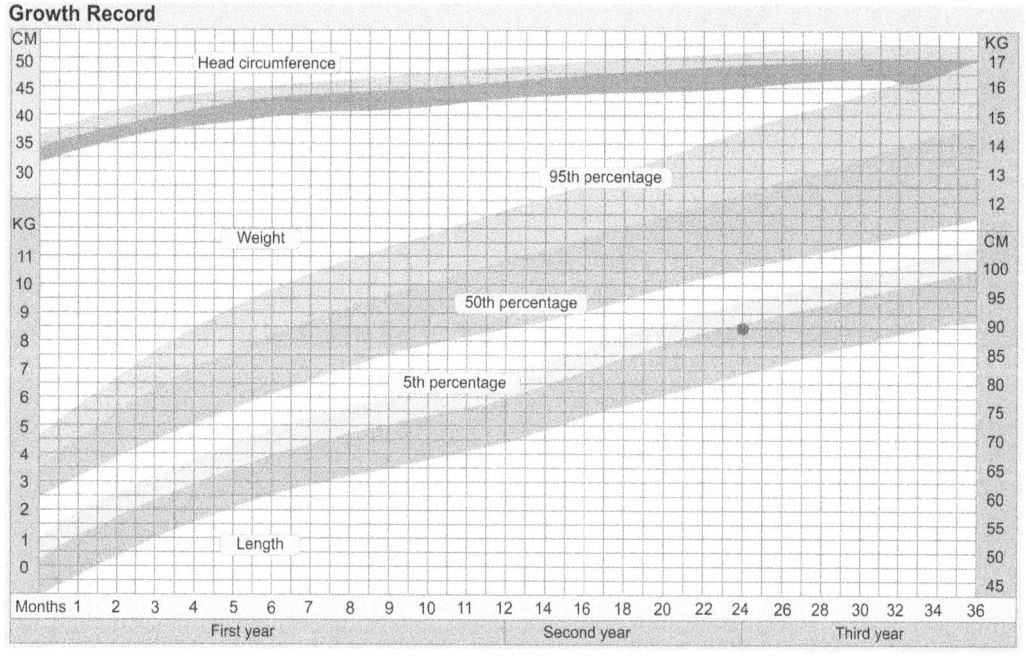

Fig. 1: 2 years → 8.5 kg (12 kg) → 70%.

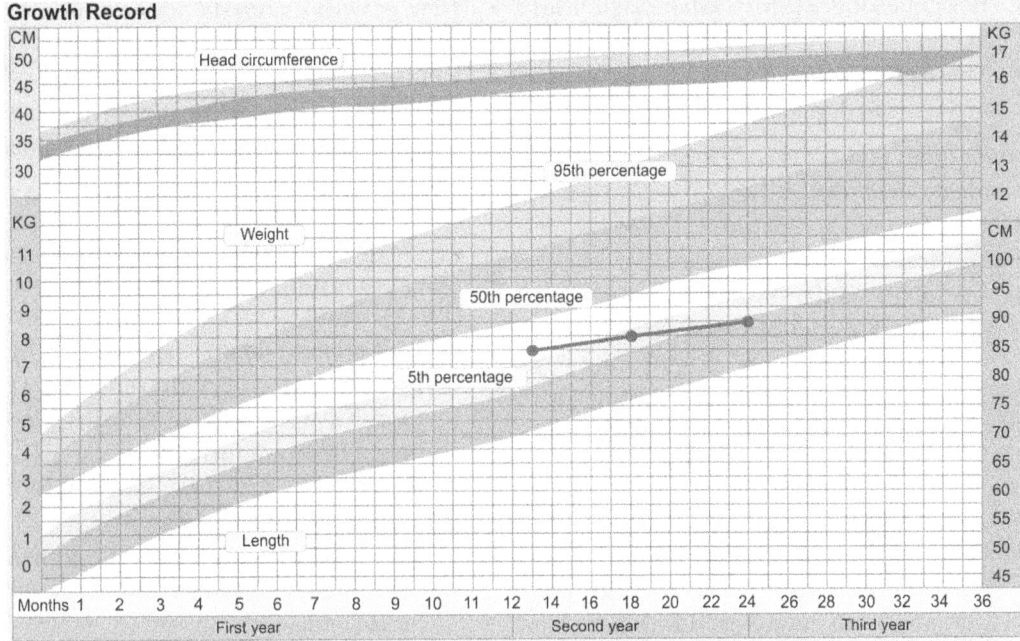

Fig. 2: A child <3 years of age whose weight is <3rd percentile for age, on more than one occasions.

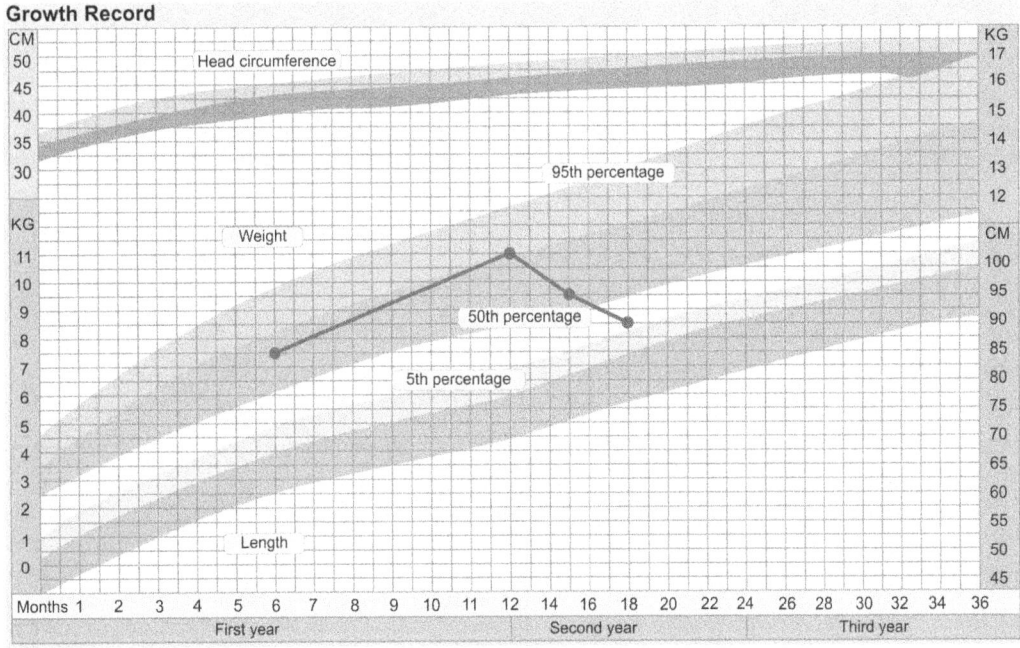

Fig. 3: A child <3 years of age whose weight crosses two major percentiles downward on a standard growth chart.

- Body mass index (BMI) <5th percentile for age and gender.
- These criteria may be extended up to age of 5 years in developing countries.

Some other conditions, different from FTT, should be identified:
- Emaciation: Excessive loss of body fat
- Wasting: Loss of muscle mass
- Cachexia: Only skin and bones. It is commonly associated with tuberculosis (TB) and malignancy. Tumor necrosis factor (TNF), interferon gamma, and interleukin-6-like inflammatory cytokines appear to play a role for cachexia.

Normal variants:
- Birth weight or birth length of an infant does not necessarily reflect their growth potential, but relate predominantly to maternal nutrition.
- Deceleration of growth is seen in first 3–6 months.
- New growth channels are assumed by 13 months of age.
- Familial (genetic) factors:
  - Weight and height are proportionately below the third percentile and follow the growth curves, though below it.
  - No organic cause
  - Skeletal age is equal to chronological age.
- Preterm and intrauterine growth restriction (IUGR) infants:
  - Well preterm infants exhibit catch-up growth, head circumference by 18 months, weight by 24 months, and height by 40 months **(Fig. 4)**.
  - Overall, 35% of IUGR infants do not exhibit catch-up growth.
  - 3% of normal population has a growth curve below the third percentile for height or age.

Red flags for FTT:
- Psychological history: Abnormal family dynamics

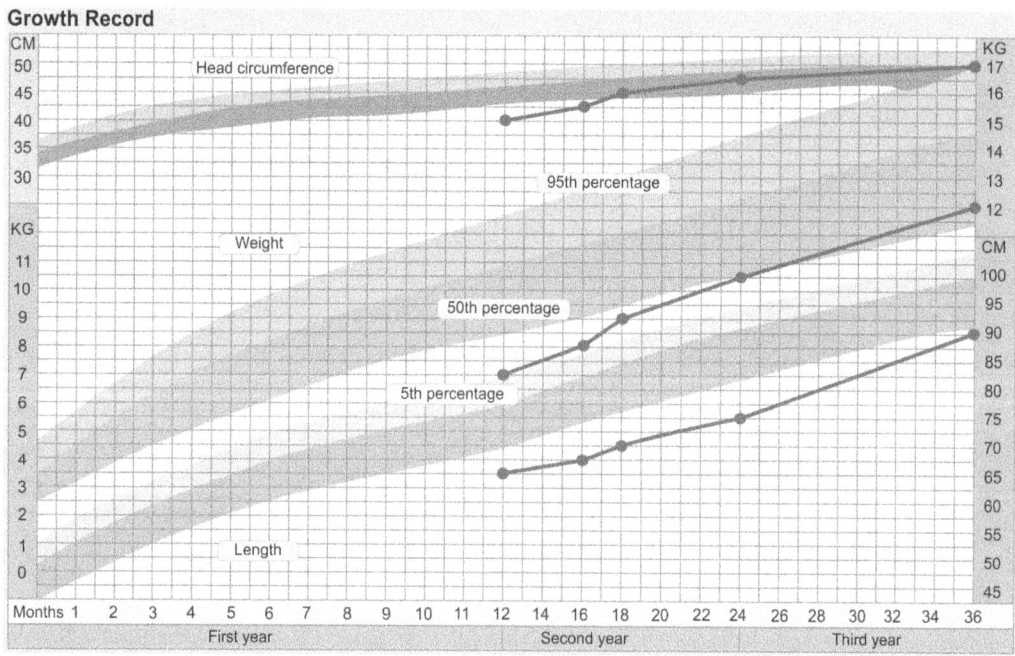

Fig. 4: Catch up growth in preterms, head circumference by 18 months, weight by 24 months and height by 40 months.

- Clinical findings suggestive of suspected child abuse like unusual injuries, recurrent injuries, etc.
- Emotional deprivation

HISTORY

- *Age at onset:*
  - Early infancy: Feeding problems, IUGR, intrauterine infections, renal tubular acidosis (RTA), and inborn error of metabolism (IEM).
  - Beyond infancy: Chronic infections [TB, human immunodeficiency virus (HIV)], eating disorders, silent organ disease like cystic fibrosis (CF), chronic kidney disease, inflammatory bowel disease (IBD), celiac disease, interstitial lung disease (ILD), etc.
- Previous weight and height records will indicate onset and magnitude of the problem.
- *Antenatal history:*
  - Pregnancy-induced hypertension (PIH)
  - Poor weight gain during pregnancy
  - IUGR on ultrasono scan
  - Fever and infections during pregnancy
- *Birth weight and length:*
  - IUGR
  - Risk of being slow grow
  - Hypoglycemia in neonatal period (hypopituitarism)
- *Feeding history/dietary history:*
  - Lactation failure
  - Diluted formula
  - Faulty feeding practice
  - Not growing well despite good appetite (diabetes mellitus, CF)
  - Eating disorder in adolescents
- *Stool pattern:*
  - Fatty (oily) stool in CF
  - Malodor in celiac disease
  - Bulky stool containing undigested food in giardiasis
  - Repeated episodes of blood in stool in IBD
- Urinary tract infection
- *Dyspnea/easy fatigability:*
  - ILD
  - Cardiomyopathy
  - Congenital heart disease (CHD)
  - RTA
  - IEM.

PHYSICAL EXAMINATION

- Well looking/sick looking
- *Vitals:*
  - Tachypnea, low SPO_2.
  - Hypertension: Renal or cardiac condition
  - Tachycardia, tachypnea, recurrent lower respiratory tract infection (LRTI), and CHD
- Prolonged fever (chronic infections like TB, HIV)
- Pallor
- Growth monitoring (growth chart)
- Nutritional assessment
- Skin pigmentation, petechiae
- Clubbing (CF, celiac disease, IBD, ILD, etc.)
- Abdominal distention (celiac disease)
- Ascites
- Hepatosplenomegaly
- Lymphadenopathy [TB, HIV, TORCH (toxoplasmosis, other agents, rubella, cytomegalovirus, and herpes simplex)]
- *Syndromic features:*
  - Short stature, micropenis (hypopituitarism)
  - Short female (Turner syndrome)
  - Hypertelorism, cataracts, high-arched palate, clinodactyly, skin changes, and abnormal dermatoglyphics
  - CHD.

With detailed history and thorough physical examination, categorization of child with FTT like well looking or sick looking, condition with increased calories requirement or deffective utilization of calories, malabsorption syndrome, psychosocial reasons, follow the algorithms to locate the cause **(Figs. 5, 6 and 7)**.

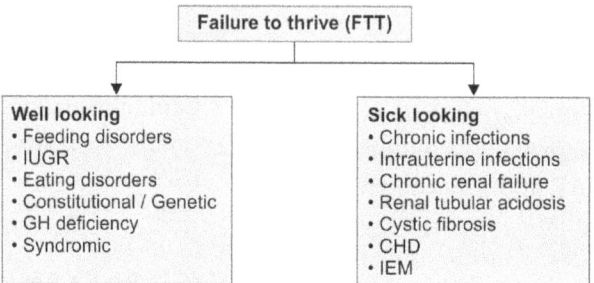

Fig. 5: FTT with look (well/sick looking).
(CHD: congenital heart disease; GH: growth hormone; IEM: inborn error of metabolism; IUGR: intrauterine growth restriction)

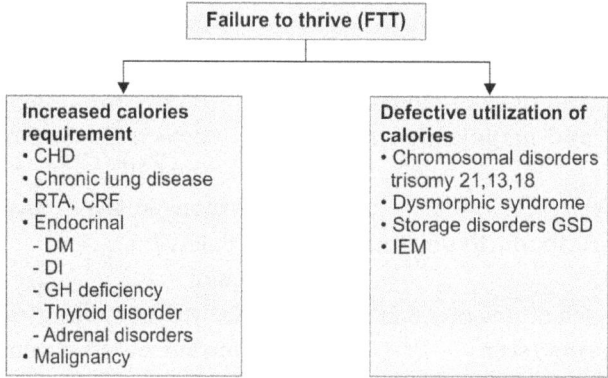

Fig. 6: FTT with increased requirement or defective utilization of energy.
(CHD: congenital heart disease; CRF: chronic renal failure; DI; diabetes insipidus; DM: diabetes mellitus; GH: growth hormone; GSD: glycogen storage disease; IEM: inborn error of metabolism; RTA: renal tubular acidosis)

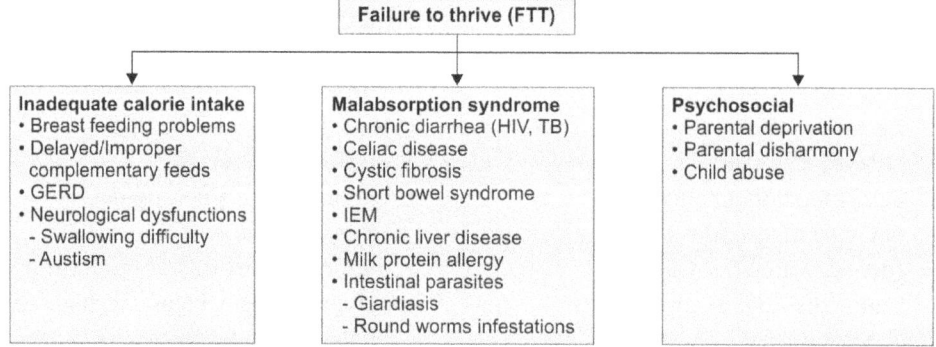

Fig. 7: FTT with inadequate calory intake, malabsorption syndrom and psychosocial conditions.
(GERD: gastroesophageal reflux disease; HIV: human immunodeficiency virus; IEM: inborn error of metabolism; TB: tuberculosis)

Fatigue

INTRODUCTION

Children often complain of fatigue. Complaint of fatigue indicates a general state of decreased endurance for, or interest in, activities. It is generally associated with lack of energy, tiredness, and sleepiness. Usually, fatigue is for simple reasons like because of a busy day, lack of sleep, or excessive physical activities. They need more rest to get better. But, when a child complains all the time and fatigue starts to get in the way of activities they usually enjoy, it could be a sign of problem. The neonates may present with excessive sleepiness, lethargy, feeding issues like prolonged feeding time (>30 minutes), suck-rest-suck cycle, etc.

COMMON CAUSES OF FATIGUE

- *Physiological:*
  - Inadequate rest
  - Excessive exercise/activities
  - Insufficient calorie intake
- *Infections:*
  - Tuberculosis
  - Viral infections [Epstein–Barr virus (EBV), human immunodeficiency virus (HIV)]
  - Hepatitis
  - Brucellosis
  - Autoimmune disorders
- Anemia
- Obesity
- Malnutrition
- Chronic hypoxemia (sarcoidosis, interstitial lung disease, etc.)
- *Central nervous system (CNS) causes:*
  - Tuberculous meningitis (TBM)
  - Encephalitis
  - Myasthenia gravis
  - Myopathy
  - Peripheral neuropathy
- *Endocrinal causes:*
  - Hypothyroidism
  - Hyperthyroidism
  - Adrenocortical insufficiency
- *Cardiac causes:*
  - Congestive heart failure
  - Decreased perfusion
  - Pericarditis
  - Myocarditis
  - Cardiomyopathy
  - Constrictive pericarditis
- *Connective tissue disorders:*
  - Juvenile rheumatoid arthritis
  - Systemic lupus erythematosus (SLE)
  - Dermatomyositis
- *Renal causes:*
  - Chronic renal failure
  - Uremia
  - Renal tubular acidosis
  - Bartter syndrome
- *Metabolic causes:*
  - Hypoglycemia
  - Hypoxemia
  - Hyponatremia
  - Hypokalemia

GASTROINTESTINAL DISORDERS
- Inflammatory bowel diseases
- Chronic liver disorders
- *Parasitic diseases:*
  - Roundworm infestation
  - Hookworm infestation
  - Chronic malaria
  - Kala-azar
  - Giardiasis
- Chronic fatigue syndrome may be associated with chronic infestations, chronic organ dysfunctions, malignancy, etc.
- *Drugs:*
  - Antihistamines
  - Anticonvulsants
  - Opiates.

38 Feeding Issues

INTRODUCTION

- Feeding issues are very common in daily pediatric practice, especially in infants and toddlers.
- To observe the actual act of feeding the child, is the best way to understand the feeding issue. Another alternate is to have the video clip of feeding the child.
- Feeding issues can be categorized as follows; it will help to understand the cause of feeding issue and can be managed accordingly.
  - Faulty technique of feeding
  - Mismanaged feeding
  - Difficulty in feeding
  - Functional feeding problem.

Pointers indicating feeding problem or disorder:
- Refuses to eat or drink
- Preference of breast
- Cries or fusses when feeding
- Arching of back
- Stiffness on feeding
- Falls asleep or is not alert while feeding
- Prolonged feeding time (>30 minutes)
- Suck–Rest–Suck cycle
- Drools a lot, coughs or gags while feeding
- Has problems of chewing and swallowing
- Difficulty in swallowing or mouthful
- Choking on feeding
- Has trouble breathing while eating or drinking
- Frequently spits up or vomits
- Hoarseness of voice after or during feeding
- Not gaining weight.

CLASSIFICATION OF FEEDING DISORDERS

- Functional immaturity (preterm, low birth weight (LBW), gastroesophageal reflux (GERD), regurgitation)
- Structural abnormalities [cleft palate, choanal atresia, large tongue, tracheo-esophageal fistula (TOF)]
- Neurological conditions (cerebral palsy, VII nerve palsy, spinal muscular atrophy (SMA), post diphtheritic cranial nerve palsy, and muscular dystrophy)
- Cardiology conditions (congestive heart failure)
- Respiratory conditions (severe respiratory distress)
- Metabolic dysfunctions
- Behavioral issues (fussy child, autism, etc.)
- Mixed problems.

FAULTY TECHNIQUE OF BREAST FEEDING

Proper technique of breast feeding is important to avoid feeding problems.
- *Proper position of baby:*
  - Make sure that baby is wrapped properly in a cloth.
  - Baby's whole body is supported and not just neck or shoulders.
  - Baby's head and body are in one line without any twist in the neck.

- Baby's body turned toward the mother. Abdomen of the baby and the mother touching each other.
- Baby's nose is at the level of nipple.
- *Signs of good attachment (latching):*
  - The baby's mouth is wide open.
  - Most of the nipple and areola in the mouth, only upper areola is visible and not the lower one.
  - The baby's chin touches the breast.
  - The baby's lower lip is everted.
- *Effective sucking:*
  - Baby suckles slowly and pauses in between to swallow (suck, suck, suck, and swallow). One may see throat cartilage and muscles moving and hear the gulping sounds of milk being swallowed.
  - Baby's cheeks are full and not hollow on retracting during sucking.

PROBLEMS IN BREASTFEEDING

- Inverted nipple
- Sore nipple (cracked nipple)
- Breast engorgement
- Breast abscess
- Not enough milk.

MISMANAGED FEEDING

- Underfeeding
- Highly diluted formula [crying, failure to thrive (FTT)].
- Overfeeding (forceful feeding) (regurgitation, vomiting, excessive crying, obesity)
- Bottle feeding [increased incidences of infections—Acute diarrhoeal disease (ADD) and respiratory tract infection (RTI), otitis media, and aerophagia]
- Bottle addiction.

DIFFICULTY IN FEEDING

- *Structural abnormalities:*
  - Cleft lip and cleft palate (aspiration, repeated RTIs).
  - TOF (choking, aspiration, and RTIs)
  - Large tongue
  - Small oral cavity (Pierre Robin syndrome)
  - Choanal atresia (especially bilateral choanal atresia).
- *Cardiac conditions (congestive heart failure, left to right shunts):*
  - Prolonged feeding time (>30 times)
  - Suck-Rest-Suck cycle
- *Respiratory conditions:*
  - Severe respiratory distress [acute laryngotracheobronchitis (ALTB), bronchiolitis, and hypoxemia]
  - Nasal foreign body
- *Gastrointestinal conditions:*
  - GERD
  - Intestinal colic
  - Aerophagia
  - Constipation
- *Neurological conditions:*
  - Cerebral palsy (difficulty in sucking, swallowing, mouth fullness, and occasionally choking)
  - Anterior horn cell disorders (poliomyelitis, SMA)
  - Neuromuscular junction disorders (myasthenia gravis)
  - Polyneuropathy [(Guillain-Barré syndrome (GBS)]
  - 25–50% of neurological conditions and up to 80% of those with developmental disabilities have feeding problems.

COMPLICATIONS OF FEEDING PROBLEMS

- Malnutrition
- Dehydration
- Aspiration pneumonia
- Lung infection
- Speech, cognition, and behavioral problems.

39 Fever of Short Duration

INTRODUCTION

Fever of short duration is the most common symptom in daily outdoor pediatric practice. Parents expect immediate diagnosis and prompt control of fever, as against this, it is almost impossible for a treating person to diagnose cause of fever in initial period of 3–4 days (barring some exceptions such as acute tonsillitis, acute lymphadenitis, and bacillary dysentery). This leads to unnecessary laboratory investigations, use of irrational antibiotics, and combination of antipyretics due to pressure effect of parents and fear of missing serious illness.

SERIOUS CONDITION PRESENTING WITH FEVER

The first step is to look for red flag conditions which require immediate attention and prompt management. The common conditions are as follows:

- Altered sensorium/drowsiness/irritability/bulging anterior fontanelle (AF)/signs of meningeal irritation present [central nervous system (CNS) infections]
- Fever in <3 months, particularly neonates
- Poor perfusion (impending shock)
- Increased work of breathing (tachypnea, indrawings, and sounds)
- Petechial/purpura spots [dengue hemorrhagic fever (DHF), sepsis, meningococcemia, rickettsial, etc.]
- Faucial membrane (diphtheria)
- Toxic child, keeping neck flexed, drooling of saliva (retropharyngeal abscess)
- *Immunocompromised child:*
  - Malignancy and on antimalignant therapy
  - Human immunodeficiency virus (HIV)
  - Primary immunodeficiency disorders
  - Severe acute malnutrition
  - Nephrotic syndrome and on steroid therapy
- Abdominal guarding/rigidity (acute appendicitis, peritonitis, intestinal perforation, ruptured abscess, etc.).

DIFFERENTIATION OF VIRAL AND BACTERIAL INFECTIONS

- *Viral infections:*
  - Presents with high fever at the onset.
  - Usually subsides by day 3–4.
  - During the interfebrile period, child appears nearly normal.
  - Affects the entire system [upper respiratory tract infection (URTI) + lower respiratory tract infection (LRTI)] or multiple systems [respiratory system (RS) and gastrointestinal (GI) system].
  - History of (H/o) contact with similar infection in family and community clinches the diagnosis of viral etiology.
  - Good response to antipyretic (paracetamol).
  - Complete blood count (CBC) is noncontributory; leukocytosis and polymorphonuclear reaction may be seen in initial period.

- *Bacterial infections:*
  - Often starts with mild to moderate fever and gradually reaches to peak by day 4–5.
  - During interfebrile period, child looks toxic or sick (no normal activity and appetite reduced).
  - Gets localized by day 3–4 (pneumonia and meningitis); pathology may get localized, but clinical manifestations are not obvious [enteric fever and urinary tract infection (UTI)].
  - Poor response to antipyretic (paracetamol)
- Consideration of following points is important in deciding the cause of fever of short duration:
  - Age
  - Host (immunocompetent/immunocompromised)
  - Vaccination status
  - Epidemiology
  - Community acquired or nosocomial
- Patient with prolonged fever may harbor occult infections such as enteric fever, UTI, osteomyelitis, septic arthritis, and tuberculosis or have inflammatory or oncogenic conditions.
- Kawasaki disease should be considered among children with prolonged fever, especially fever for >5 days and no response to antibiotics. Careful evaluation for other stigmata associated with Kawasaki disease is always rewarding.
- Looking like viral fever, prolonged for some weeks may be Epstein–Barr virus (EBV) (infectious mononucleosis)
- In a diagnosed case of dengue fever, persistent fever may be due to immune-mediated mechanism.
- In diagnosed conditions such as enteric fever, dengue fever, and tuberculosis, development of new episode of fever with fast deterioration, organomegaly, lymphadenopathy and bicytopenia, think of hemophagocytic lymphohistiocytosis (HLH).

HOW DOES COMPLETE BLOOD COUNT HELP?

- More of negative predictive value
- Gives baseline value of hemoglobin (Hb) and different cell line
- Peripheral smear examination may confirm malaria; however, negative smear does not rule out it.
- Presence of abnormal cells, band cells, atypical lymphocytes, and blast cells may be an important clue.
- Extremes of counts, absolute neutrophil count (ANC), absolute lymphocyte count (ALC), and marked thrombocytopenia may indicate specific condition.
- Two or more cell lines affected (HLH and leukemia)
- Clinical correlation is mandatory.

INTERPRETATION OF COMPLETE BLOOD COUNT IN SHORT DURATION OF FEVER

WBC	Polymorphs	Lymphocytes	Eosinophils	Platelets	Hb	Probable disease
↑↑	↑↑	↓	↓/0	N	N	Acute bacterial infection
N/↓	↓	↑	↓/0	N	N	Typhoid
N/↓	↓	↑	↓	N/↓	N	Acute viral infection
↓↓	↑	↓	N	↓	N/↑	Dengue
↓/N	N	N	N/↑	↓	↓	Malaria

(Hb: hemoglobin; N: Normal; 0: Zero; WBC: white blood cell)

Fever of Short Duration

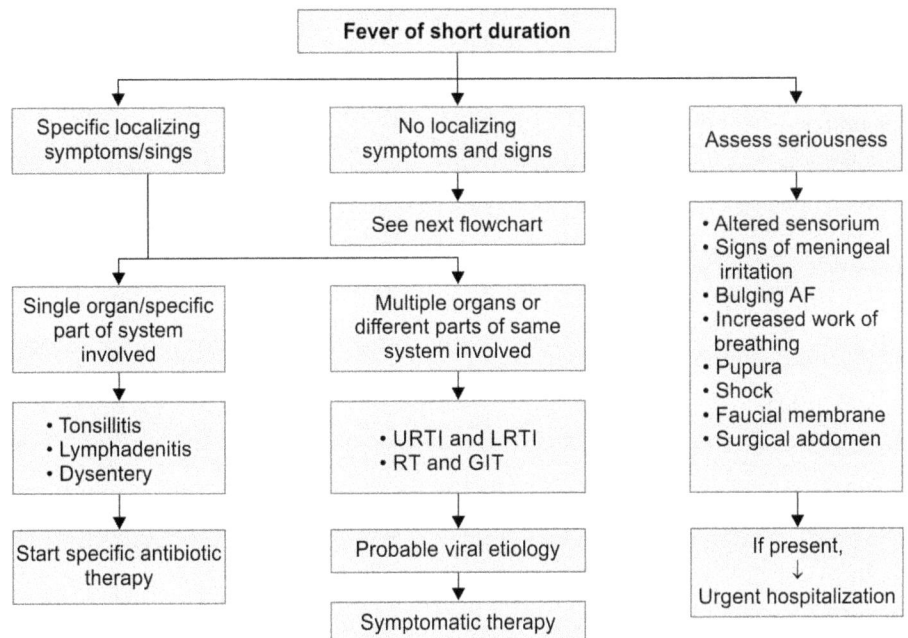

(AF: anterior fontanelle; LRTI: lower respiratory tract infection; URTI: upper respiratory tract infection)

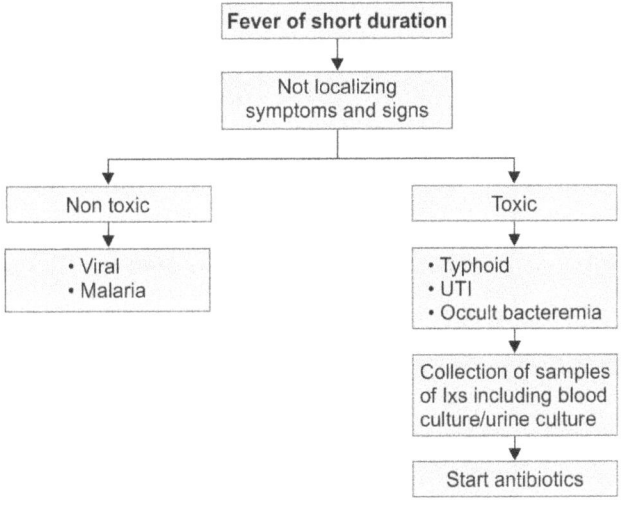

(Ixn: investigations; UTI: urinary tract infection)

COMMON CAUSES OF FEVER OF SHORT DURATION

- Viral infections
- Bacterial infections
- Malaria
- Enteric fever
- Dengue fever
- UTI
- Occult bacteremia
- Kawasaki disease

- *Toxin-mediated:*
  - Toxic shock syndrome
  - Staphylococcal scalded skin syndrome
- *Malignancy:*
  - Leukemia
  - Lymphoma
  - Neuroblastoma
- Endocrinal-like hyperthyroidism
- Drug-induced
- Heat stroke
- Others like HLH, macrophage activation syndrome
- Vaccine-associated fever.

40 Fever with Skin Rash

INTRODUCTION

The skin is the largest organ of the human body with many vital functions. It has been observed that about 30–40% of children seen in pediatric office practice, present with dermatological problems. Many a time, skin condition offers a visual clue to the underlying systemic disorder. Skin over the entire body has to be examined including palms, soles, and mucosa. Examination of hairs and nails is also important.

- Fever with rash is a common clinical scenario in pediatric practice. Skin rash is an important marker for several conditions.
- Most occasions, it is benign, viral exanthema, and self-limiting. But, it can be due to potential serious conditions such as meningococcemia, leukemia, Kawasaki disease, juvenile idiopathic arthritis (JIA), and systemic lupus erythematosus (SLE).
- Skin rash is the mirror of many internal ailments which may manifest as rashes.
- It should be evaluated as:
  - Age of the child
  - Type of skin rash
  - Onset and duration
  - Static, progressive, and recurrent
  - Site of beginning, progress, and pattern of distribution
  - Associated other symptoms such as fever, itching, and edema; manifestations of involvement of other systems
  - History of (H/o) drug, travel, and food; H/o similar disorder in family and community; H/o insect bite, etc.
- *Types of skin rashes:*
  - Macules are flat lesions of altered color of skin.
  - Papules are raised, flat, topped lesions with <5 mm in size.
  - Nodules are >5 mm in size with raised rounded configuration.
  - Vesicles are fluid-filled lesions <5 mm in size.
  - Bullae are fluid-filled lesions >5 mm in size.
  - Pustules are raised, pus-filled lesions.
  - *Petechiae* is bleeding into skin, non-blanchable, and pinhead size, 2 mm.
  - *Purpura* is superficial bleeding skin lesion, 2–5 mm in size. Skin lesions are called dry purpura and mucosal purpura is wet purpura. Wet purpura is considered as serious condition.
  - *Ecchymosis* is deep bleeding skin lesion, >5 mm in size.
- *Day of appearance of rash in a febrile child and likely condition:*
  - Day 1 → Varicella
  - Day 2 → Scarlet fever
  - Day 3 → Smallpox
  - Day 4 → Measles
  - Day 5 → Typhus fever
  - Day 6 → Dengue fever
  - Day 7 → Typhoid
- *First to sixth diseases (fever with rash):*
  - First → Rubeola (measles)
  - Second → Scarlet fever
  - Third → Rubella

- Fourth → Filatov-Duke's disease
- Fifth → Erythema infectiosum (slapped cheek syndrome) (parvovirus B19)
- Sixth → Roseola (exanthem subitum) [human herpes virus 6 and 7 (HHV 6 and 7)].

MEASLES

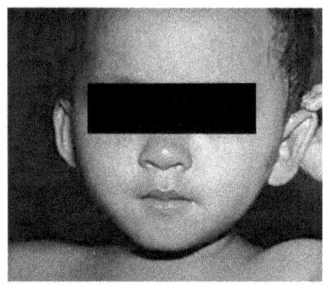

- Highly contagious
- *Prodromal:* Acute onset of high-grade fever, cough, coryza, rhinitis, conjunctivitis, malaise, and anorexia
- *Enanthematous:* Koplik's spots—on 3rd or 4th day of fever, on buccal mucosa at premolar level, like grain of sand
- *Exanthematous:* Rashes on 4th day—behind the ears, face, neck, near hairline → all over body, 5 days
- *Recovery:* Rashes disappear after 5 days in sequence in which they had appeared—postmeasles staining—desquamation of skin.
- *Incomplete (modified) measles:* In children with passively acquired antibody such as infants who received blood products or immunoglobulins, may develop a subclinical form of measles. The rash may be indistinct, brief or rarely and entirely absent. Likewise, some individuals who have received the vaccine, when exposed to measles, may have a rash but few other symptoms. Persons with modified measles are not considered highly contagious.
- *Hemorrhagic measles (black measles):* It is a severe form of measles disease. It manifests as hemorrhagic skin eruptions and may be fatal. Thrombocytopenia may be present.
- *Atypical measles:* Atypical measles syndrome is an altered expression of measles. It begins suddenly with high fever, headache, cough and abdominal pain. The rash may appear early, 1–2 days later, often beginning on the limbs. Edema of hands and feet may occur. Pneumonia is common and may persist for 3 months or more.

VARICELLA (CHICKENPOX)

- Pox means any disease characterized by formation of pustules on the skin that leave pock (small indentation or pit) marks when healed.
- Big pox (Great pox) → Syphilis
- Smallpox → Variola
- Chickenpox → Varicella
- Chickenpox means like chicken peas (garbanzo beans). It is a type of legume.

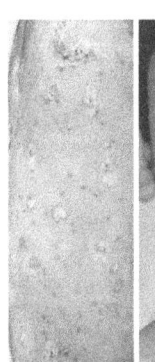
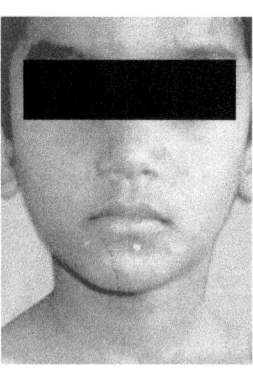
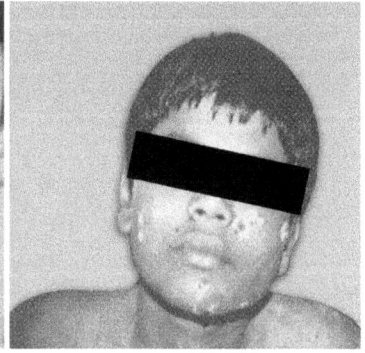

- Peak age 5–10 years
- Rash appears after 24–48 hours of prodromal symptoms.
- Intensely pruritic erythematous macules, first on trunk → rapidly spreads to face and extremities → lesions evolve into papules, clear fluid-filled vesicles, clouded vesicles, and then crusted vesicles.
- Pleomorphic skin lesions are characteristic.
- Number of lesions may be (10–1,500) (most of patients have lesions around 300)
- Break through chickenpox lesions <50.

Congenital Varicella Syndrome

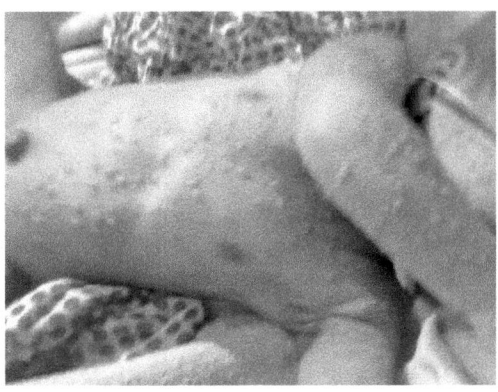

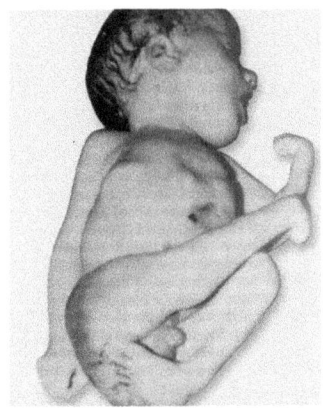

- Maternal varicella in first trimester → 2% risk of congenital varicella
- Cicatricial skin scarring, limb hypoplasia, digital defects, retinitis, cataract, and cortical atrophy.

Neonatal Varicella

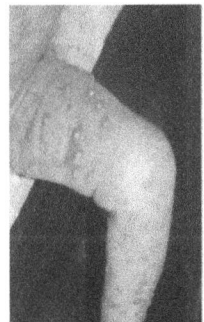
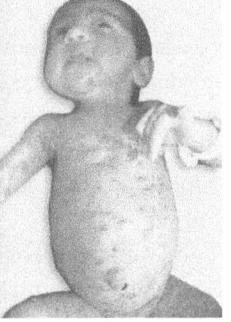

If mother develops varicella 5 days before 2 days after delivery, severe and often fatal neonatal varicella may result (risk 17–30%) (mortality 30%).

HERPES ZOSTER

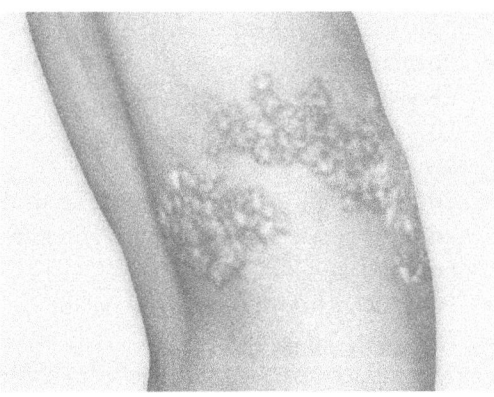

- Vesicular lesions clustered within one or two adjacent dermatomes
- Begins with burning pain, with clusters of skin lesions in a dermatomal pattern
- Low-grade fever, localized pain, hyperesthesia, and pruritus are common symptoms in children.
- Complete resolution within 1–2 weeks
- Increased risk of herpes zoster in:
  - Children who acquire varicella in first year of life
  - Mothers who have varicella infection in third trimester of pregnancy.

RUBELLA (GERMAN MEASLES) (3-DAY MEASLES)

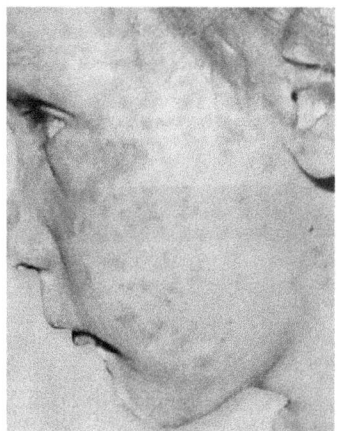

- It was initially recognized as resembling measles and was closely studied by German physicians. Later on, it was continued to be called as German measles.
- Postnatal infection with rubella → mild disease
- Low-grade fever, sore throat, red eyes, and headache
- Suboccipital, posterior auricular, and anterior cervical lymph nodes (LN) are enlarged
- Petechial hemorrhages on soft palate
- Rashes for 3 days
- Thrombocytopenia, arthritis, encephalitis, and progressive rubella panencephalitis are known complications.

Congenital Rubella Syndrome

- Maternal rubella infection in first trimester (embryogenesis) → defects in 90% of the off springs
- Nerve deafness (single most common)
- Congenital heart disease (CHD) [patent ductus arteriosus (PDA), pulmonary stenosis, and septal defects]
- Cataract
- Salt and pepper retinopathy
- Microcephaly
- Hepatosplenomegaly
- Thrombocytopenia
- Rubella vaccine to all girls is most effective preventive measure for congenital rubella syndrome.

INFECTIOUS MONONUCLEOSIS EPSTEIN–BARR VIRUS

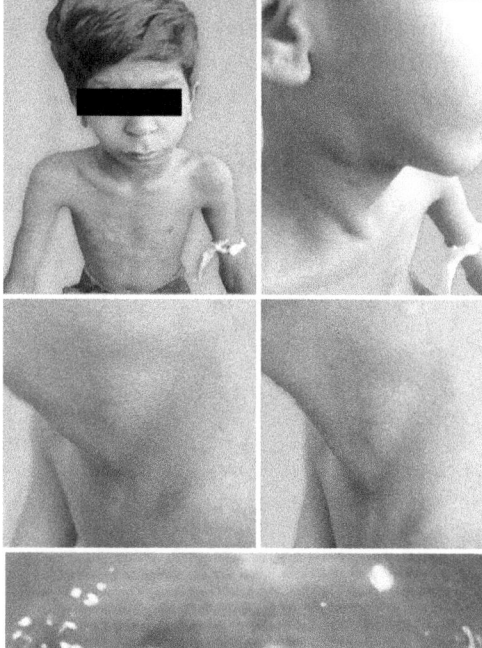

- Fever of long duration, malaise, fatigue, sore throat, and abdominal pain
- Marked pharyngotonsillitis, periorbital edema, generalized tender lymphadenopathy, and hepatosplenomegaly
- Soft splenomegaly is the characteristic, ruptured spleen following trivial injury is known.
- Epitrochlear LN is almost pathognomonic.
- Macular rash, precipitated or aggravated by ampicillin/amoxicillin

- Infectious mononucleosis is named because of the mononuclear lymphocytosis with atypical lymphocytes that accompany the clinical syndrome.
- It is also called as kissing disease due to transmission of Epstein–Barr virus (EBV) by oral kissing in adolescents.
- It was called as glandular disease due to lymphadenopathy.
- EBV infection can occur without manifestations of disease, while infectious mononucleosis means clinical manifestations of EBV infections.
- Transmission by:
  - Exposure to saliva
  - Oral kissing in adolescents
  - Blood transfusion
  - Bone marrow transplantation
  - No spread by droplets, fomites, or sexual contact
- Pharyngitis is often associated with whitish or gray-green exudates having an offensive odor.

ERYTHEMA INFECTIOSUM (FIFTH DISEASE)

- Parvovirus B19
- 5–15 years of age
- Prodromal symptoms → Rash of "slapped cheek" appearance → spreads to trunk and extremities.

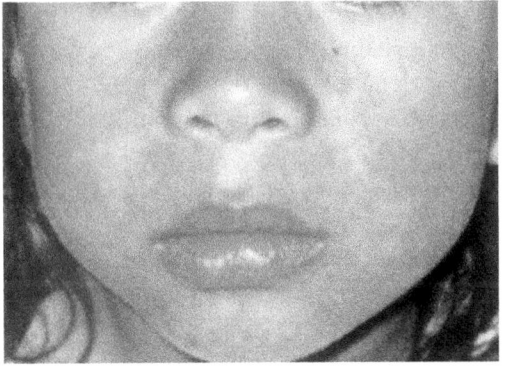

- Complications like arthropathy, idiopathic thrombocytopenic purpura (ITP), aseptic meningitis, transient aplastic crisis in patients with chronic hemolytic anemia, HLH, hydrops fetalis, and myocarditis

HAND-FOOT-AND-MOUTH DISEASE

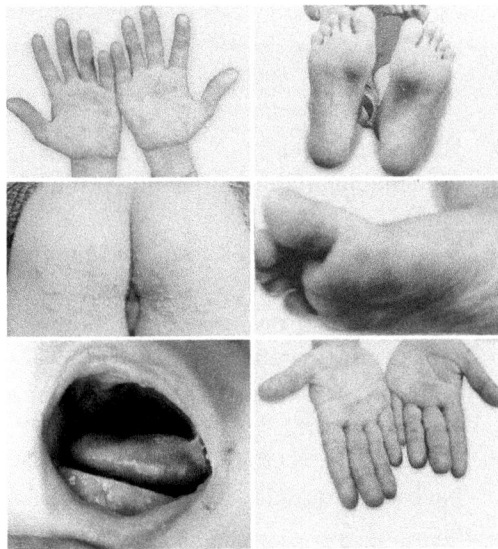

- Frequently caused by coxsackievirus A 16, also by enterovirus 71, coxsackie A virus 5, 7, 9 and 10.
- Mild illness, with or without low-grade fever
- Inflamed oropharynx, scattered vesicles on tongue, buccal mucosa, palate lips may ulcerate
- Maculopapular, vesicular and/or pustular lesions over hands, feet, buttocks, and groins
- Hand-foot-and-mouth disease by enterovirus 71 is frequently severe, neurological disease, pulmonary hemorrhage, shock, and rapid death.

DENGUE FEVER

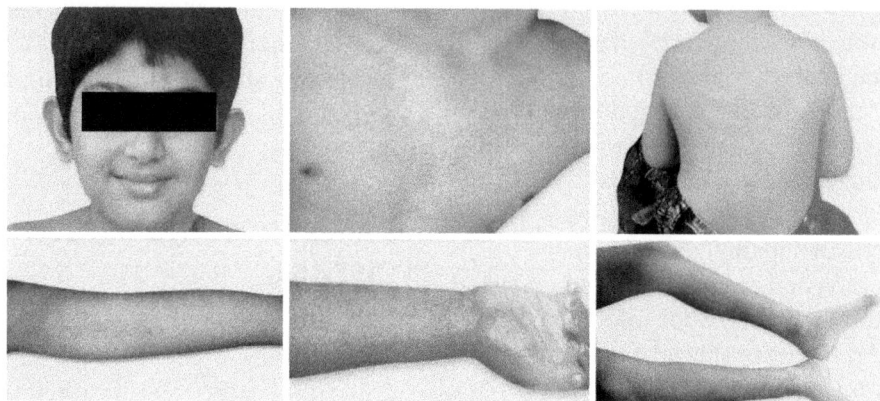

- High-grade fever
- Blanchable erythematous flush (measly look)
- Swollen face, injected eyes, and redness of ears
- Maculopapular rash may develop on the top of erythematous flush.
- Catarrh, typical characteristic of respiratory virus is missing.
- Headache, retro-orbital pain, photophobia, backache, myalgia, arthralgia, anorexia, etc.
- Petechiae spots and mucous membrane bleeding (nose, gum, and conjunctiva) may be seen.

CHIKUNGUNYA

- Chikungunya named is derived from stooped position of the patient due to severe arthralgia in a case of chikungunya.
- Chikungunya is the mosquito-borne arboviral disease.
- It is transmitted to human through day-biting mosquitoes, *Aedes aegypti*, and *Aedes albopictus*. Some cases of blood-borne transmission also have been reported. Fetomaternal transmission has been documented during pregnancy mainly in perinatal period.

- Sudden onset of fever with polyarthralgia more often bilateral symmetric pattern, myalgia, headache, fatigue and skin rashes are common symptoms. Fever may rise up to 104°F and may be associated with rigors. Fever may last up to 7 days.
- *Atypical and severe manifestations:*
  - Vesiculobullous skin lesions and hyperpigmentation
  - Febrile seizures
  - Meningoencephalitis
  - Guillain–Barré syndrome (GBS)
  - Encephalopathy
  - Cerebellar syndrome
  - Myocarditis and arrhythmias
  - Acute renal failure
  - Bleeding dyscrasias
- *Chikungunya in neonates and infants:*
  - High-grade fever
  - Irritability
  - Generalized hyperpigmentation
  - H/o chikungunya to mother or family member

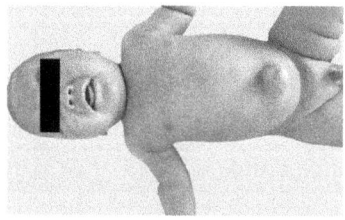

SCARLET FEVER

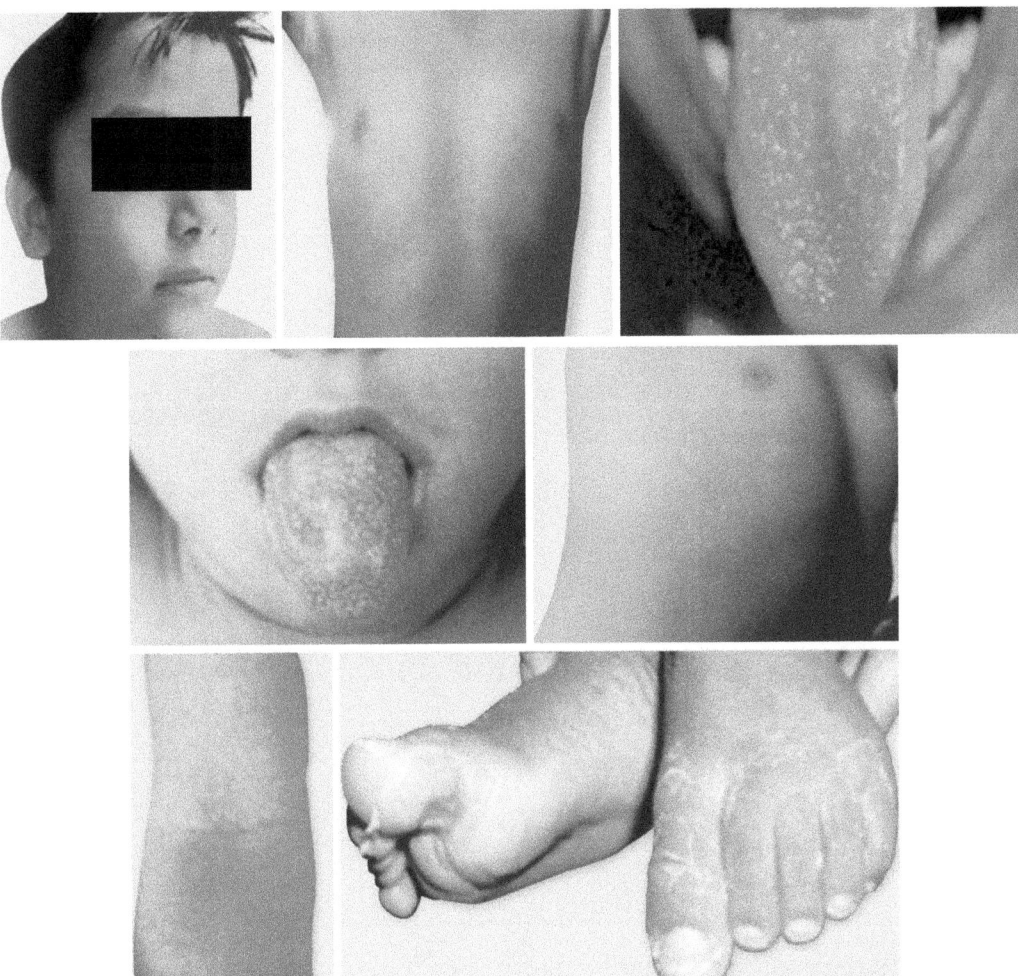

- Upper respiratory tract infection (URTI) by group A streptococci
- Fever, exudative pharyngitis, and erythematous rash
- An exotoxin (erythrogenic toxin)-mediated disease
- Sudden onset of fever, throat pain, malaise, and headache
- Rash appears within 24–48 hour after onset of symptoms.
- Often begins around the neck, spreads over trunk, and extremities
- Diffuse, fine papular, erythematous eruption → bright red discoloration of skin, blanching on pressure
- Often more intense along the creases of elbows, axillae, and groin
- Goose-pimple appearance of skin, feels rough
- Desquamation starts after 3–4 days
- White and red strawberry appearance of tongue.

KAWASAKI DISEASE

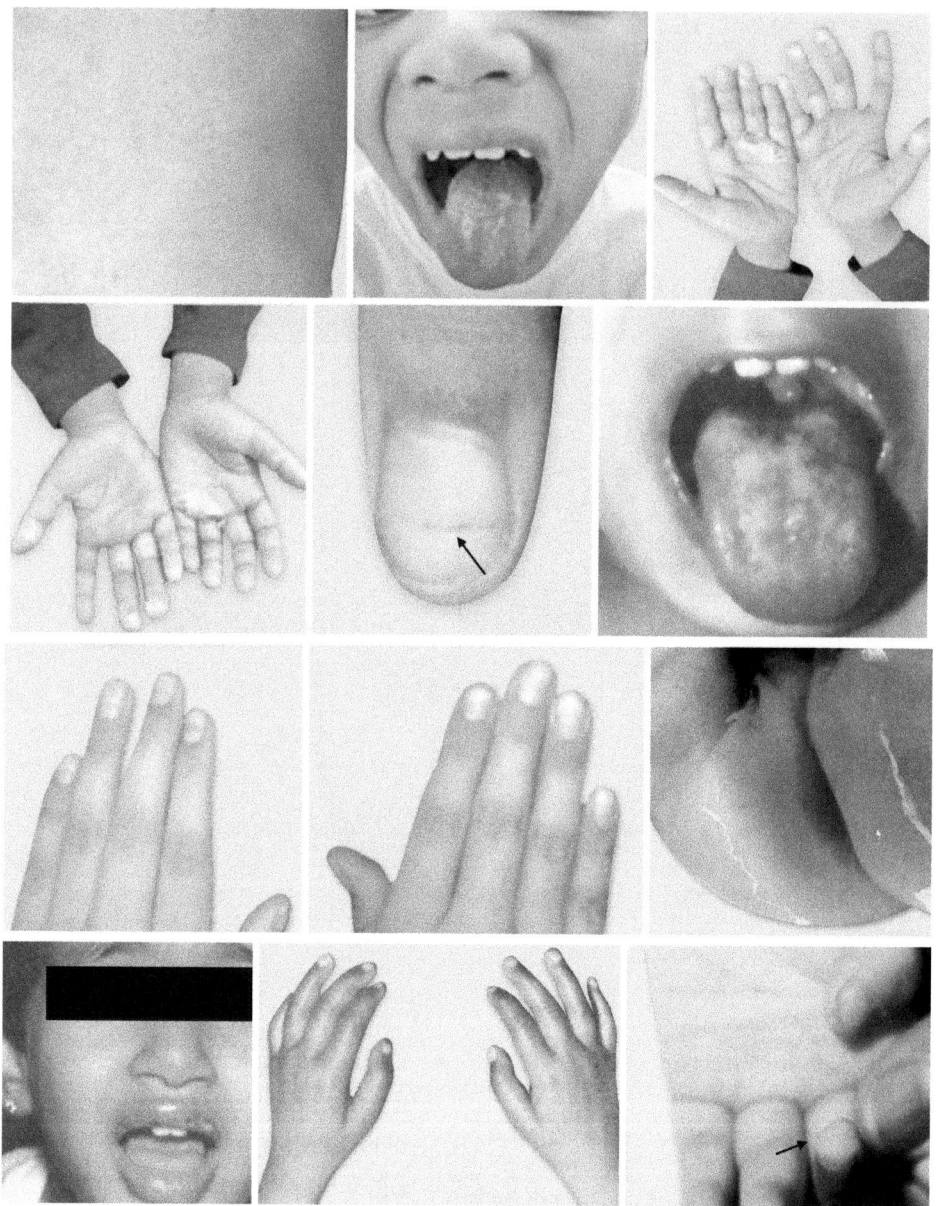

Classic Clinical Criteria

- Age <5 years
- High-grade fever, >5 days duration, no response to antibiotics
- Acute erythema of palms and soles
- Edema of hands and feet
- Bilateral bulbar conjunctival injection, without exudate.
- Erythema of oral and pharyngeal mucosa
- Strawberry tongue
- Dry, cracked lips without ulcerations

- Maculopapular, erythema multiforme (EM), and scarlatiniform rashes.
- Perineal desquamation is pathognomonic.
- Periungual desquamation of fingers and toes, begins 1–3 weeks after onset of illness
- Lymphadenopathy.

RICKETTSIAL DISEASES

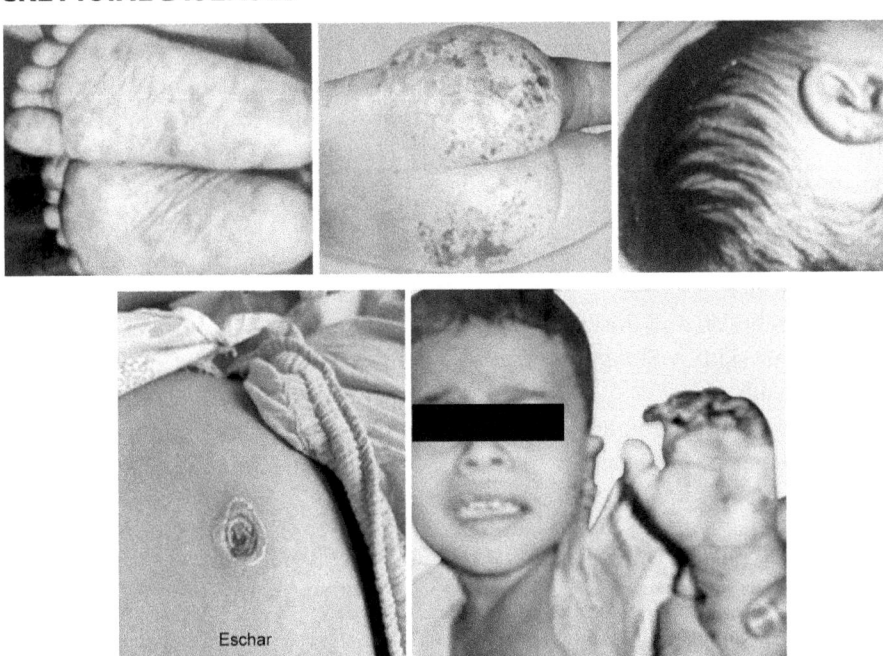

Eschar

- Rash is initially discrete.
- Pale, rose red, blanching, macules or maculopapular over extremities including ankles, wrists, lower limbs → petechial or hemorrhagic, sometimes palpable purpura → ecchymosis → necrotic → Gangrene of digits, toes, ear lobes, scrotum, nose, and entire limb.
- Painless eschar may be seen at initial site of tick attachment and regional lymphadenopathy.

NECROTIZING FASCITIS

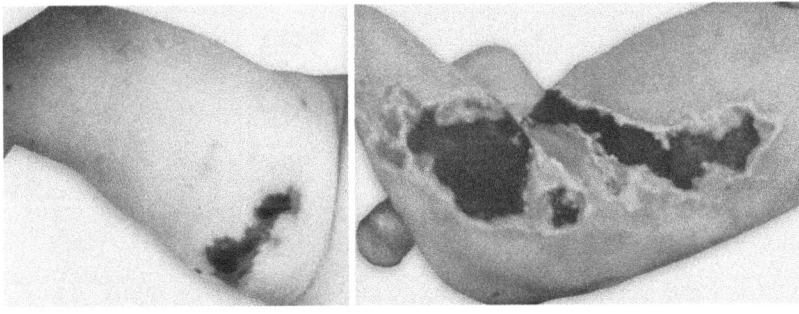

- Streptococcal pyogenes is most common organism, may be polymicrobial.
- May result from secondary bacterial infection following varicella.
- Acute, rapidly progressive, severe, deep-seated infection of subcutaneous tissues → extensive and rapidly spreading necrosis of superficial and deep fascia → Gangrene of the skin and underling structures.
- Diffuse, erythematous swelling, and associated with agonizing pain
- More common at extremities
- May follow cut, burns, penetrating injuries, blunt trauma, etc.
- Skin becomes bluish and dusky → Bullae → Gangrenous skin → Slough of skin → Shock and Death
- Prompt, appropriate antibiotics + Surgical debridement may be lifesaving.

MENINGOCOCCEMIA

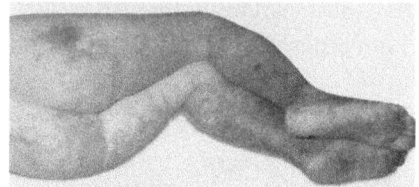

- Maculopapular rash, which is indistinguishable from rashes seen after viral infections is common.
- As disease progresses, cold hands or feet and abnormal skin color may be important sign.
- Nonblanching or petechial rash in >80% cases
- Purpura fulminans develops in severe disease.
- Meningococcal, meningitis, shock, acidosis, adrenal hemorrhage, and renal failure are fatal complications.

SYSTEMIC ONSET JUVENILE IDIOPATHIC ARTHRITIS

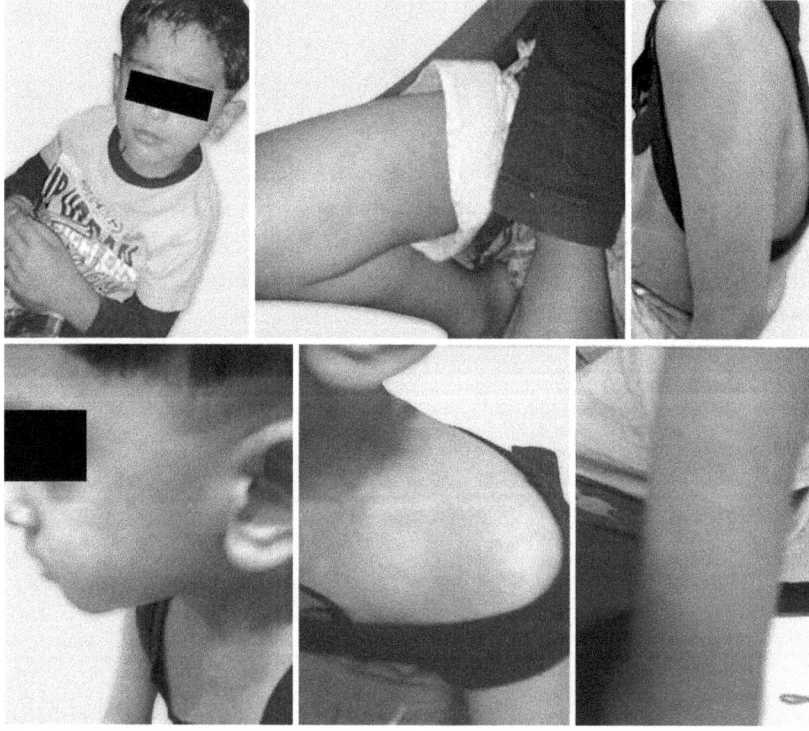

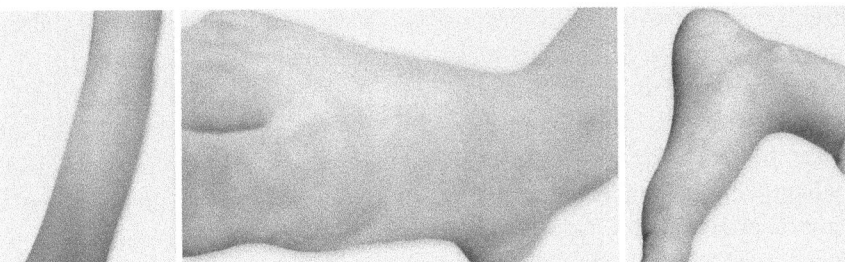

- Fever >39°C (102.2°F) for >2 weeks, with a rapid return to normal or subnormal temperature
- Each febrile episode is frequently accompanied by a characteristic faint, erythematous, and macular rash.
- The evanescent (quickly fading and vanishing) salmon-colored lesions, classic for systemic-onset juvenile idiopathic arthritis (SOJIA), are linear or circular, 2–5 mm in size, often distributed in groups, over the trunk and proximal extremities.
- Nonpruritic and migratory, lasting for <1 hour
- Koebner phenomenon (cutaneous hypersensitivity) is often present.
- Heat and warm bath evokes reappearance of the rash.
- Hepatosplenomegaly and lymphadenopathy in >70% patients
- Arthritis may develop later on after several weeks or months
- Serositis may be present.

SYSTEMIC LUPUS ERYTHEMATOSUS

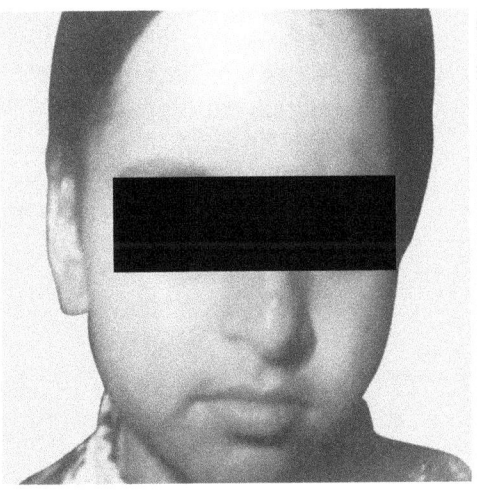
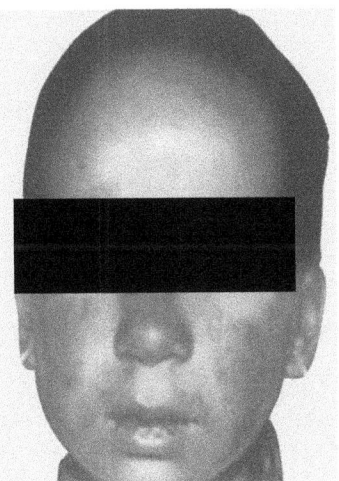

- Fever, fatigue, hematologic abnormalities, arthralgia or arthritis, skin rash, and renal disease are more common in children.
- Skin manifestations are frequently present:
  - Malar butterfly rash is hallmark of SLE, involving cheeks and nasal bridge, erythematous bluish to scaly patches. It develops over malar eminences, crosses the nasal bridge and spares the nasolabial folds.
  - Rash may be photosensitive, extend to sun-exposed areas.

- Mucous membrane involvement causes vasculitic erythema, painless ulcers over palatal and nasal mucosa.
- Vasculitis lesions appearing over palms, fingers and soles in form of erythematous macular eruptions.
- Purpura, urticaria, and Raynaud phenomenon are other skin manifestations.
- Frontal baldness is characteristic feature of SLE.
  - Discoid lupus lesions may be present in 5–10% patients. Discoid lupus, named after its coin-shaped appearance, is an erythematous rash that primarily affects face, ears, and scalp, although upper extremities, upper chest, and back may be affected.

HENOCH–SCHÖNLEIN PURPURA

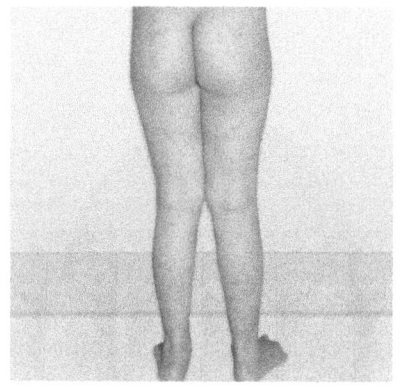

- Most common vasculitis in children
- It is small-vessel vasculitis.
- Henoch–Schönlein purpura (HSP) is an immunoglobulin A (IgA)-mediated dysregulated immune response to antigen as suggested by the deposition of IgA.
- Non thrombocytopenic and palpable purpura (inflammation makes it palpable)
- The skin lesions are more common over lower extremities and buttocks in ambulatory children, and sacrum along with buttocks and ears in infants as gravity causes immune complexes to deposit and incite inflammation in dependent areas.
- There may be an abundance of rash at the pressure points, especially on the extensor aspect of the knees in crawling infants.
- Edema may develop over face, scalp, and extremities due to inflammation.
- Transient arthralgia or arthritis may develop.
- Pain in abdomen (due to vasculitis), vomiting, hematemesis, melena, and bleeding per rectum are common features of HSP. It may mimic as an acute surgical abdomen.
- Renal involvement is common.
- Intussusception, intestinal perforation, and torsion of testis are serious complications.

JUVENILE DERMATOMYOSITIS

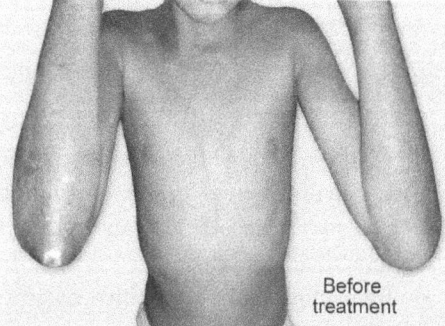

Before treatment

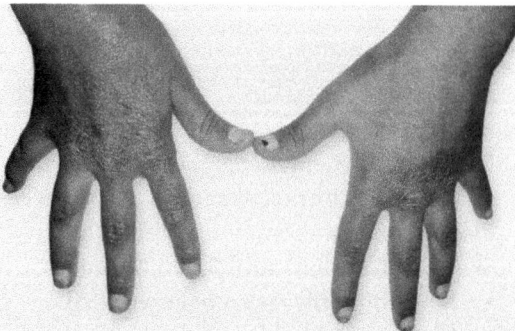

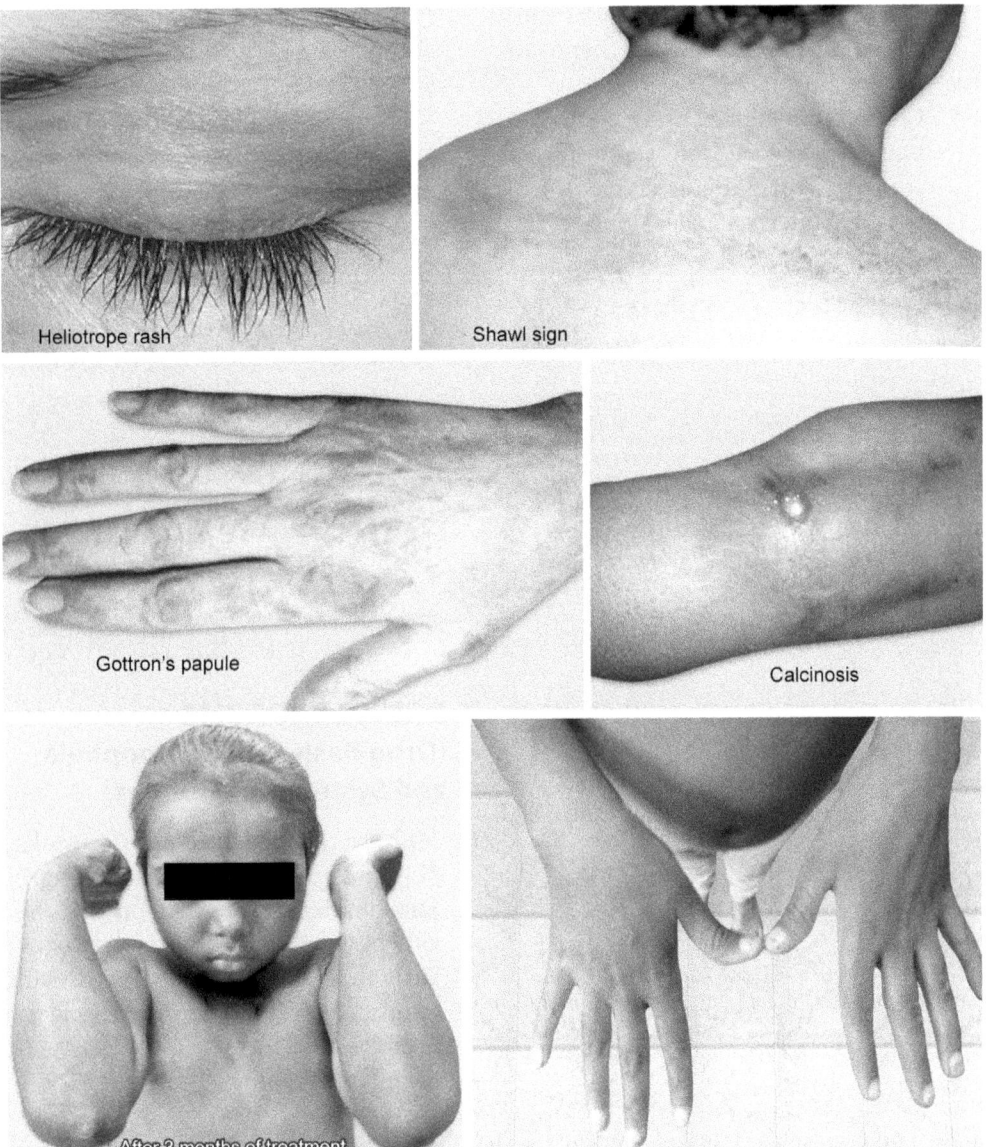

- Uncommon, chronic inflammatory, multisystem disease, affecting predominantly skin striated muscles
- Most common inflammatory myopathy in children.
- Girls are more commonly affected than the boys.
- Symmetrical proximal muscle weakness, heliotrope rash, and Gottron's papules over the knuckles and elbows are characteristics of the disease.
- Mucocutaneous involvement:
  - *Heliotrope rash:* It is discoloration of upper eyelids as a violaceous and purple coloration.
  - Malar rash may develop
  - Periorbital edema

- Skin may thin out—atrophy of subcutaneous structures with hypo- or hyperpigmentation.
- Gottron's papules are shiny, erythematous plaques occurring over the extensor surfaces of the joints, common over proximal interphalangeal joints of the hands, and extensor surfaces of elbows and knees.
- *Calcinosis:* Dystrophic calcinosis may occur in subcutaneous plaques or nodules.
- Acanthosis nigricans and lipodystrophy are other manifestations.

ERYTHEMA NODOSUM

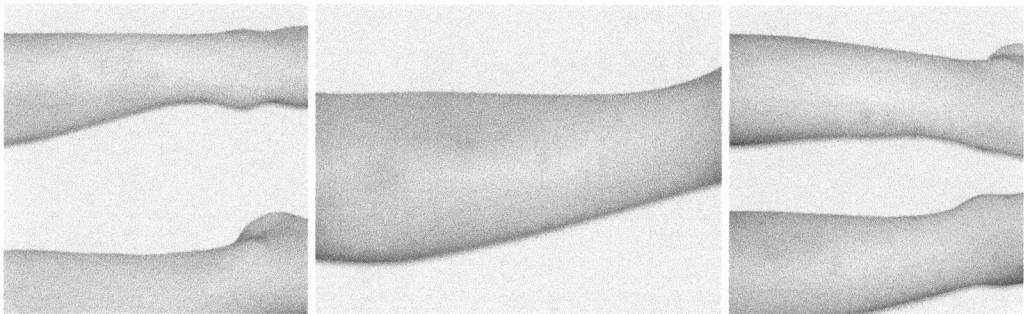

- Pretibial, tender, and erythematous nodules
- Hypersensitive reaction resulting from infections, inflammatory disease, and drug

Causes of Erythema Nodosum	
Infections	• Group A streptococcal (GAS) pharyngitis • Tuberculosis • Histoplasmosis
Inflammatory disease	• Inflammatory bowel disease (IBD) • Sarcoidosis
Drugs	• Sulfonamides • Phenytoin

DRESS SYNDROME
(Drug Rash, with Eosinophilia and Systemic Symptoms)

- Multisystem reaction after 4 weeks of starting phenytoin, carbamazepine, phenobarbitone, or primidone
  Other drugs like antibiotics can also cause:
- Skin rash identical to EM, Stevens-Johnson (SJ) syndrome, or toxic epidermal necrolysis (TEN)
- Lymphadenopathy
- Fever
- Hepatic, renal and pulmonary involvement
- Leukocytosis
- Eosinophilia.

41 CHAPTER

Fever without Focus

INTRODUCTION

Fever without Focus (FWF) in a child is defined as a rectal temperature of 38°C (100.4°F) or higher as the only presenting complaint. There is acute onset of fever and duration is short (less than a week). There is no any sign or symptom of localization. FWF is a diagnostic challenge especially in children less than 36 months of age because of high risk for occult bacteremia and serious bacterial infections.

- *Definition:* Fever without focus (FWF) or fever without localizing signs is defined as an acute febrile illness (less than a week) in which the etiology of fever is not apparent after a thorough history and physical examination. A rectal temperature >38°C (100.4°F) is defined as fever.
- As the etiology of this entity and risk of serious bacterial infection (SBI) is variable in different age groups, they are classified as follows:
  - Neonates (up to 1 month of age)
  - Infants 1–3 months of age
  - Infants 3–36 months of age
- When an infant less than 3 months of age presents with FWF, it is a very common dilemma to the treating clinician whether the baby needs hospitalization or can be managed as an outdoor patient; investigations should be performed immediately or can be postponed; empirical antibiotics should be started or may be decided later on.
- We are more concerned with this group as immunologically they are weak because of their immature immune system. Moreover, the incidence of occult bacteremia and SBIs in these babies is significantly high. SBI may be in form of occult bacteremia, bacterial meningitis, urinary tract infection (UTI), pneumonia, osteomyelitis, and septic arthritis, and all these conditions initially may not show localization on clinical examination.
- They have very limited number of symptoms and signs of infections and those too are nonspecific. Therefore, it is clinically difficult to differentiate between non-serious conditions such as dehydration fever, viral infections, and serious SBIs.
- If SBIs are missed clinically, not investigated for confirmation of their presence and not managed with intravenous (IV) antibiotics promptly, it results in disastrous with high mortality and significant permanent sequelae.

Therefore, a prudent clinician should follow the standard protocol as follows: As the risk of SBI is variable and etiological agents are different, they can be divided in two groups: (1) Neonates (up to 1 month of age) and (2) 1–3 months of age.

NEONATES (UP TO 1 MONTH OF AGE) WITH FEVER WITHOUT FOCUS

- When neonates present with FWF and a sick or toxic appearance, there is no dilemma to the treating clinician and parents, on the need of immediate hospitalization and management.
- But, neonates with FWF who are well looking (alert, active, and taking breast feeding) present big dilemma to parents as well as the medical personnel for hospitalization.
- As immunologically, they are weak due to their immature immune system and incidence of SBIs is as high as 15–20%, they require appropriate, prompt action. They should be hospitalized immediately and proper work up should be performed for SBIs.
- *Common organisms for neonatal sepsis:* In India, common organisms for neonatal sepsis are *Escherichia coli*, *Klebsiella*, and *Staphylococcus aureus*. *Haemophilus influenzae* B, and *Streptococcus pneumoniae* are other organisms. *Listeria monocytogenes* and perinatally acquired herpes simplex virus (HSV) have also been implicated. Malaria remains a possibility in endemic area and may be transplacentally transmitted.
- *Investigations for neonatal sepsis:* After hospitalization, investigations for neonatal sepsis should be performed before starting antibiotics.
  - Blood samples are collected for complete blood count (CBC) including total and differential counts, absolute neutrophil count, peripheral smear examination for band cells, C-reactive protein (CRP), and blood culture.
  - Urine sample is collected for routine examination as well as culture with absolute aseptic precautions.
  - Lumbar puncture and collection of cerebrospinal fluid (CSF) for routine examination and culture is mandatory to rule out meningitis before starting the antibiotics.
  - Tests for malaria, dengue fever, and corona viral infection should be performed, if indicated looking at the epidemic and endemic situation in the area.
  - Chest X-ray may help to exclude pneumonia.
- *Interpretation of investigations for neonatal sepsis:*
  - Leukopenia (leukocyte count <5,000/cu.mm) is commonly seen rather than leukocytosis (leukocyte count >15,000/cu.mm in 3-day-old neonates).
  - Absolute neutrophil count >1,500/cu.mm and ratio of immature to total neutrophils (I:T ratio) >0.2 are considered as more reliable indicators.
  - CRP >1 mg/dL is an important marker for neonatal sepsis.
  - If first CRP is negative, it should be repeated after 12–24 hours. If two CRP tests are negative, it almost excludes neonatal sepsis.
  - CRP has better negative predictive value than positive predictive value. It means if CRP is twice negative, neonatal sepsis is almost excluded and alternate diagnosis should be considered. But, only positive CRP means not necessarily neonatal sepsis, it should be correlated with other parameters also. In nutshell, to start the antibiotics based on only positive CRP is not justified.
  - Out of all these markers of neonatal sepsis, total leukocyte count <5,000/cu.mm, raised I:T ratio (>0.2) and positive CRP (>1 mg/dL) are best

indicators for neonatal sepsis. If any two out of these three markers are positive, consider neonatal sepsis.
- CSF and urine examination (including cultures) are important investigations, not to miss bacterial meningitis and UTI.
- If bacterial meningitis and UTI remain undiagnosed and treated partially, it will cause damage to respective organs resulting in serious complications and sequelae.

Management

- After obtaining samples for necessary investigations, IV empirical antibiotics should be initiated at the earliest with combination of ampicillin and/or cefotaxime and amikacin. It can be modified according to isolation of organisms from culture.
- Minimum duration of antibiotics for neonatal sepsis is 7–10 days. It should be IV for 3 weeks in a case of bacterial meningitis and 4–6 weeks for skeletal infections.

FEVER WITHOUT FOCUS IN INFANTS 1–3 MONTHS OF AGE

- In infants, 1–3 months of age, FWF is commonly due to viral illness. Still, SBI remains one of the possibilities in 5–20% of this group.
- The common bacterial infections in this group are UTI, pneumonia, otitis media, and skin and soft tissue infections. Among all these, UTI is most common in both the groups, sick-looking and well-looking.
- The most common organisms are *E. coli*, *S. pneumoniae*, *S. aureus* and *H. influenzae*.

Investigations and Management

Infants of this age group with FWF need to be categorized as high or low risk for SBI by certain criteria as laid down in **Table 1**. Decision for hospitalization and further line of treatment can be taken based on it.

TABLE 1: Criteria for low risk for SBI in 1–3 months of age with FWF.

	Philadelphia protocol	Pittsburg guidelines	Rochester criteria	Boston criteria
General appearance	Well	Well	Well	Well
Physical examination	Normal	Normal	Normal	Normal
WBC/mm^3	<15,000	5,000–15,000	5,000–15,000	<20,000
Immature to total (I:T) neutrophil ratio absolute band count (mm^3)	<0.2	<1,500	<1,500	
Urine examination	<10 WBC/HPF No bacteria or Gram stain	9 WBC/mm^3, no bacteria or Gram stain	<10 WBC/HPF	Negative leukocyte esterase
CSF cell count	<8 WBC/mm^3 No bacteria or Gram stain	5 WBC/mm^3 No bacteria or Gram stain		<10 WBC/mm^3
Chest X-ray (CXR)	No infiltrates	No infiltrates		
Stool examination	No RBC, few or no WBC	5 WBC/HPF with diarrhea	<5 WBC/HPF if diarrhea	

(CSF: cerebrospinal fluid; FWF: fever without focus; HPF: high power field; RBC: red blood cell; WBC: white blood cell)

- *High risk for SBI:*
  - Febrile infant <3 months of age with lethargy, decreased activity, refusal of feeds, increased work of breathing (tachypnea, chest indrawing and grunting), mottled cool extremities and/or irritability should be hospitalized immediately and management should be started promptly. In this category, investigations as suggested in neonates with FWF should be performed and IV antibiotics should be started.
- *Low risk for SBI:*
  - In well looking infants who have previously been healthy and with low risk criteria, investigations should be obtained and the child sent home.
  - Parents should be advised to follow-up after 24 hours or earlier on deterioration.
  - Antibiotic therapy should be planned after reports confirm sepsis.
  - Meanwhile, at any age, if the child deteriorates, the baby should be hospitalized, samples should be collected for investigations, and empirical antibiotics started.
  - Prior to initiation of antibiotics in the event of clinical deterioration, lumbar puncture is always mandatory.
  - If the baby becomes afebrile and reports for sepsis are negative, antibiotic therapy should be stopped and only symptomatic therapy is indicated.
- Low risk in 1–3 months old children with fever without localizing signs (FWLS).

MANAGEMENT ALGORITHM OF INFANTS LESS THAN 3 MONTHS OF AGE

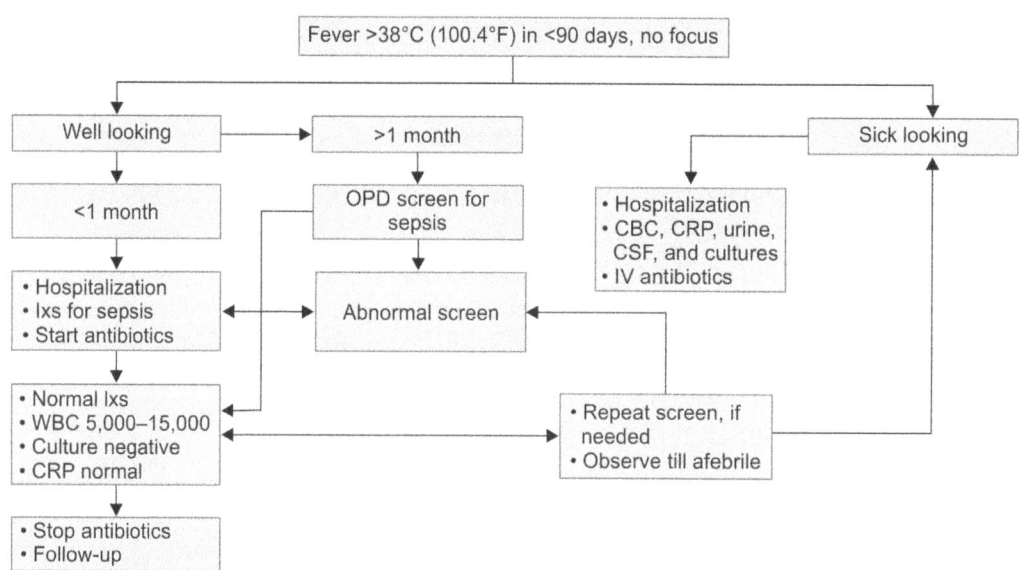

(CBC: complete blood count; CRP: C-reactive protein; CSF: cerebrospinal fluid; IV: intravenous; Ixs: investigations; WBC: white blood cell).

FEVER WITHOUT FOCUS IN 3–36 MONTHS OLD CHILDREN

- Viral infections are most common.
- SBI can also occur due to *S. pneumoniae*, *Neisseria*, and *H. influenzae*.
- Risk factors for SBI in this group include:
  - Rectal temperature >39°C
  - WBC count >15,000/cu.mm
  - Raised erythrocyte sedimentation rate (ESR) and CRP
- Rectal temperature >40°C and WBC count >25,000/cu.mm indicate a high probability of SBI.
- Most common bacterial infections include otitis media, pneumonia, sinusitis, UTI, osteomyelitis, bacterial meningitis, etc.
- In this age group, child with rectal temperature >40°C or WBC count >15,000/cu.mm, obtain samples for investigations including blood culture and start antibiotics.

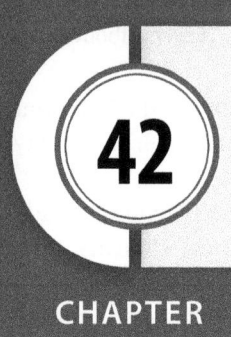

Floppy Infant

CHAPTER 42

INTRODUCTION

Floppy infant is a well-recognized entity in pediatrics. An organized approach is essential for its proper evaluation.

The word "floppy" can be used to mean:
- Decreased muscle tone (hypotonia)
- Decreased muscle power (weakness/paresis)
- Laxity of ligaments and increased range of joint mobility

But "floppy infant" is considered in terms of hypotonia.

ESSENTIAL BASIC FACTS TO UNDERSTAND FLOPPY INFANT

- Muscle tone is the resistance of the muscle to stretch. It refers to the state of muscle tension or contraction.
- Clinicians test two types of tones:
  - *Phasic tone:* Rapid contraction in response to a high-intensity stretch. It is also called monosynaptic reflex or deep tendon reflex (DTR).
  - *Postural tone:* It is defined as prolonged contraction of antigravity muscles in response to low-intensity stretch of gravity.

  It is also defined as continuous and passive partial contraction of the muscles due to minimal continuous motor electrical discharges. It helps to maintain the posture.
  - When postural tone is depressed, the trunk and limbs cannot maintain themselves against gravity and the infant appears floppy (hypotonic).
- The maintenance of normal tone requires intact central and peripheral nervous system.
- Hypotonia occurs in disorders of cortex, basal ganglia, cerebellum, spinal cord, nerves, and muscles.

TYPES OF HYPOTONIA

- *Hypotonia can be divided into two broad groups:*
  - *Central hypotonia:* The supraspinal conditions include brain, brain stem, and cervical spinal function. It also includes basal ganglia and cerebellum.
  - *Periphery nervous system hypotonia (motor unit hypotonia):*
    - Anterior horn cell [poliomyelitis and spinomuscular atrophy (SMA)]
    - Peripheral nerve (neuropathy)
    - Neuromuscular junction (myasthenia gravis)
    - Muscle [myopathies like Duchenne muscular dystrophy (DMD)]
- Central nervous system (CNS) accounts for 60–80% of hypotonic causes while peripheral nervous system accounts for 15–20%.

WHEN TO SUSPECT FLOPPY INFANT (FIGS. 1A TO C)

- Mother feels her baby is loose—floppy.
- Slips from hands

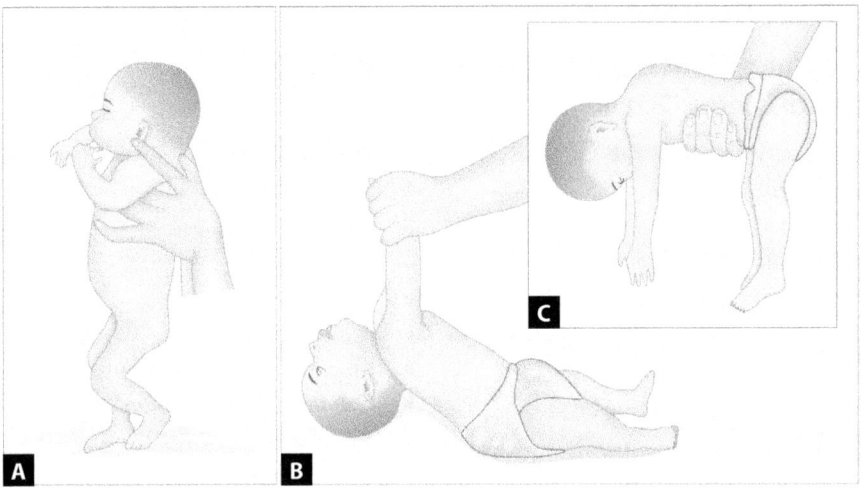

Figs. 1A to C: Assessment of hypotonia. (A) Axillary suspension; (B) Traction response; and (C) Ventral suspension.

- Less movements of limbs
- Frog-like position
- Baby is alert, but remains inactive.
- Delayed motor development.

CLINICAL EVALUATION

- Age of onset (congenital/acquired), mode of onset, presenting complaints, and progress
- History regarding pregnancy and neonatal period:
  - Consanguinity
  - Previous fetal losses
  - Less fetal movements (SMA)
  - Polyhydramnios
  - Breech presentation
  - History of (H/o) hypoxic ischemic encephalopathy (HIE)
- H/o respiratory difficulty or ventilator support in neonatal period
- Weak cry
- Poor feeding
- Congenital talipes equinovarus (TEV), joint dislocation, and contractures
- Prepare family pedigree for three generations
- Delayed motor milestones
- Fatigability
- Frequent falls
- Difficulty in getting up from floor, ascending, and descending stairs
- Problems in dressing and reaching above the head.
- H/o repeated pneumonias and lower respiratory tract infections (LRTIs)
- Dysmorphic facial features
- Ptosis and ophthalmoplegia

NEUROLOGICAL ASSESSMENT

- Posture and spontaneous movements
- Head size
- Elicitation of floppiness
- Pull to sit (traction): Head leg
- Ventral suspension: Inverted "U" shape
- Vertical suspension: Slipping through
- Scarf sign: Elbow can easily be brought well beyond the midline before encountering resistance.
- DTR:
  - Brisk or clonus (central cause)
  - Diminished or absent (peripheral motor system cause).

CLINICAL FEATURES

Clinical Features Suggestive of Hypotonia of Central Origin

- Predominantly axial weakness
- Fisting of hands
- Brisk DTR and brisk jaw jerk
- Scissoring on vertical suspension
- Global delayed development
- Dysmorphic facial features.

Clinical Features Suggestive of Hypotonia of Peripheral Origin

- *Anterior horn cell:*
  - Hypotonia
  - Flaccidity
  - Decreased or absent DTR
  - Decreased power, e.g., poliomyelitis and SMA
- *Peripheral nerves:*
  - Tingling and numbness
  - Gloves and stocking type
  - More distal involvement
  - Decreased/absent DTR
  - Loss of power
- *Neuromuscular junction:*
  - Weakness increases with exercise
  - Fatigability (fluctuating)
  - Facial muscles are more involved.
  - Diplopia
  - Ptosis
  - Ophthalmoplegia, e.g., myasthenia gravis
- *Muscles:*
  - Proximal muscles are more involved
  - Difficulty in getting up from floor
  - Problems in ascending and descending stairs
  - Difficulty in raising upper extremities above the head, while removing clothes or combing the hairs.

CENTRAL CAUSES OF FLOPPY INFANT

- *Encephalopathies:*
- HIE
- Hypoglycemia
- Brain trauma
- Inborn errors of metabolism
- *Genetical and chromosomal disorders:*
  - Prader-Willi syndrome
  - Trisomy 21, 13, and 18
  - Lowe syndrome (oculocerebrorenal syndrome).
  - Familial dysautonomia
- *Metabolic causes:*
  - Rickets
  - Renal tubular acidosis
- *Miscellaneous:*
  - Cerebellar disorders
  - Ehlers-Danlos syndrome.

PERIPHERAL CAUSES OF A FLOPPY INFANT

- Spinomuscular atrophy
- Paralytic poliomyelitis
- Polyneuropathies
- *Neuromuscular junction disorders:*
  - Myasthenia gravis
  - Botulism
  - Magnesium toxicity
  - Aminoglycoside toxicity
- *Muscular disorders:*
  - DMD
  - Dermatomyositis
  - Becker's myopathy
  - Steroid-induced myopathy
  - Hypothyroidism.

43 Gait Disorders

INTRODUCTION

In simple terms, gait abnormality means problem with walking. One should know normal gait to understand its abnormality. To decide the type of abnormality, gait examination is very important. Gait abnormalities may be due to musculoskeletal disorders, various central nervous system diseases like cerebral palsy, hemiplegia, cerebellar disorders, extrapyramidal diseases, myopathies and spinal cord disorders. Methodological evaluation is essential.

- *Definition:* Series of rhythmical, alternating movements of the trunk and limbs which

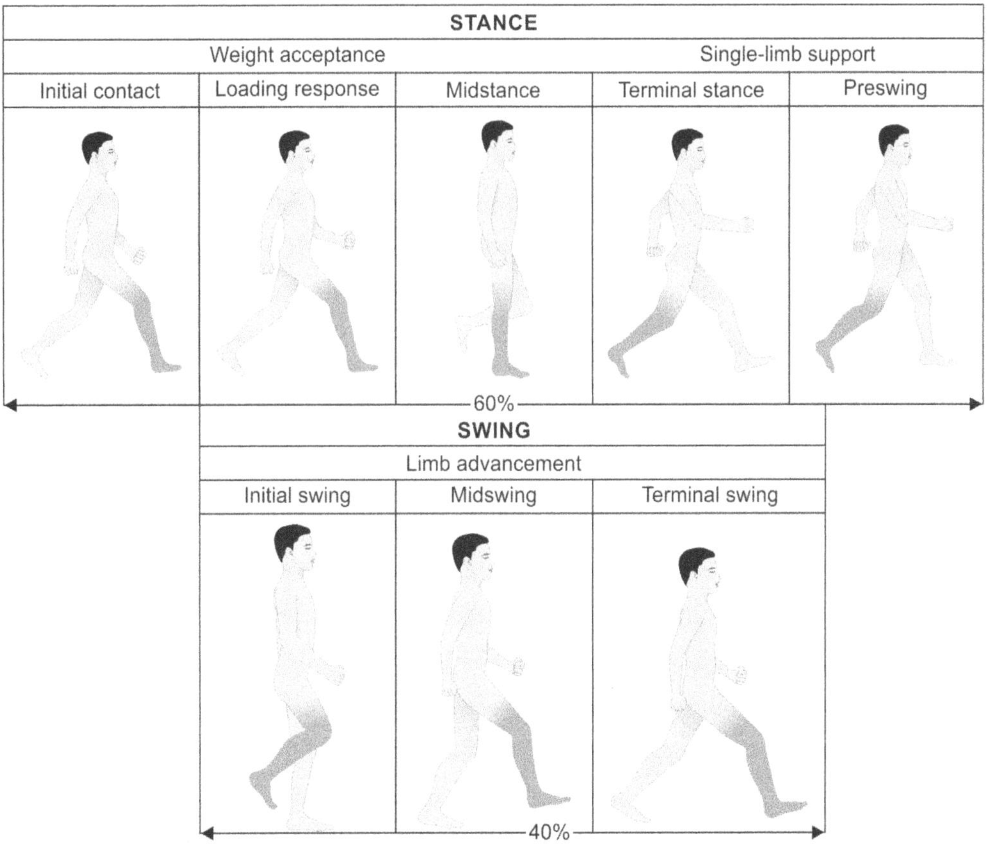

STANCE				
Weight acceptance			Single-limb support	
Initial contact	Loading response	Midstance	Terminal stance	Preswing

— 60% —

SWING		
Limb advancement		
Initial swing	Midswing	Terminal swing

— 40% —

- result in the forward progression of the center of gravity, and thereby forward movement of body.
- Human walking follows a repetitive pattern called the gait cycle. The gait cycle can be divided into two phases: (1) the stance phase when the lower limb is in contact with the ground and (2) the swing phase when the limb is lifted off in order to advance the body forward. Stance phase accounts for 60% of the gait cycle and the swing phase contributes about 40%.
- *Phases of gait cycle (eight-phase model):*

  Stance phase (60%)
  1. Initial contact
  2. Loading response
  3. Midstance
  4. Terminal stance
  5. Preswing

  Swing phase (40%)
  6. Initial swing
  7. Midswing
  8. Terminal swing

- Gait examination is very important in assessment of neurological and musculoskeletal disorders. It reveals involvement of various parts of the nervous system such as cerebral cortex, extrapyramidal system, cerebellum, and lower motor neuron (LMN) lesions such as Guillain–Barré syndrome (GBS), myopathies, muscular dystrophy, and neuropathy. It also helps for analysis of various musculoskeletal disorders.
- It is important to observe the child walking and sometimes running for a distance of a few feet. Also, watch how he is getting up from floor and climbing the stairs.
- Thorough clinical observations of gait, careful history taking focused on gait, and physical, neurological, and orthopedic examinations are basic steps in categorization of gait disorders and serve as a guide for necessary investigations and therapeutic interventions.
- *Abnormality in gait may be caused by:*
  - Pain
  - Joint and muscle range of motion limitation
  - Muscular weakness/paralysis
  - Neurological involvement [upper motor neuron (UMN), LMN]
  - Leg length discrepancy
- *Antalgic gait (limping gait):*
  - Limping gait is due to painful limb. Limp is adopted to avoid pain on weight bearing structures.
  - Stance phase is shortened.
  - Common causes: Fractures, tendinitis, and arthritis
- *Ataxic gait (reeling gait) (tandem gait):*
  - Most common manifestation of cerebellar damage
  - Often the first clinical sign of cerebellar disease
  - Wide base
  - Cannot follow walking path in a straight line, but instead veers in different directions, giving the appearance of stumbling or drunkenness
  - Falls to the side of lesion
  - Frequent falling
  - Sometimes, a high steppage gait pattern is also seen.
- *Hemiplegic gait (circumduction gait):*
  - With spastic type of hemiplegic leg:
    - Hip into extension, adduction, and medial rotation
    - Knee in extension and unstable
    - Ankle in a drop foot with ankle plantar flexion and inversion (in both stance and swing phases)
  - In order to clear the foot from the ground, the hip and knee should flex.
  - But the spastic muscles would not allow the hip and knee to flex for the floor clearance.
  - So the patient hikes hip and brings the affected leg by making a half circle,

circumducting the leg. Hence, the gait is known as "circumductory gait".
- No reciprocal arm swing
- Step length tends to be lengthened on the affected side and shortened on the normal side.

- *Scissoring gait:*
  - Results from spasticity of bilateral adductor muscles of hip
  - One leg crosses directly over the other with each step like crossing the blades of the scissor.
  - Commonly seen in children with cerebral palsy of spastic diplegia type, arthrogryposis, etc. Scissoring gait is commonly seen in preterm babies with cerebral palsy.

- *High stepping gait (stamping gait):*
  - It is seen in patients with foot drop and weakness of foot dorsiflexion.
  - There is an attempt to lift the leg high enough during walking so that foot does not drag on the floor.
  - On bringing the foot to the ground, toes touch first and then heel. It results in high stepping gait. Due to sudden sound, it is also called as stamping gait.
  - It is due to paralysis of the common peroneal nerve.
  - It is seen in peripheral neuropathies, lesions of cauda equine, etc.

- *Trendelenburg gait:*
  - It results due to weakness of gluteus medius muscle. It is called "Trendelenburg gait" or "lurching gait" when one side is affected.
  - The person shifts the trunk over the affected side during stance phase.
  - When right gluteus medius or hip abductor is weak, it causes two things:
    - The body leans over the left leg during stance phase of the left leg.
    - Right side of the pelvis will drop when the right leg leaves the ground and begins swing phase.
  - Shifting the trunk over the affected side is an attempt to reduce the amount of strength required of the gluteus medius to stabilize the pelvis.
  - Causes:
    - Weak abductors [poliomyelitis, Duchenne muscular dystrophy (DMD)]
    - Congenital dislocation of hip joint
    - Perthes disease.

- *Waddling gait (duck gait):*
  - Bilateral paralysis of gluteus medius muscle causes waddling or duck gait.
  - The patient lurches to both sides while walking.
  - The body sways from side to side on a wide base with excessive shoulder swing.
  - It is seen in muscular dystrophies such as DMD and spinomuscular atrophy (SMA).

- *Short limb gait:*
  - Shortening <1.5 cm compensated by pelvic tilt and shortening up to 5cm compensated by equines
  - Shortening >5 cm, the patient dips his body on that side

- *Toe walking (equinus gait):*
  - May be normal in children up to age of 2 years
  - It is seen in children with spastic cerebral palsy and DMD.

- *Festinate gait (short shuffling gait)— (Parkinson's gait):*
  - Seen in Parkinson's disease
  - Because of rigidity, all the joints will go for a flexion position with spine stooping forward.
  - This posture displaces the center of gravity anteriorly.

- So in order to keep center of gravity within limits, the patient will walk with small, shuffling steps.
- Due to loss of voluntary control over the movement, the patient loses balance and walks faster as if he is chasing the center of gravity. Therefore, it is called "festinate gait". It is also called "shuffling gait" due to his shuffling steps.

44 Growth Charts

INTRODUCTION

We, pediatricians, care for growing children as against physicians who look after adult patients who have completed their growth. So, it is mandatory that a pediatrician measures weight, length/height, and head circumference periodically in every child under his care and plots the readings on a standard growth chart, interprets the findings, and derives the conclusion. We should communicate to the parents regarding growth of the child and necessary actions should be suggested, if indicated. Growth charts provide several vital information, besides merely physical growth.

ANTHROPOMETRY

Accurate measurement of weight, length (by an infantometer, up to the age of 2 years; **Fig. 1**), or height (by a stadiometer beyond the age of 2 years; **Figs. 2A and B**) and head circumference is an important first step for proper evaluation of growth of the child by using growth charts.

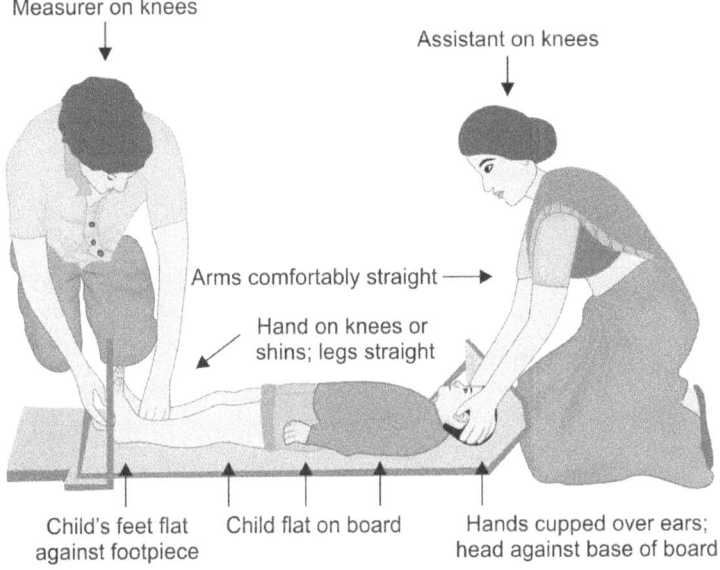

Fig. 1: Measurement of length by an infantometer in children less than 2 years.

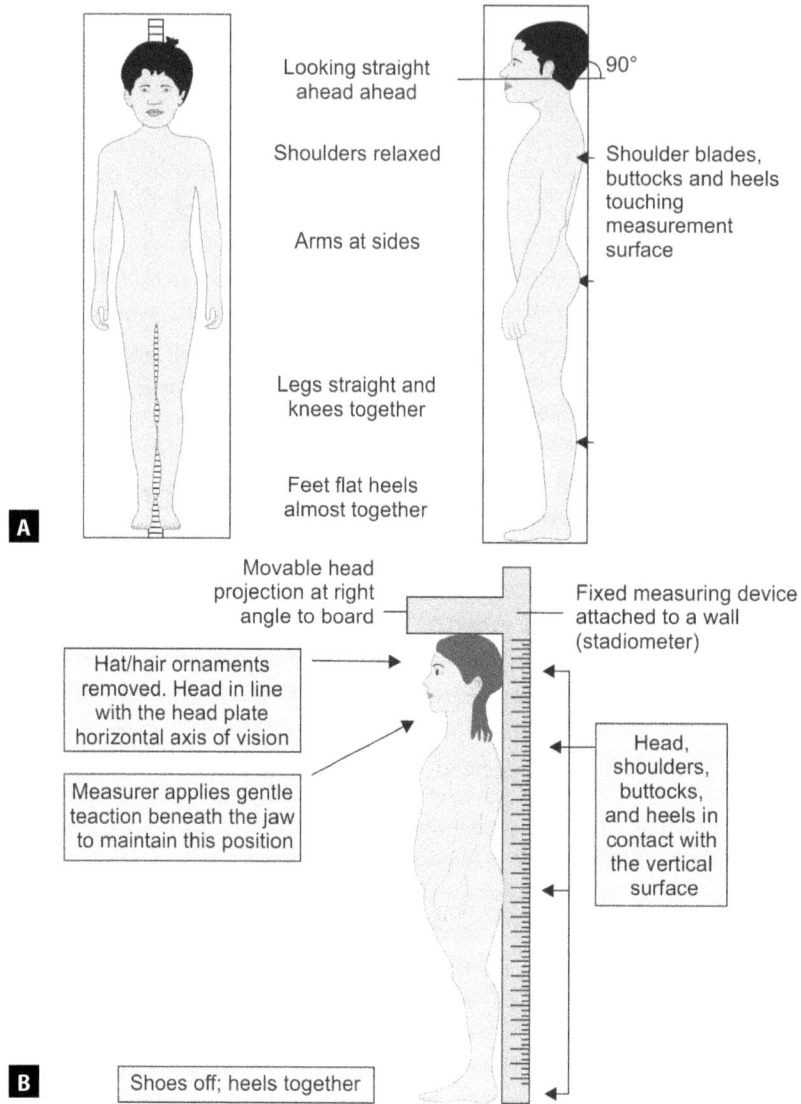

Figs. 2A and B: Measurement of height by a stadiometer beyond the age of 2 years.

AVAILABLE GROWTH CHARTS

- *WHO growth charts (standard growth charts):* These are prescriptive and define how the population should grow given optimal nutrition and optimal health.
- *Reference growth charts (Agarwal and Khadilkar growth charts):* These are descriptive and prepared from a population, thought to be growing under the best circumstances.

  These growth charts represent how children are growing and not how they should grow.
- *Disease-specific growth charts:* Disease-specific (special) growth charts are designed for certain conditions like achondroplasia, Turner syndrome, Down syndrome, etc.

STEPS FOR PLOTTING ON A GROWTH CHART

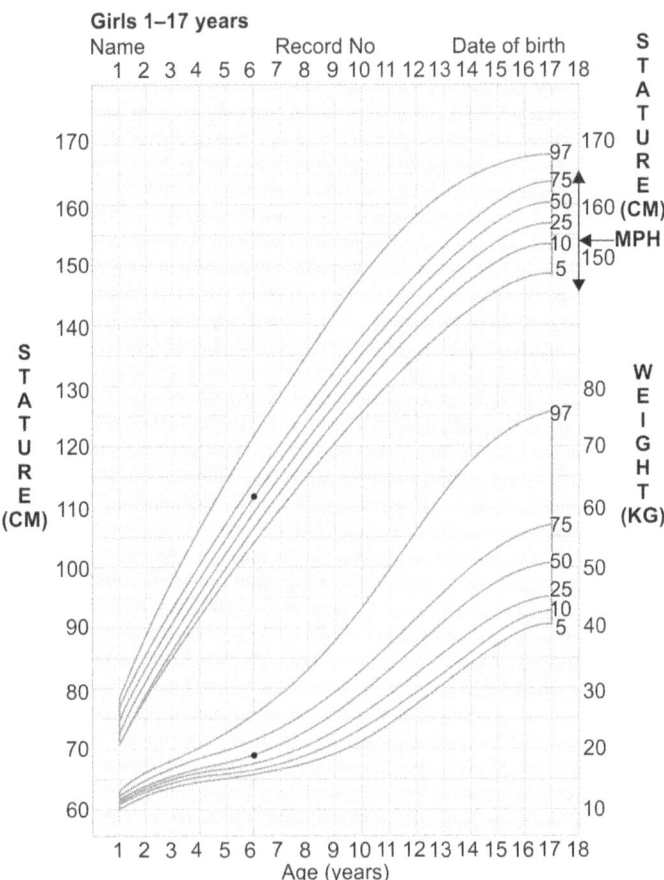

Adapted from 1. Agarwal DK et al. Physical and sexual growth pattern of affluent Indian children from 5–18 years of age. Indian Pediatrics.1992;29:1203.
2. Agarwal DK, Agarwal KN. Physical growth in affluent Indian children birth to 6 years. Indian Pediatrics. 1994;31:377. Dept of endocrinologist Lucknow.

Step 1
Measure height and weight accurately

Step 2
Select an appropriate growth chart, **pink for girl and blue** for boys
Plot height and weight on the growth chart
Make a small dot on the chart do not circle it for example 6-years-old girl height 112 cm, weight 18 kg

Step 3
Height and weight percentile
Height percentile-50th
Weight percentile-50th

Step 4
Calculate **midparental height**

Boys MPH = $\frac{FH+MH+13}{2}$

Girls MPH = $\frac{FH+MH-13}{2}$

In this case,
Father 170 cm
Mother 150 cm

MPH = $\frac{170+150-13}{2}$ = 153.5 cm

Plot at 18 year

Step 5
Calculate **target height** (6.5 cm on either side of mid parental height)
Target range–147.5–159.5 cm

Growth Charts

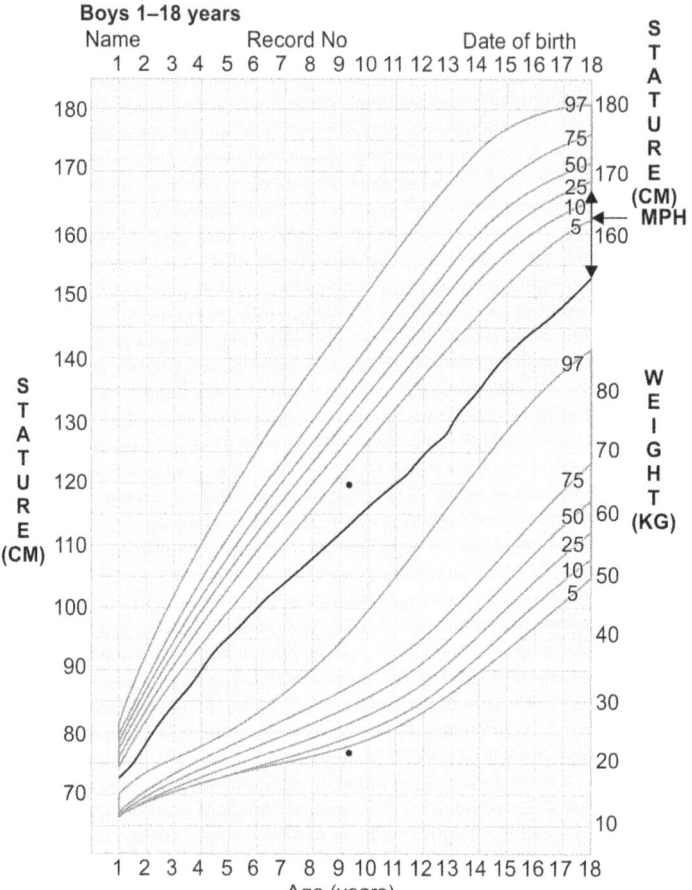

Adapted from 1. Agarwal DK et al. Physical and sexual growth pattern of affluent Indian children from 5–18 years of age. Indian Pediatrics.1992;29:1203.
2. Agarwal DK, Agarwal KN. Physical growth in affluent Indian children birth to 6 years. Indian Pediatrics. 1994;31:377. Dept of endocrinologist Lucknow.

Step 6
Construct 3rd **percentile** for the family. For example 9 years 3 months old boy.
Height 118 cm, Weight 18 kg
MPH 160 cm, target range (154–166 cm)
Height <15th percentile
Weight <15th percentile
Draw an imaginary line upto the lower point of TH–this constitutes the third percentile
Interpretation
Child is growing in target range, what next?

Step 7
Monitor **growth velocity**

$$GV = \frac{\text{Change in height}}{\text{Change in time in years}}$$

After 6 months, child is 121 cm
GV = 121–118/0.5 = 6 cm/year = normal GV

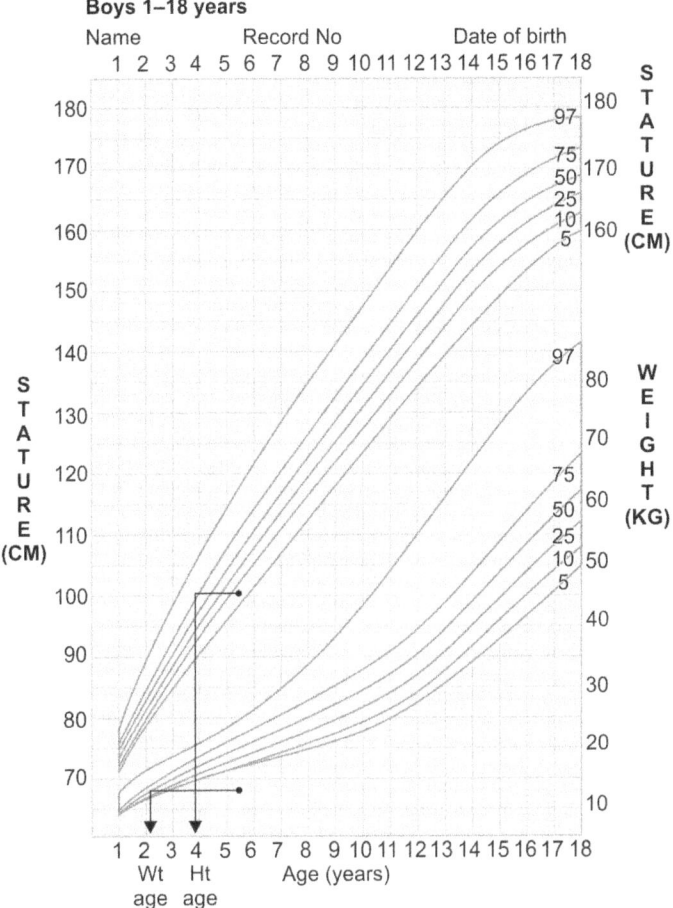

Adapted from 1. Agarwal DK et al. Physical and sexual growth pattern of affluent Indian children from 5–18 years of age. Indian Pediatrics.1992;29:1203.
2. Agarwal DK, Agarwal KN. Physical growth in affluent Indian children birth to 6 years. Indian Pediatrics. 1994;31:377. Dept of endocrinologist Lucknow.

Step 8
Calculate **height age** and weight age 5.5 years old boy, height 99 cm, weight 12 kg
Draw a horizontal line from the dot to the 50th percentile and then droop a line vertically down
Note the age which corresponds to this height age 4 years weight age 2.5 years

Equation
CA > HA > WA
CA chronological age (actual age)
HA height age
WA weight age

Growth Charts

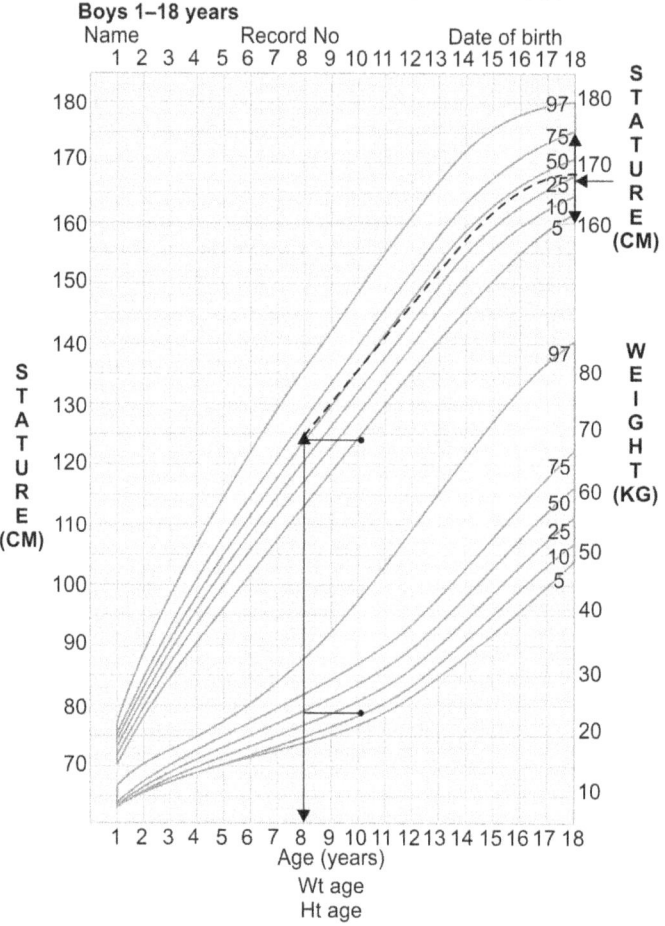

Interpretation
Child is thin and short
Weight more affected than height
Chronic illness or malnutrition (Ix accordingly)

Boys 1–18 years

Adapted from 1. Agarwal DK et al. Physical and sexual growth pattern of affluent Indian children from 5–18 years of age. Indian Pediatrics.1992;29:1203.
2. Agarwal DK, Agarwal KN. Physical growth in affluent Indian children birth to 6 years. Indian Pediatrics. 1994;31:377. Dept of endocrinologist Lucknow.

10-year-old boy height 123 cm, weight 23 kg
MPH 168 cm (162–174 cm)
Height age 8 years
Weight age 8 years
Equation
HA = WA < CA

Step 9
Bone age should be done BA 8 years

Equation
HA = WA = BA < CA
Projected from BA, the child will grow in his target range

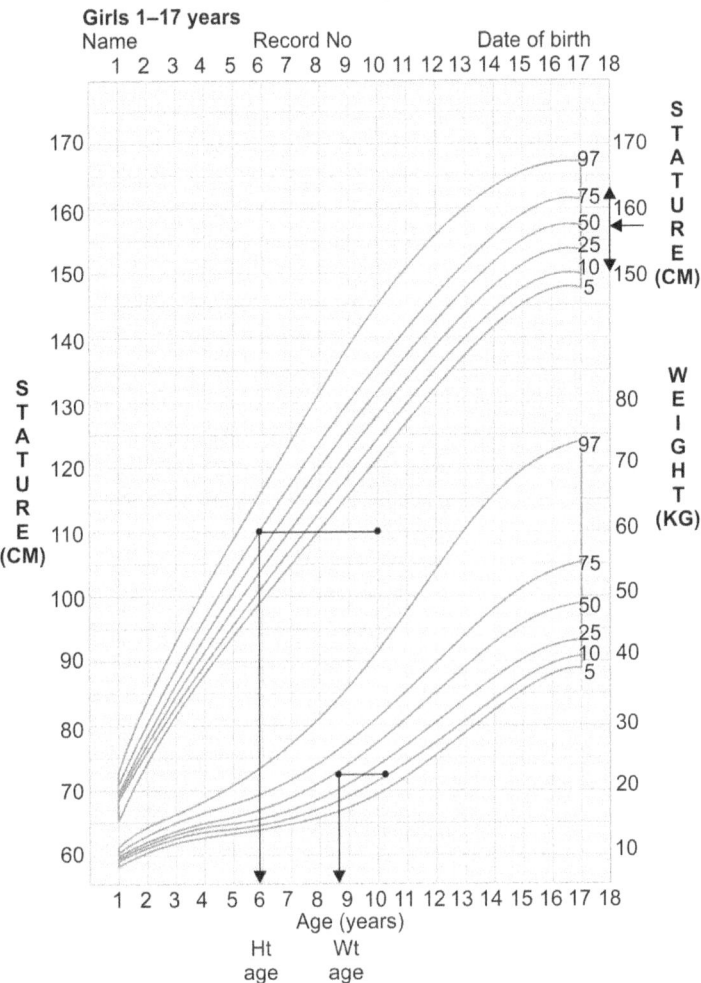

Interpretation
Constitutional delay of growth

Adapted from 1. Agarwal DK et al. Physical and sexual growth pattern of affluent Indian children from 5–18 years of age. Indian Pediatrics.1992;29:1203.
2. Agarwal DK, Agarwal KN. Physical growth in affluent Indian children birth to 6 years. Indian Pediatrics. 1994;31:377. Dept of endocrinologist Lucknow.

10-year-old female
Height 110 cm, weight 22 kg
MPH 157 cm (151–1163 cm)
Height age 5.75 years
Weight age 8.5 years
Chronological age 10 years
Equation
HA < WA < CA
Bone age 5.5 years
BA = HA < WA < CA

Growth Charts

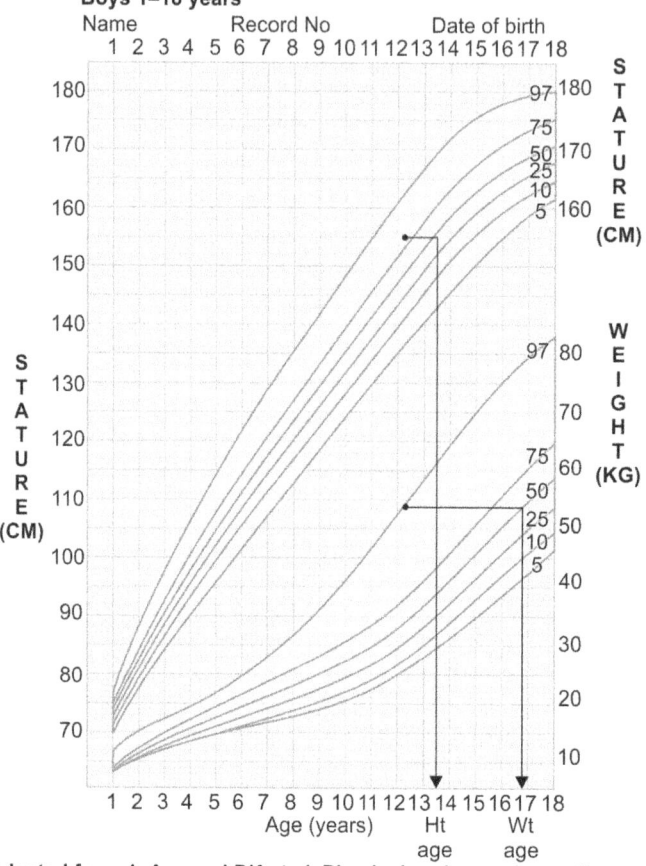

Interpretation
Height is more affected than weight
Endocrine cause is likely (Ix accordingly)
Boys 1–18 years

Adapted from 1. Agarwal DK et al. Physical and sexual growth pattern of affluent Indian children from 5–18 years of age. Indian Pediatrics.1992;29:1203.
2. Agarwal DK, Agarwal KN. Physical growth in affluent Indian children birth to 6 years. Indian Pediatrics. 1994;31:377. Dept of endocrinologist Lucknow.

12 years 3 months old boy
Weight 55 Kg (97th percentile)
Height 155 cm (75th–97th percentile)
Height age 13.5 years
Weight age 16.75 years

Equation
WA > HA > CA
Child is tall and overweight
Weight > hight

Step 10
Calculate BMI

$$BMI = \frac{\text{Weight in kg} = 22.9}{(\text{Height in mt})^2}$$

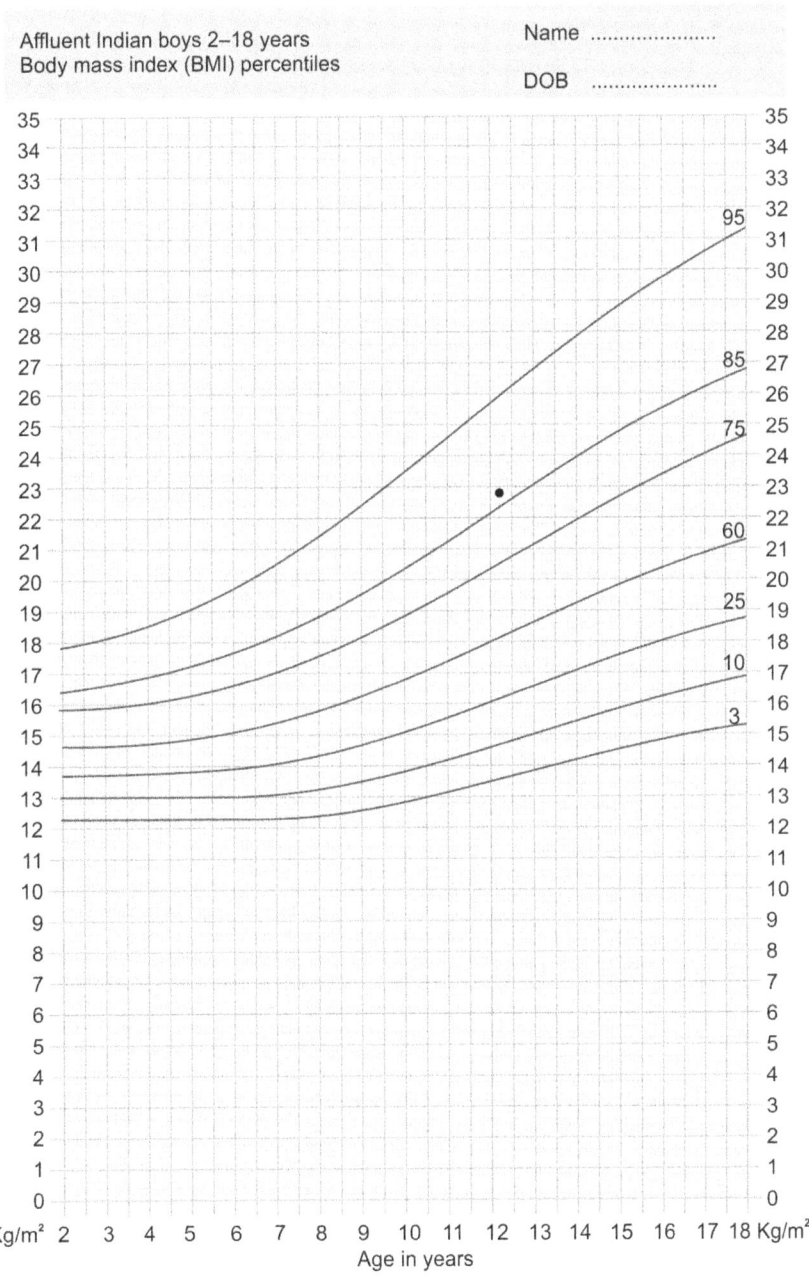

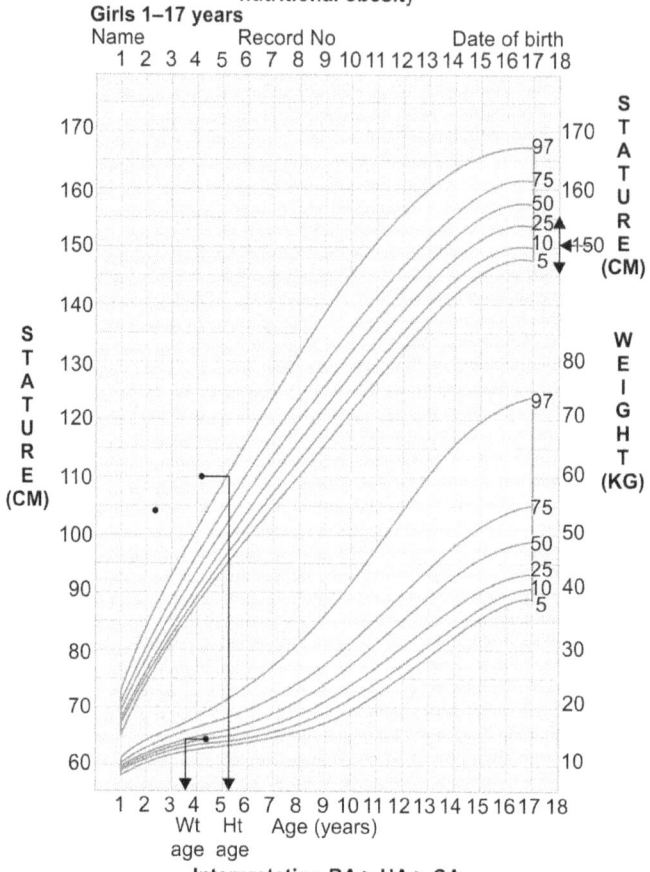

Interpretation
Weight > height, BMI – overweight
nutritional obesity

Adapted from 1. Agarwal DK et al. Physical and sexual growth pattern of affluent Indian children from 5–18 years of age. Indian Pediatrics.1992;29:1203.
2. Agarwal DK, Agarwal KN. Physical growth in affluent Indian children birth to 6 years. Indian Pediatrics. 1994;31:377. Dept of endocrinologist Lucknow.

4.5-year-old female
Height 110 cm (75th–97th percentile)
Weight 15 kg (10th–25th percentile)
MPH 150 cm (10th percentile)
Height age 5.5 years
Weight age 3.75 years

Equation
HA > CA > WA
Tall for family

Step 11
Pubertal status B3A1P1 bone age 6.5 years
Equation BA > HA > CA > WA

INTERPRETATION OF GROWTH CHARTS AND THEIR CLINICAL APPLICATION

- *How to define time of onset of disease and duration of disease?*
  - Quite often, illness starts with subtle symptoms that may be present for few weeks or months prior to the onset of major complaints. Parents may often miss these and therefore seek medical advice only when the child is obviously symptomatic. However, the growth chart may pick up this as an asymptomatic but unwell phase. Thereby, it also reveals the exact duration of illness, even if the symptoms seem to be relatively of recent origin.
- *How to define persistent or recurrent, progressive or nonprogressive disease?*
  - Recurrent viral infections or hyperactive airway diseases are very common in our daily practice. The treating physician and parents are concerned for missing some underlying disease. Demonstrating a normal growth pattern would rule out underlying serious disease and help in reassuring the parents. It would also avoid unnecessary laboratory and radiological investigations.
  - Growth faltering indicates some continuous chronic (progressive) disease.
- *Abnormal growth patterns and suggesting conditions:*
  - Significant faltering of weight by >2 SD (standard deviation) in a short time is referred to failure to thrive (FTT). The height is not affected. It suggests acute deterioration of health. FTT indicates serious rapidly progressive disease such as inborn errors of metabolism (IEM), immune deficiency, cystic fibrosis, and multidrug-resistant (MDR) tuberculosis.
  - Faltering of both weight and length/height, but weight faltering is more than that of length/height which suggests long-standing malnutrition (chronic malnutrition). It may be due to deficient intake of food or secondary to an underlying pathology like malabsorption, chronic infection, or chronic organ dysfunction.
  - When there is faltering of height, but not weight (weight for height may be good), it is referred to as stunting without wasting. It is called short stature, likely due to a hormonal problem such as growth hormone deficiency or hypothyroidism, skeletal dysplasia like achondroplasia, chromosomal abnormalities, or growth pattern like familial short stature or constitutional delay of growth and puberty.
  - Regular growth charting can pick up upward deviation of weight and that may suggest obesity. In this situation, timely intervention would be rewarding. Once obesity has set in, it is very difficult to revert the process. If both weight and height have gone up equally, it means that the child is tall and obese. It is always due to exogenous factors like unhealthy diet and poor exercise.
- *Charting the growth of a child from day 1 is mandatory:*
  - If the growth of the child gets affected later on, past records are very useful to the study pattern of growth, on set of deceleration of growth, etc.
  - Serial measurements of head circumference and plotting them on growth chart may be helpful to suspect

microcephaly, hydrocephalus, and other abnormalities of brain growth like megalencephaly. Regular follow-up of head circumference in the first 2 years of life is very essential.

- *Catch-up growth in preterm and intrauterine growth restriction (IUGR) babies:* Growth parameters follow different velocities in infants born after full term, preterm and IUGR babies. Preterm infants start catching up growth parameters in the first year, IUGR infants catch up much slower and may not catch up weight to normal, especially symmetrical IUGR babies. Head circumference catches up normal first, followed by length, and weight is the last to catch up to normal. This is achieved by 2 years of age in most.

45 Gynecomastia

INTRODUCTION

The proliferation of mammary glandular tissues in the male is called gynecomastia. It should be differentiated from pseudogynecomastia, which is the result of accumulation of adipose tissues in the area of breast. It is also called adipomastia or lipomastia. Pseudogynecomastia is commonly seen in overweight (obese) males. True gynecomastia is characterized by the presence of a palpable fibroglandular mass 0.5-1 cm in diameter that is located concentrically beneath the nipple and areolar region. Glandular tissue feels firm or grainy, while adipose tissue feels soft.

Gynecomastia is caused by an altered balance between estrogens and androgens. It may be in form of increased estrogens, decreased androgens, or increased sensitivity of breast tissue to estrogens.

PHYSIOLOGIC GYNECOMASTIA

Physiologic gynecomastia occurs during three phases of life: 1. Neonatal; 2. Pubertal; and 3. Elderly (>60 years of age).

Neonatal Gynecomastia

- Transient gynecomastia occurs in 60-90% of male newborns secondary to exposure to estrogens during pregnancy.
- Breast development may be asymmetrical and galactorrhea (secretion of milk from breast) is seen in approximately 5%.
- Most cases resolve within 4-8 weeks of birth, but a few can last as long as 12 months.
- It should not be massaged or squeezed as it may lead to mastitis or breast abscess formation.

Puberty Gynecomastia

- During early puberty to midpuberty, up to 70% of males develop various degrees of subareolar hyperplasia of the breasts.
- Incidence peak at 14 years of age, at Tanner stage of 3-4 with testicular volume of 5-10 mL.
- Physiologic pubertal gynecomastia may involve only one breast. It may cause enlargement of both breasts at disproportionate rates or at different tissues.
- Tenderness of the breast is common, but transitory.
- Spontaneous regression is common within a few months, rarely persists beyond 2 years.
- Significant psychological distress may occur, especially in obese males with relatively large breasts.

Elderly

The third age range in which physiological gynecomastia is frequently seen is during older age (>60 years).

Like the gynecomastia of obesity, the gynecomastia of aging may partly result from increased aromatase activity, causing increased conversion of androgens to estrogens.

■ PATHOLOGIC GYNECOMASTIA

Pathologic gynecomastia is due to an increase in the circulating and/or local breast tissue ratio of estrogen to androgen.

- Gynecomastia of prepubertal onset, associated with systemic disorders or hypogonadism, discharge, hard fixed tissue or increasing in size should be considered as pathologic.
- The underlying cause must be confirmed by necessary investigations and treated appropriately.
- Breast cancer in male is known, but extremely rare.
- Weight loss may be needed.
- Emotional distress should be addressed.
- Medical therapy may be offered, if regression does not occur. Surgery is definitive.

■ PATHOLOGICAL CAUSES OF GYNECOMASTIA

- *Exogenous sources of estrogens:*
  - Very small amount of estrogens can cause gynecomastia.
  - Accidental exposure may occur by inhalation, percutaneous absorption, or ingestion.
  - Common sources of estrogen include oral contraceptive pills and oral or transdermal estrogen preparations.
- Herbal preparations, food supplements, estrogen-containing creams (for cosmetic purpose), etc., are known sources of estrogens.
- Alcohol, heroin, anabolic steroids for body building, amphetamines, marijuana, etc., have been linked with gynecomastia.

Common Pathological Causes of Gynecomastia

- *Estrogen-secreting tumors:*
  - Leydig cell tumor
  - Sertoli cell tumor
  - Adrenocortical tumor
- *Androgen deficiency:*
  - Primary hypogonadism:
    - Klinefelter syndrome
    - Testicular injury (mumps, trauma, and radiation)
    - Drugs like methotrexate and vincristine
  - Secondary hypogonadism:
    - Hypothalamic-pituitary disease/surgery/radiation, e.g., craniopharyngioma
    - Abnormal testosterone synthesis due to drugs such as ketoconazole, spironolactone, metronidazole, and cimetidine
    - Abnormal testosterone action due to androgen insensitivity syndromes
    - Hyperthyroidism
    - Chronic liver diseases
    - Drugs.

Halitosis

CHAPTER 46

INTRODUCTION

The term "halitosis" means an offensive odor of the breath, also called malodorous breath. It is a very common complaint by parents in pediatric outdoor patients.

POINTS ON HISTORY TAKING

- Acute or chronic
- Eating habits (chocolates, garlic, onion, etc.)
- Care of orodental hygiene
- History of sore throat, rhinorrhea, sneezing, sinusitis, foreign body in nose, etc.
- History of dyspepsia and ulcers in the month over tongue or gums
- Family history of halitosis.

POINTS ON PHYSICAL EXAMINATION

- Look for orodental condition.
- Check for chronic sinusitis, postnasal drip, chronic tonsillitis, diphtheria, etc. Halitosis with chronic suppurative lung disease, lung abscess, and bronchiectasis should be kept in mind and focus examination is important.

Poor Orodental Hygiene

- Very common
- Look for dental abscess, dental caries (which may entrap the food debris), gingivitis, stomatitis, etc.
- Failure of habit of brushing teeth and washing mouth after having meals, chocolates, and icecream is an important cause for poor orodental hygiene.

Chronic Rhinitis

- Atrophic and allergic chronic rhinitis may be responsible for halitosis.
- Fetor is often a remarkable feature of atrophic rhinitis. It is often taken cognizance by the relatives or the examiner.
- The patient may be unaware of it because of anosmia.
- Dryness and obstruction of nose with formation of crusts in nasal cavities are other features.
- Nasal mucosa appears congested and atrophic.
- The nostrils may be widened.

Foreign Body in the Nose

- Halitosis along with unilateral blood-stained nasal discharge and manifestations of nasal obstruction highly suggest a foreign body in the nose.
- The common nasal foreign bodies are beads, nuts, crayon, plastic, button, cell, etc.
- Sneezing, local comfort, purulent, malodorous or blood discharge, and cellulitis in the surrounding areas are other features.
- The nasal foreign body is located anteriorly in the beginning, but later on it is forced

deeper way back in the nose due to repeated attempts by the child to remove it.

INFECTIONS

- *Vincent's angina:*
  - Common in chronically ill and malnourished children
  - Caused by usual oral flora and heavy overgrowth of fusiform bacilli and spirochetes
  - Severe fetid odor, fever, malaise, and oral lesions consisting of gray necrotic membrane and tiny ulcers over tender, congested gingivae are characteristic features.
- Chronic tonsillitis
- Diphtheria
- Infectious mononucleosis.

BRONCHIECTASIS

- Halitosis is a prominent feature of bronchiectasis.
- Persistent or recurrent cough, productive of copious, mucopurulent sputum which is foul smelling; changes in cough and expectoration with postural variations are the characteristic of bronchiectasis. Cyanosis, clubbing, and hemoptysis are other features.

LUNG ABSCESS

- Halitosis and foul-smelling sputum are common features of lung abscess.
- Fever, persistent cough, hemoptysis, chest pain, and clubbing are common features of lung abscess.

OTHER CAUSES OF HALITOSIS

- Onion, garlic, and spicy foods
- Dyspepsia
- Mouth breathing
- Cirrhosis of liver
- Certain poisoning like lead, mercury, iodine.

Headache

INTRODUCTION

Headache is one of the most common symptoms in pediatric office practice. Absence of a methodological approach along with cursory history and clinical examination in the practice may result in a serious outcome. If it is not evaluated carefully, serious conditions like raised intracranial pressure and space-occupying lesions (SOLs) may be missed. At the same time, asking for computed tomography (CT) scan of brain liberally without proper clinical evaluation is also not justified. Therefore, detailed history and thorough clinical examinations are the key to rational management of headache. Investigations are required in very few patients with headache to confirm the diagnosis and further management.

LOOK FOR RED FLAGS

- Look for conditions requiring immediate attention and management and they are:
  - Early morning headache (may be relieved following vomiting) and gradually developing as progressive headache suggests raised intracranial pressure due to hydrocephalus, space-occupying lesions, etc.
  - Hyperacute headache and fast neurological deterioration indicate intracranial hemorrhage.
  - Fever, headache, vomiting, and signs of meningeal irritation suggest central nervous system (CNS) infections like acute bacterial meningitis (ABM), tuberculous meningitis (TBM), encephalitis, etc.
- Associated systemic features like fever and myalgia may be due to dengue fever and leptospirosis. Fever, headache, marked pallor, and enlarged spleen may be due to falciparum malaria.
- Headache may arise from pain-sensitive structures
  - Brain and ependyma are pain insensitive.
  - Vascular sinuses, large vessels, and dura are intracranial pain-sensitive structures.
  - Following development of intracranial pathology, there is inflammation, displacement of structures, injury or traction to the pain-sensitive structures, leading to headache or facial pain.
  - Extracranial pain-sensitive structures are skin, subcutaneous tissues, and teeth.
- Most of the pain signals of head and face area are mediated through the trigeminal nerve and upper cervical nerves.
- Headache in infancy may present as irritability or head banging.
- Headache that disrupts sleep should be thoroughly investigated.
- Any headache which interferes with the activity and performance in school must be assessed properly.

TYPES OF HEADACHE

- *Acute:*
  - Viral infections [upper respiratory tract infection (URTI), influenza-like illness]
  - Malaria
  - Leptospirosis
  - Dengue fever
  - Meningitis
  - Intracranial hemorrhage
  - Localized infections like sinusitis, dental origin, temporomandibular joint pain etc.
- *Acute recurrent:* Migraine, tension headache
- *Chronic progressive:* Raised intracranial pressure (ICP), SOL, hydrocephalus, TBM, brain abscess, etc.
- *Chronic nonprogressive:* Chronic migraine, hypertension, etc.

COMMON CAUSES OF HEADACHE

- Viral infections: Dengue fever, chikungunya etc.
- Malaria
- Cluster headache
- Tension headache
- Headache during fever (vasodilatation due to fever)
- CNS infections:
  - ABM
  - TBM
  - Encephalitis [herpes simplex virus (HSV), Japanese encephalitis (JE), post chickenpox, etc.]
- SOLs
- Sinusitis
- Acute otitis media
- Tooth infection
- Trauma
- Postlumbar puncture
- Refractive error

IMPORTANT HISTORY-TAKING POINTS FOR HEADACHE

- *Onset:*
  - Hyperacute: Intracranial hemorrhage
  - Acute and recurrent: Migraine, cluster headache
  - Chronic: Tension headache, psychogenic
  - Early morning and progressive: Raised ICP
- *Location:*
  - Generalized: CNS infections, raised ICP, hypertension
  - Localized: Frontal headache in sinusitis and refractive errors, temporal headache in migraine, occipital headache in hypertension, headache around orbit in cluster headache.
- *Duration and frequency:*
  - Episodic headache in migraine and cluster headache
  - Chronic and daily in tension headache
  - Slowly progressive in raised ICP.
- *Character:*
  - Pulsative and throbbing headache in migraine
  - Dull and boring in tension headache
  - Thunder scalp headache, worst, intolerable headache in subarachnoid hemorrhage
  - Unilateral headache in classical migraine
- *Precipitating and aggravating factors:*
  - Episodes of migraine are precipitated by stress, sleep deprivation, hunger, certain foods containing coca, bright-light, loud noise, etc.
  - Headache due to raised ICP is aggravated by coughing and straining and decreases by an episode of vomiting
- *Functional impairment:*
  - A patient of migraine likes to take rest in dark room without noise.

- In case of tension headache, the patient continues to work and it does not disturb the sleep.
- *Associated factors:*
  - Nausea, vomiting, photophobia, and visual aura are common with migraine headache
  - Fever, headache, and vomiting may be due to CNS infections
  - Projectile vomiting, altered sensorium, and bradycardia are common with raised ICP
  - Nasal discharge, nasal blocks, and URTI indicate sinusitis.
- Refractive error is a rare cause of headache.
- Family history is common in migraine.
- Bradycardia and hypertension are seen in raised ICP.

Hearing Loss

INTRODUCTION

Hearing loss and deafness is a major problem for various health, educational, and social reasons. Unfortunately, recognition of deafness or hearing loss often occurs late, compounding the difficulties for child and family. Having realization of the gravity of this problem and its consequences, the importance of universal newborn screening is understood. Some centers have started universal newborn screening for hearing and others perform in high-risk babies with history of prematurity, birth asphyxia, neonatal hyperbilirubinemia, central nervous system (CNS) infections, metabolic disorders, etc. All patients with suspected hearing loss require appropriate testing to decide the nature (conductive, sensorineural, and mixed) and extent of the loss. Early treatment is essential, as is early habitation for those whom the hearing loss is not reversible.

CONGENITAL HEARING LOSS

About one-third to one-half of congenital hearing loss is genetic, of which 15–30% may be syndromic. Universal newborn screening programs allow diagnosis and thereby habilitation of deaf children at a much younger age, dramatically increasing the likelihood of their developing meaningful communication skills.

Causes of Congenital Hearing Loss

- *Congenital infections:*
  - Congenital rubella [cataract, sensorineural deafness, and patent ductus arteriosus (PDA)]
  - Cytomegalo viral infection
  - Toxoplasmosis
  - Congenital syphilis
- Bacterial meningitis
- Prematurity
- *Metabolic causes:*
  - Hypoglycemia
  - Hyperbilirubinemia (kernicterus)
  - Hypercholesterolemia
  - Mucopolysaccharidosis
- *Ototoxic medications:*
  - Aminoglycosides (gentamicin, amikacin, streptomycin)
  - Quinine
- *Temporal bone anomaly:*
  - Middle ear anomaly
  - Dilated vestibular aqueduct
  - Peritympanic fistula
- Nonsyndromic hereditary congenital deafness
- *Syndromic hereditary congenital deafness:*
  - Alport syndrome (nephritis, hearing loss)
  - Apert syndrome (craniofacial dysostosis)
  - Crouzon syndrome
  - Waardenburg syndrome (white forlock, telecanthus, colored iris, confluent eyebrows)

- Pendred syndrome (euthyroid goiter)
- Oto-palato-digital syndrome (cleft palate, stubby-clubbed digits)
- Congenital aural atresia
- Treacher Collins syndrome
- Turner syndrome
- Klippel–Feil malformation
- Down syndrome, Edward syndrome, Patau syndrome
- LEOPARD syndrome.

CAUSES OF ACQUIRED HEARING LOSS

- *Conductive deafness:*
  - External auditory canal foreign body
  - Middle ear effusion
  - Tympanic membrane perforation
  - Cholesteatoma
  - Ossicular erosion or fixation
  - External auditory canal stenosis
  - Middle ear tumor
- *Sensorineural deafness:*
  - Bacterial meningitis
  - Mumps
  - Autoimmune diseases (vasculitis, scleroderma)
  - Acoustic trauma (noise induced)
  - Ototoxic drugs:
    - Aminoglycosides (gentamicin, amikacin, kanamycin, and streptomycin)
    - Diuretics like frusemide
    - Quinine
    - Chloroquine
    - Cytotoxic drugs
  - Temporal bone fracture
  - Peritympanic fistula
  - Cerebellopontine angle tumor
  - Vestibular schwannoma (associated with neurofibromatosis)
  - Meniere disease.

Hematuria

INTRODUCTION

Children presenting with hematuria is a frightening situation for the child, parents, and a clinician. Defining category of hematuria is necessary for proper evaluation and further workup.

HEMATURIA

Hematuria is defined as the presence of five or more red blood cells (RBCs) per high-power field in multiple centrifuged urine examinations.

Gross Hematuria

Child is brought with red-colored urine. Dipstick test is performed first. If dipstick test is positive, it indicates true hematuria or hemoglobinuria (usually caused by severe intravascular hemolysis) or myoglobinuria from rhabdomyolysis (due to muscle trauma or strenuous exercise). True hematuria is confirmed by microscopic demonstration of RBCs.

A negative dipstick test indicates red-colored urine due to other causes like pigments in foods, ingestion of beetroot and urates, porphyria or drugs like rifampicin, pyridium, nitrofurantoin, sulfasalazine, etc.

Microscopic Hematuria

More than 5 RBCs/cu.mm on microscopic examination of urine denotes hematuria.

Transient Hematuria

Fever, infections like pneumonia, enteric fever, exercise, and trauma are common causes for transient hematuria and they are benign and do not require any further investigations.

Persistent Hematuria

Persistent presence of RBCs in the urine with or without other cellular deposits and recurrent macroscopic hematuria are classified in the category of persistent hematuria which indicates renal disease.

Symptomatic Hematuria

Associated symptoms such as fever, burning, micturition, oliguria, edema, hypertension, etc., always indicate underlying disease and need detailed evaluation.

Asymptomatic Hematuria

It can be macroscopic or microscopic and may be the sole abnormality. History and physical examination may not provide any clue. Important causes include—hypercalciuria, nephrocalcinosis, immunoglobulin A (IgA) nephropathy, hydronephrosis, coagulation disorders, sickle cell disease renal vein thrombosis, Wilms tumor, renal tuberculosis, collagen vascular disease, urolithiasis, arteriovenous malformations, etc. Ultrasonographic examination of abdomen will identify some of them, and other conditions may be revealed on specific investigations. Some patients require long-term follow-up to identify benign or slowly progressive diseases. A patient with an unidentified cause for persistent or recurrent microscopic hematuria may require renal biopsy.

Glomerular and Extraglomerular Hematuria

- Bright-red urine, visible clots, or crystals with normal appearance of RBCs suggest the site of bleeding from the urinary tract (extraglomerular).
- Cola-colored urine, presence of RBC casts, and dysmorphic RBCs suggest glomerular origin.
- For identification of dysmorphic (deformed) RBCs, phase-contrast microscopic examination is required. Presence of >20% dysmorphic RBCs suggests glomerular hematuria.
- Presence of proteinuria indicates glomerular origin hematuria.

COMMON CAUSES OF HEMATURIA

Glomerular

- Acute glomerulonephritis (GN) [(most common poststreptococcal glomerulonephritis (PSGN)]
- Membranous and membranoproliferative GN
- Focal segmental GN
- IgA nephropathy
- Rapidly progressive GN
- Hemolytic uremic syndrome (HUS)
- Alport syndrome
- Goodpastures syndrome.

Extraglomerular

- Urinary tract infection
- *Drugs:*
  - Nonsteroidal anti-inflammatory drugs (NSAIDs) like Nimesulide, Ibuprofen, and Mefenamic acid
  - Cyclophosphamide
- Urolithiasis
- Hypercalciuria
- Wilms tumor
- Renal vein thrombosis
- Urethral foreign body
- Cystic kidney disease
- Vascular malformations.

Systemic Disorders

- Henoch–Schonlein purpura (HSP)
- Systemic lupus erythematosus (SLE)
- Infective endocarditis
- Sickle cell disease (papillary necrosis)
- Coagulation disorders
- Disseminated intravascular coagulation (DIC)
- Anticoagulant therapy.

Hemoptysis

INTRODUCTION

- Hemoptysis is defined as the coughing-up of blood or blood-streaked sputum from the respiratory tract.
- It is a common symptom in adults, but it is rare in children.
- It is categorized as massive and non-massive depending upon the amount of blood loss. Blood loss of >200 mL/day is categorized as massive hemoptysis and is considered as life threatening.
- It is important to differentiate hemoptysis from hematemesis. The differentiation may not always be easy. The following points may help to differentiate hemoptysis from hematemesis.

	Hemoptysis	*Hematemesis*
Appearance of blood	Bright red and frothy	Coffee ground mixed with food
Preceding symptoms	• Cough • Tickling sensation in throat	Vomiting
Associated symptoms	• Cough • Expectoration • Fever • Known case of rheumatic heart disease (RHD) (mitral stenosis)	• Abdominal pain • Vomiting • Known case of portal hypertension
Following day/days	Rusty sputum	Melena: Tarry, black, sticky, and offensive stool
Reaction of blood	Alkaline	Acidic

TYPES OF HEMOPTYSIS

Hemoptysis can be of two types:
1. *True hemoptysis:* Hemorrhage from the lungs, bronchial tree, and trachea
2. *Pseudohemoptysis:* Bleeding from nose, mouth, pharynx, and larynx.

COMMON CAUSES OF HEMOPTYSIS

- *Pseudo-hemoptysis:*
  - Trauma in mouth, pharynx, and larynx
  - Pharyngitis
  - Mouth ulcers
  - Scurvy (spongy gums)
  - Malignancy of mouth, pharynx, and larynx (in adults).
- True hemoptysis:
  - *Respiratory causes:*
    - Pneumonia
    - Tuberculosis cavitary lesion
    - Bronchiectasis
    - Lung abscess
    - Cystic fibrosis

- Pulmonary embolism
- Foreign body aspiration
- Fungal lung infections.
- *Cardiovascular causes:*
  - Mitral stenosis
  - Left ventricular failure (pulmonary edema)
  - Pulmonary hypertension
  - Bacterial endocarditis (pulmonary embolism)
  - Arteriovenous (A-V) malformation.
- *Immunologic causes:*
  - Goodpasture syndrome
  - Wegener's granulomatosis
  - Polyarteritis nodosa.
- *Bleeding disorders:*
  - Immune thrombocytopenic purpura
  - Leukemia
  - Anticoagulant therapy
- *Miscellaneous causes:*
  - Following procedures like bronchoscopy, lung biopsy
  - Endotracheal intubation
  - Drugs (anticoagulants)
  - Functional and malingerer.

51 Hepatomegaly

CHAPTER

INTRODUCTION

Liver is the second largest organ in the body, the first being the skin. In infants, liver may be palpable 3 cm and in older children 2 cm below the right costal margin at midclavicular line. The conditions like chronic asthma and emphysema are known to give erroneous impression of hepatomegaly due to pushed down liver. Rickets can also give false impression of hepatomegaly due to visceroptosis. The span of liver is more reliable to assess the size of liver.

- *Important points on examination of liver:*
  - Size (span of liver at midclavicular line)
  - Shape (symmetric/asymmetric enlargement)
  - Consistency (soft, firm, hard)
  - Surface (smooth, nodular, irregular)
  - Edge (rounded, sharp)
  - Tender/nontender
  - Pulsatile/nonpulsatile
  - Rub
  - Bruit
- *Span of liver:* Span of liver is measured from upper border (decided by percussion) to lower border (decided by palpation) in centimeters at midclavicular line. Span of liver at different ages is as follows:

Age	Liver span in cm
At birth →	5.5–6 cm
2 months →	5 cm

Contd...

Contd...

Age	Liver span in cm
1 year →	6 cm
2 years →	6.5 cm
3 years →	7 cm
4 years →	7.5 cm
5 years →	8 cm
6–12 years →	9 cm
Adolescents and adults →	10–15 cm

- *Classification of hepatomegaly:*
  - Mild: <4 cm
  - Moderate: 4–7 cm
  - Massive: >7 cm
- *Hepatobiliary microanatomy:* There are major four components of liver, namely hepatocytes, reticuloendothelial (RE) cells (Kupffer cells), biliary tract, and portal venous circulation. There are specific characteristics with involvement of each component, which gives an important clue to decide the cause of hepatomegaly.
  - Features of hepatocyte involvement:
    - Hepatomegaly (usually soft and tender)
    - May be sick looking child
    - Raised hepatic enzymes [serum glutamic-pyruvic transaminase (SGPT) and serum glutamic-oxaloacetic transaminase (SGOT)]
    - Jaundice
    - Ascites, edema (due to hypoalbuminemia)

- Bleeding manifestations [prolonged prothrombin time (PT) and activated partial thromboplastin time (aPTT)]
- Encephalopathy
- Features of RE cells (Kupffer cells) involvement:
  - Hepatomegaly (firm and nontender)
  - May be associated with splenomegaly and lymphadenopathy
  - No jaundice or ascites
  - Hepatic enzymes (SGPT, SGOT), PT, and albumin are not altered.
  - Common conditions of hepatomegaly with involvement of RE cells are malaria, enteric fever, tuberculosis, collagen disorders, etc.
- Features of involvement of biliary tract:
  - Marked jaundice
  - Itching is common (scratch marks may be present).
  - Clay-colored stools
  - Dark yellow urine
  - Serum alkaline phosphatase and gamma-glutamyl transferase (GGT) are significantly raised.
- Features suggesting disorder of portal venous circulation (portal hypertension):
  - Presinusoidal: Splenomegaly, may be history of hematemesis. No hepatomegaly, no ascites
  - Postsinusoidal: Enlarged liver and spleen, may be signs of hepatic failure, ascites, etc.
- Postsinusoidal: Hepatomegaly, ascites, and engorged neck veins in constrictive pericarditis

COMMON CAUSES OF HEPATOMEGALY

- *Hepatomegaly in neonates:*
  - Intrauterine infections:
    - Cytomegalovirus (CMV)
    - Rubella
    - Herpes simplex
    - Toxoplasmosis
    - Congenital syphilis
    - Malaria
    - Parvo virus
    - Varicella
  - Neonatal septicemia
  - Neonatal hepatitis
  - Extrahepatic biliary atresia
  - Erythroblastosis fetalis
  - Congestive cardiac failure
  - Galactosemia
  - Wolman disease
  - Alpha-1 antitrypsin deficiency
  - Inspissated bile syndrome
  - Hemangioma of liver
- *Hepatomegaly in infancy and childhood:* Hepatomegaly commonly occurs due to various mechanisms like inflammation, proliferation of cells, congestion, obstruction, infiltration, and excessive storage.
  - Inflammation:
    - Viral hepatitis [hepatotropic viruses like A, B, C, Epstein–Barr virus (EBV), and cytomegalovirus (CMV)]
    - Malaria
    - Tuberculosis
    - Enteric fever
    - Human immunodeficiency virus (HIV)
    - Kala-azar
    - Drugs like isoniazid (INH), rifampicin, pyrazinamide, valproate, and acetaminophen.
    - Autoimmune hepatitis
    - Collagen disorders like systemic lupus erythematosus (SLE)
    - Brucellosis liver abscess: Leptospirosis
  - Proliferation of cells:
    - Proliferation of hematopoietic cells in thalassemia, sickle cells like hemolytic anemia

- Tumors like hepatoblastoma and hepatoma
- Proliferation of Kupffer cells
- Hemangioma
- Histiocytosis
- Metabolic and storage disorders:
  - Galactosemia
  - Glycogen storage disorders
  - Gaucher disease
  - Niemann-Pick disease
  - Wolman disease
  - Mucopolysaccharidosis
  - Wilson disease
  - Hemochromatosis
- Vascular congestions:
  - Congestive heart failure
  - Budd–Chiari syndrome
  - Veno-occlusive disease
- Biliary obstruction:
  - Biliary atresia
  - Alagille syndrome
  - Cystic fibrosis
  - Inspissated bile syndrome
  - Primary sclerosing cholangitis
- Malignant disorders:
  - Lymphoma
  - Leukemia
  - Histiocytosis
  - Neuroblastoma
- Reye's syndrome.

CHAPTER 52

Hepatosplenomegaly

INTRODUCTION

Liver and spleen are organs of the reticuloendothelial (RE) system. Enlargement of both of them indicates a disorder involving RE system, which may be due to infection, metabolic, or malignant conditions. Hepatosplenomegaly associated with other symptoms, such as fever, lymphadenopathy, jaundice, and anemia, gives an important clue about its etiology.

HEPATOSPLENOMEGALY WITH PALLOR

Hemolytic anemia is the most common condition in children presenting with hepatosplenomegaly, rather splenohepatomegaly. Presentation in infancy, history of repeated blood transfusions, hemolytic facies, and family history of anemia are points suggesting congenital hemolytic anemia. Acquired hemolytic anemia like malaria and autoimmune hemolytic anemia presents as an acute condition with fever. Infectious, metabolic, malignancy, and collagen disorders are the other conditions presenting with hepatosplenomegaly and pallor.

- *Hematological disorders:*
  - Thalassemia
  - Sickle cell disease
  - Hereditary spherocytosis
  - Autoimmune hemolytic anemia
- *Infections:*
  - Malaria
  - Infective endocarditis
  - Enteric fever
  - Kala-azar
  - TORCH (toxoplasmosis, rubella, cytomegalovirus, and herpes simplex virus) infections in newborns.

HEPATOSPLENOMEGALY WITH JAUNDICE AND ANEMIA

- *Infections:*
  - Malaria
  - Kala-azar
- *Hematological:*
  - Spherocytosis
  - Sickle cell
  - Thalassemia
- Wilson disease.

HEPATOSPLENOMEGALY WITH FEVER

- *Infections:*
  - Malaria
  - Enteric fever
  - Bacterial endocarditis
  - Brucellosis
  - Infectious mononucleosis
  - Disseminated tuberculosis
  - Human immunodeficiency virus (HIV)
- *Malignancy:*
  - Leukemia
  - Lymphoma

- *Collagen disorders:*
  - Systemic lupus erythematosus (SLE)
  - Juvenile idiopathic arthritis
  - Juvenile dermatomyositis.

HEPATOSPLENOMEGALY WITH LYMPHADENOPATHY WITH OR WITHOUT FEVER

- *Infections:*
  - HIV
  - Epstein–Barr virus (EBV)
  - Disseminated tuberculosis
  - Brucellosis
  - Congenital infections in newborns
- *Collagen disorders:*
  - SLE
  - Juvenile rheumatoid arthritis (JRA)
- *Malignancy:*
  - Leukemia
  - Lymphoma
  - Histiocytosis
- Drug like phenytoin
- Hemophagocytic lymphohistiocytosis (HLH)
- DRESS (drug reaction with eosinophilia and systemic symptoms) syndrome.

HEPATOSPLENOMEGALY WITH ICTERUS

- *Infections:*
  - Hepatitis
  - Enteric fever
  - Malaria
  - EBV
  - Leptospirosis
  - TORCH infections
  - Neonatal hepatitis
  - Tuberculosis (antituberculous drugs, lymph node causing obstruction at sphincter of Oddi)
- *Hematological disorders:*
  - Spherocytosis
  - Autoimmune hemolytic anemia
  - Sickle cell disease
- *Malignancy:* Icterus may be due to obstruction by lymph node.
- *Metabolic diseases:*
  - Galactosemia
  - Tyrosinemia
  - Alpha-1 antitrypsin deficiency
  - Cirrhosis of liver (in later stages)
  - Drugs (antituberculous drugs, antiepileptic drugs).

HEPATOSPLENOMEGALY WITH BLEEDING MANIFESTATIONS

- *Infections:*
  - Dengue fever
  - Leptospirosis
  - Septicemia
  - Disseminated intravascular coagulation (DIC)
  - TORCH infections in newborns
- *Hematological diseases:*
  - Immune thrombocytopenia (ITP)
  - Hypersplenism
  - Malignancy (leukemia, lymphoma)
  - Metabolic disorders (Gaucher disease, Niemann–Pick disease)
- *Hepatosplenomegaly with ascites:*
  - Cirrhosis
  - Malignancy
  - Disseminated or abdominal tuberculosis
  - Congestive cardiac failure (CCF).

Hoarseness of Voice

INTRODUCTION

Hoarsness occuring at all ages, including neonatal period, is a frequent problem encountered in pediatric practice. Hoarsness is a sign of laryngeal disorder. The abnormal quality of the voice is usually the result of changes in the mass of the vocal cords, disorders that interfere with the approximatin of the edges of cords or some compressing effect from outside. Detailed history and physical examination reveal the cause in most cases.

VOICE MECHANISM

Speaking and singing involve a voice mechanism that is composed of three subsystems. Each subsystem is composed of different parts of the body and has specific roles in voice production.

Subsystems	Voice organs	Role in sound production
Air pressure system	Diaphragm, chest muscles, ribs, abdominal muscles, and lungs	Provides and regulates air pressure to cause vocal folds to vibrate
Vibratory system	Larynx, vocal cords	Vocal folds vibrate, changing air pressure to sound waves producing "voice sound" described as a "buzzy sound" varies with pitch of sound
Resonating system	Vocal tract, pharynx, oral cavity, and nasal cavities	Changes the "buzzy sound" into a person's recognizable voice

HOARSENESS OF VOICE

In hoarseness of voice, the voice is breathy, raspy or strained, softer in volume, or lower in pitch. The child may feel scratchy throat. Hoarseness is often a symptom of problems in the vocal cords of the larynx.

Clinical Evaluation

- Onset:
  - Acute onset in viral infections, foreign body, trauma, etc.
  - Gradual onset in conditions associated with weakness of laryngeal muscles like cretinism, myasthenia gravis, Werdnig-Hoffmann disease, etc.
- Duration:
  - Acute laryngitis is common in viral infections, diphtheria, trauma, instrumentation, etc.
  - Chronic hoarseness of voice may be due to laryngeal web, gastroesophageal reflux disease (GERD), cretinism, mucopolysaccharidosis, laryngeal polyp, cyst, hemangioma, etc.
- Hoarseness of voice following prolonged crying, shouting, or singing, may be due to exhaustion of vocal cords.

- History of trauma to larynx as a part of birth injury should be evaluated in a newborn. It is more common in forceps delivery.
- History of intubation or instrumentation should be confirmed.
- Hoarseness of voice in a floppy infant may be due to hypothyroidism, myasthenia gravis, Werdnig-Hoffmann disease, etc.
- Any history of foreign body should be asked for.
- An infant presenting with high-grade fever, sick looking, and hoarseness of voice should be looked for laryngeal diphtheria.

Laryngitis
- It is one of the most common causes of hoarseness
- Acute nondiphtheritic laryngitis (infectious group) is almost always viral in etiology.
- It is characterized by a peculiar brassy or croupy cough, usually accompanied by inspiratory stridor, hoarseness of voice, and varying degrees of respiratory distress.
- It can be in the form of acute laryngotracheobronchitis (ALTB), acute epiglottitis, acute spasmodic laryngitis, etc.
- Acute diphtheritic laryngitis is characterized by fever, toxic look, noisy breathing, progressive stridor, and hoarseness of voice. The severity of respiratory distress depends upon the extent of obstruction caused by the membrane.

Congenital Laryngeal Anomalies
- Laryngeal web causes weak, hoarse cry, stridor, and respiratory distress.
- Laryngeal mass or cyst may cause obstruction and hoarseness of voice.
- Laryngeal hemangioma is known to cause hoarseness and obstruction.

Trauma to Larynx
- Birth injury may cause dislocation of cricothyroid or cricoarytenoid articulations, leading to hoarseness along with wheezing.
- Another mechanism by which birth injury may produce hoarseness is through recurrent laryngeal nerve paralysis during forceps delivery.
- Instrumentation and intubation are known to cause trauma and hoarseness of voice.

Overusing of Voice
Excessive crying, shouting and singing are known for overuse of voice and exhaustion of vocal cords resulting in hoarseness.

Foreign Body
Laryngeal foreign body may be life-threatening. It may cause hoarseness, stridor, and dyspnea. Severe manifestations may be in the form of cyanosis and hemoptysis.

Other causes:
- Vocal cord nodules, polyps, and cysts are benign growths within or along with vocal folds. Vocal nodules are called "singer's nodules".
- GERD is known to cause hoarseness of voice.
- Neurological conditions like Parkinson's disease, stroke, etc., are known to cause hoarseness.
- *Weakness of laryngeal muscles:*
  - Cretinism
  - Myasthenia gravis
  - Werdnig-Hoffmann disease.

54 Hypertension

INTRODUCTION

The measurement of blood pressure (BP) should be an integral part of physical examination of the child. Every child over the age of 3 years should have his BP measured once a year and during every visit to the doctor during adolescence. The BP should be measured in all the four limbs. It should be measured in every neonate before the discharge.

Hypertension in children is defined as BP that is at or above the 95th percentile for children who are the same sex, age, and height as the patient **(Table 1 and 2)**.

Accurate measurement of BP in children is the great challenge. To obtain the correct reading, following points to be kept in mind:

- The appropriate size of the BP cuff must be used.
- The width of the rubber inflatable bladder should be approximately 40% of the arm circumference midway between the olecranon and the acromion. This should result in a cuff that encircles 80–100% of the circumference of the extremity and covers two-thirds of the length of the upper arm, a narrow cuff results in an elevated reading.
- If the BP is taken in the sitting position, the arm should be supported at the level of the heart.
- Fear, agitation, apprehension, and other emotional factors, in addition to heat and exercise, may cause elevations in BP.
- Repeated readings may be necessary to confirm hypertension. Secondary hypertension (75–80%) is more common in children, most common being renal origin. Essential hypertension, once considered as rare in children, is on rising trend recently, mainly due to obesity and syndrome X.

COMMON CAUSES OF HYPERTENSION IN NEONATES

- Renal artery thrombosis
- Renal artery stenosis
- Congenital renal malformations
- Acute kidney injury
- Coarctation of aorta
- Aortic thrombosis.

COMMON CAUSES OF HYPERTENSION IN CHILDREN

- *Renal causes:*
  - Postinfectious glomerulonephritis (PIGN)
  - Pyelonephritis
  - Reflux nephropathy
  - Renal artery abnormalities such as stenosis, arteritis, aneurysm, fibromuscular dysplasia, and thrombosis

- Interstitial nephritis
- Henoch–Schönlein purpura
- Renal trauma
- Hydronephrosis
- Hemolytic uremic syndrome
- Renal vein thrombosis
- Renal stones
- Nephrotic syndrome
- Hypoplastic kidney
- Wilms tumor
- Neuroblastoma
- Renal tuberculosis
- Polycystic kidney disease
- *Endocrinal causes:*
  - Adrenogenital syndrome
  - Cushing syndrome
  - 17α-hydroxylase deficiency
  - 11β-hydroxylase deficiency
  - Pheochromocytoma
  - Primary aldosteronism
  - Chromic nephropathy (diabetes mellitus)
  - Hyperparathyroidism
  - Hypo-/hyperthyroidism
- *Cardiovascular causes:*
  - Coarctation of aorta
  - Takayasu disease (pulseless disease)
  - William syndrome
- *Neurologic causes:*
  - Seizures
  - Guillain–Barré syndrome
  - Familial dysautonomia
  - Increased intracranial pressure (ICP)
  - Poliomyelitis
- *Collagen vascular diseases:*
  - Systemic lupus erythematosus (SLE)
  - Dermatomyositis
  - Scleroderma
  - Polyarteritis nodosa
- *Drug-induced hypertension:*
  - Corticosteroids
  - Oral contraceptive pills (in adolescents)
  - Anabolic steroids
  - Sympathomimetic (including eye and nasal drops)
- *Miscellaneous causes:*
  - Postsurgical
  - Acute pain
  - Hypernatremia
  - Burns
  - Heavy metal poisoning (lead, mercury)
  - Hypercalcemia
  - Sickle cell disease
  - Tuberous sclerosis
  - Malignancies
  - Acute intermittent porphyria
  - Neurofibromatosis
  - Malignant hyperthermia
- Essential hypertension (obesity).

TABLE 1: Blood Pressure (BP) Levels for Boys by Age and Height Percentile.

Age (yr)	BP percentile	Systolic BP (mm Hg)							Diastolic BP (mm Hg)						
		Height percentile							Height percentile						
		5th	10th	25th	50th	75th	90th	95th	5th	10th	25th	50th	75th	90th	95th
1	50th	80	81	83	85	87	88	89	34	35	36	37	38	39	39
	90th	94	95	97	99	100	102	103	49	50	51	52	53	53	54
	95th	98	99	101	103	104	106	106	54	54	55	56	57	58	58
	99th	105	106	108	110	112	113	114	61	62	63	64	65	66	66
2	50th	84	85	87	88	90	92	92	39	40	41	42	43	44	44
	90th	97	99	100	102	104	105	106	54	55	56	57	58	58	59
	95th	101	102	104	106	108	109	110	59	59	60	61	62	63	63
	99th	109	110	111	113	115	117	117	66	67	68	69	70	71	71
3	50th	86	87	89	91	93	94	95	44	44	45	46	47	48	48
	90th	100	101	103	105	107	108	109	59	59	60	61	62	63	63
	95th	104	105	107	109	110	112	113	63	63	64	65	66	67	67
	99th	111	112	114	116	118	119	120	71	71	72	73	74	75	75
4	50th	88	89	91	93	95	96	97	47	48	49	50	51	51	52
	90th	102	103	105	107	109	110	111	62	63	64	65	66	66	67
	95th	106	107	109	111	112	114	115	66	67	68	69	70	71	71
	99th	113	114	116	118	120	121	122	74	75	76	77	78	78	79
5	50th	90	91	93	95	96	98	98	50	51	52	53	54	55	55
	90th	104	105	106	108	110	111	112	65	66	67	68	69	69	70
	95th	108	109	110	112	114	115	116	69	70	71	72	73	74	74
	99th	115	116	118	120	121	123	123	77	78	79	80	81	81	82
6	50th	91	92	94	96	98	99	100	53	53	54	55	56	57	57
	90th	105	106	108	110	111	113	113	68	68	69	70	71	72	72
	95th	109	110	112	114	115	117	117	72	72	73	74	75	76	76
	99th	116	117	119	121	123	124	125	80	80	81	82	83	84	84
7.	50th	92	94	95	97	99	100	101	55	55	56	57	58	59	59
	90th	106	107	109	111	113	114	115	70	70	71	72	73	74	74
	95th	110	111	113	115	117	118	119	74	74	75	76	77	78	78
	99th	117	118	120	122	124	125	126	82	82	83	84	85	86	86
8	50th	94	95	97	99	100	102	102	56	57	58	59	60	60	61
	90th	107	109	110	112	114	115	116	71	72	72	73	74	75	76
	95th	111	112	114	116	118	119	120	75	76	77	78	79	79	80
	99th	119	120	122	123	125	127	127	83	84	85	86	87	87	88
9	50th	95	96	98	100	102	103	104	57	58	59	60	61	61	62
	90th	109	110	112	114	115	117	118	72	73	74	75	76	76	77

Contd...

Contd...

Age (yr)	BP percentile	Systolic BP (mm Hg)							Diastolic BP (mm Hg)						
		Height percentile							Height percentile						
		5th	10th	25th	50th	75th	90th	95th	5th	10th	25th	50th	75th	90th	95th
	95th	113	114	116	118	119	121	121	76	77	78	79	80	81	81
	99th	120	121	123	125	127	128	129	84	85	86	87	88	88	89
10	50th	97	98	100	102	103	105	106	58	59	60	61	61	62	63
	90th	111	112	114	115	117	109	119	73	73	74	75	76	77	78
	95th	115	116	117	119	121	122	123	77	78	79	80	81	81	82
	99th	122	123	125	127	128	130	130	85	86	86	88	88	89	90
11	50th	99	100	102	104	105	107	107	59	59	60	61	62	63	63
	90th	113	114	115	117	119	120	121	74	74	75	76	77	78	78
	95th	117	118	119	121	123	124	125	78	78	79	80	81	82	82
	99th	124	125	127	129	130	132	132	86	86	87	88	89	90	90
12	50th	101	102	104	106	108	109	110	59	60	61	62	63	63	64
	90th	115	116	118	120	121	123	123	74	75	75	76	77	78	79
	95th	119	120	122	123	125	127	127	78	79	80	81	82	82	83
	99th	126	127	129	131	133	134	135	86	87	88	89	90	90	91
13	50th	104	105	106	108	110	111	112	60	60	61	62	63	64	64
	90th	117	118	120	122	124	125	126	75	75	76	77	78	79	79
	95th	121	122	124	126	128	129	130	79	79	80	81	82	83	83
	99th	128	130	131	133	135	136	137	87	87	88	89	90	91	91
14	50th	106	107	109	111	113	114	115	60	61	62	63	64	65	65
	90th	120	121	123	125	126	128	128	75	76	77	78	79	79	80
	95th	124	125	127	128	130	132	132	80	80	81	82	83	84	84
	99th	131	132	134	136	138	139	140	87	87	89	90	91	92	92
15	50th	109	110	112	113	115	117	117	61	62	63	64	65	66	66
	90th	122	124	125	127	129	130	131	76	77	78	79	80	80	81
	95th	126	127	129	131	133	134	135	81	81	82	83	84	85	85
	99th	134	135	136	138	140	142	142	88	89	90	91	92	93	93
16	50th	111	112	114	116	118	119	120	63	63	64	65	66	67	67
	90th	125	126	128	130	131	133	134	78	78	79	80	81	82	82
	95th	129	130	132	134	135	137	137	82	83	83	84	85	86	87
	99th	136	137	139	141	143	144	145	90	90	91	92	93	94	94
17	50th	114	115	116	118	120	121	122	65	66	66	67	68	69	70
	90th	127	128	130	132	134	135	136	80	80	81	82	83	84	84
	95th	131	132	134	136	138	139	140	84	85	86	87	87	88	89
	99th	139	140	141	143	145	146	147	92	93	93	94	95	96	97

TABLE 2: Blood Pressure (BP) levels for girls by age and height percentile.

Age (yr)	BP percentile	Systolic BP (mm Hg)							Diastolic BP (mm Hg)						
		Height percentile									Height percentile				
		5th	10th	25th	50th	75th	90th	95th	5th	10th	25th	50th	75th	90th	95th
	90th	97	97	98	100	101	102	103	52	53	53	54	55	55	56
	95th	100	101	102	104	105	106	107	56	57	57	58	59	59	60
	99th	108	108	109	111	112	113	114	64	64	65	65	66	67	67
2	50th	85	85	87	88	89	91	91	43	44	44	45	46	46	47
	90th	98	99	100	101	103	104	105	57	58	58	59	60	61	61
	95th	102	103	104	105	107	108	109	61	62	62	63	64	65	65
	99th	109	110	111	112	114	115	116	69	69	70	70	71	72	72
3	50th	86	87	88	89	91	92	93	47	48	48	49	50	50	51
	90th	100	100	102	103	104	106	106	61	62	62	63	64	64	65
	95th	104	104	105	107	108	109	110	65	66	66	67	68	68	69
	99th	111	111	113	114	115	116	117	73	73	74	74	75	76	76
4	50th	88	88	90	91	92	94	94	50	50	51	52	52	53	54
	90th	101	102	103	104	106	107	108	64	64	65	66	67	67	68
	95th	105	106	107	108	110	111	112	68	68	69	70	71	71	72
	99th	112	113	114	115	117	118	119	76	76	76	77	78	79	79
5	50th	89	90	91	93	94	95	96	52	53	53	54	55	55	56
	90th	103	103	105	106	107	109	109	66	67	67	68	69	69	70
	95th	107	107	108	110	111	112	113	70	71	71	72	73	73	74
	99th	114	114	116	117	118	120	120	78	78	79	79	80	81	81
6	50th	91	92	93	94	96	97	98	54	54	55	56	56	57	58
	90th	104	105	106	108	109	110	111	68	68	69	70	70	71	72
	95th	108	109	110	111	113	114	115	72	72	73	74	74	75	76
	99th	115	116	117	119	120	121	122	80	80	80	81	82	83	83
7.	50th	93	93	95	96	97	99	99	55	56	56	57	58	58	59
	90th	106	107	108	109	111	112	113	69	70	70	71	72	72	73
	95th	110	111	112	113	115	116	116	73	74	74	75	76	76	77
	99th	117	118	119	120	122	123	124	81	81	82	82	83	84	84
8	50th	95	95	96	98	99	100	101	57	57	57	58	59	60	60
	90th	108	109	110	111	113	114	114	71	71	71	72	73	74	74
	95th	112	112	114	115	116	118	118	75	75	75	76	77	78	78
	99th	119	120	121	122	123	125	125	82	82	83	83	84	85	86
9	50th	96	97	98	100	101	102	103	58	58	58	59	60	61	61
	90th	110	110	112	113	114	116	116	72	72	72	73	74	75	75

Contd...

Contd...

Age (yr)	BP percentile	Systolic BP (mm Hg)							Diastolic BP (mm Hg)						
		Height percentile							Height percentile						
		5th	10th	25th	50th	75th	90th	95th	5th	10th	25th	50th	75th	90th	95th
	95th	114	114	115	117	118	119	120	76	76	76	77	78	79	79
	99th	121	121	123	124	125	127	127	83	83	84	84	85	86	87
10	50th	98	99	100	102	103	104	105	59	59	59	60	61	62	62
	90th	112	112	114	115	116	118	118	73	73	73	74	75	76	76
	95th	116	116	117	119	120	121	122	77	77	77	78	79	80	80
	99th	123	123	125	126	127	129	129	84	84	85	86	86	87	88
11	50th	100	101	102	103	105	106	107	60	60	60	61	62	63	63
	90th	114	114	116	117	118	119	120	74	74	74	75	76	77	77
	95th	118	118	119	121	122	123	124	78	78	78	79	80	81	81
	99th	125	125	126	128	129	130	131	85	85	86	87	87	88	89
12	50th	102	103	104	105	107	108	109	61	61	61	62	63	64	64
	90th	116	116	117	119	120	121	122	75	75	75	76	77	78	78
	95th	119	120	121	123	124	125	126	79	79	79	80	81	82	82
	99th	127	127	128	130	131	132	133	86	86	87	88	88	89	90
13	50th	104	105	106	107	109	110	110	62	62	62	63	64	65	65
	90th	117	118	119	121	122	123	124	76	76	76	77	78	79	79
	95th	121	122	123	124	126	127	128	80	80	80	81	82	83	83
	99th	128	129	130	132	133	134	135	87	87	88	89	89	90	91
14	50th	106	106	107	109	110	111	112	63	63	63	64	65	66	66
	90th	119	120	121	122	124	125	125	77	77	77	78	79	80	80
	95th	123	123	125	126	127	129	129	81	81	81	82	83	84	84
	99th	130	131	132	133	135	139	136	88	88	89	90	90	91	92
15	50th	107	108	109	110	111	113	113	64	64	64	65	66	67	67
	90th	120	121	122	123	125	126	127	78	78	78	79	80	81	81
	95th	124	125	126	127	129	130	131	82	82	82	83	84	85	85
	99th	131	132	133	134	136	137	138	89	89	90	91	91	92	93
16	50th	108	108	110	111	112	114	114	64	64	65	66	66	67	68
	90th	121	122	123	124	126	127	128	78	78	79	80	81	81	82
	95th	125	126	127	128	130	131	132	82	82	83	84	85	85	86
	99th	132	133	134	135	137	138	139	90	90	90	91	92	93	93
17	50th	108	109	110	111	113	114	115	64	65	65	66	67	67	68
	90th	122	122	123	125	126	127	128	78	79	79	80	81	81	82
	95th	125	126	127	129	130	131	132	82	83	83	84	85	85	86
	99th	133	133	134	136	137	138	139	90	90	91	91	92	93	93

Hypothermia

INTRODUCTION

Hypothermia is defined as core body temperature below 95°F (35°C). The reduction in body temperature reflects a negative balance between heat production, such as low metabolic state (hypothyroidism, acute severe malnutrition) and heat loss, when mechanisms to dissipate heat are exaggerated (evaporation after immersion). The body dissipates heat to environment by radiation, conduction, evaporation, and convection. The newborn and the preterm, in particular, have a large surface area to volume ratio than older children and adults, putting them at high risk of hypothermia because they may lose heat from their body surface faster than their metabolism can generate it. Wet surface, as present in the newborn, causes additional heat loss by evaporation.

COMMON CAUSES OF HYPOTHERMIA

- *In newborns:*
  - Environmental (delivered in air-conditioned rooms, winter season)
  - Hypoglycemia
  - Sepsis
  - Wet surfaces
  - Birth asphyxia
  - Intracranial hemorrhage
  - Inborn error of metabolism
  - Congenital adrenal hyperplasia
- *In children:*
  - Cold exposure (immersion, near drowning, winter season, and malnourished children)
  - Sepsis and shock
  - Central nervous system insults:
    - Meningitis, encephalitis
    - Sepsis
    - Intracranial hemorrhage
    - Craniopharyngioma
    - Cerebral malformations
  - Endocrinal causes:
    - Hypoglycemia
    - Hypothyroidism
    - Hypopituitarism
    - Addison disease
    - Anorexia nervosa
    - Diabetes mellitus
  - Severe acute malnutrition
  - Starvation
  - Drugs:
    - Paracetamol
    - Alcohol
    - Narcotics
    - Substance abuse
    - Atropine
    - Barbiturates
  - Miscellaneous:
    - Familial dysautonomia
    - Menkes kinky hair syndrome
    - Inborn errors of metabolism
    - Infusion of cold intravenous (IV) fluids
    - Burns
    - Water intoxication
    - Raynaud's phenomenon.

Impairment of Vision and Blindness

CHAPTER 56

INTRODUCTION

Impairment of vision and unilateral blindness is easily missed in children by the parents and treating medical personnel. It is mandatory for every clinician to check for vision in each child under his care. If impairment of vision is detected, proper evaluation should be performed with the help of a pediatric ophthalmologist. It is important to decide if the visual loss developed suddenly or gradual, unilateral or bilateral, affects the visual field, and associated other systemic manifestations.

COMMON CAUSES OF LOSS OF VISION AND BLINDNESS

- *Congenital blindness:*
  - *Congenital optic atrophy:* It is inherited as an autosomal recessive trait. It is evident at birth or shortly thereafter. Nystagmus is usually present.
  - *Septo-optic dysplasia:* A congenital optic nerve hypoplasia with hypopituitarism. Hypoglycemia is an important feature in the neonatal period.
  - Congenital hydrocephalus
  - Hydranecephaly
  - Porencephalic cyst involving visual cortex
  - Occipital encephalocele
  - Perinatal hypoxia
  - Congenital infections (TORCH complex)
  - Congenital cataracts
- *Traumatic causes:*
  - Chronic subdural hematoma
  - Increased intracranial pressure
- *Neurodegenerative and neurometabolic disorders:*
  - Tay-Sachs disease
  - Krabbe disease
  - Canavan disease
  - Metachromatic leukodystrophy
  - Menkes kinky hair syndrome
  - Gangliosidosis
  - Leigh disease (subacute necrotizing encephalomyelopathy)
- *Neoplastic lesions:*
  - Optic glioma
  - Craniopharyngioma
  - *Other brain tumors:* Visual defects may develop due to brain tumors depending upon their location.
- Vascular lesions (intracranial aneurysm)
- *Skeletal disease:*
  - *Osteopetrosis:* Decreased size of the cranial foramina, resulting in nerve compression. It may manifest with blindness due to compressive effect on optic nerve. Facial palsy and deafness may be other features.
  - Craniodiaphyseal dysplasia
- Retinopathy of prematurity
- Glaucoma
- *Retinitis pigmentosa:*
  - Laurence-Moon-Biedl syndrome
  - Refsum disease
  - Abetalipoproteinemia

- *Uveitis (inflammation of iris, ciliary body, and choroid):*
  - Toxoplasmosis
  - Juvenile rheumatoid arthritis
  - Sarcoidosis
  - Ankylosing spondylitis
- *Miscellaneous:*
  - Retinoblastoma
  - Retinal detachment
  - Drugs and toxins:
    - Quinine
    - Streptomycin
    - Methanol
    - Isoniazid
    - Penicillamine
    - Arsenic
  - Lymphoma (infiltration of the optic nerve)
  - Mucopolysaccharidoses
- *Sudden loss of vision:*
  - *Trauma:* Trauma to the occiput may cause sudden loss of vision. It is sudden and complete, but vision usually returns in a matter of hours.
  - *Migraine:* Vision may become blurred and distorted or may be characterized by the appearance of flashing lights; the loss may occasionally be complete. The visual loss may last for minutes or hours. The attacks may be repetitive.
  - *Optic neuritis:* Unilateral or bilateral optic or retrobulbar neuritis is a relatively common cause of sudden loss of vision. It may be following measles, mumps, varicella, Epstein–Barr virus (EBV) infection, etc.
  - *Hysterical blindness:* Pupillary response and fundus examination are normal.
  - Raised intracranial pressure
  - Cerebral embolization
  - Arterial hypotension
  - Multiple sclerosis (uncommon in children)
  - Meningitis
  - Encephalitis
  - Acute disseminated encephalomyelitis (ADEM)
  - Neuromyelitis optica
  - Systemic lupus erythematosus (SLE)
  - Cerebral venous sinus thrombosis
  - Hypoglycemia is known to cause sudden cortical blindness.

Sudden loss of vision which is reversible, usually within few hours:
- Trauma (Occiput region)
- Quinine
- Migraine
- Malignant Hypertension
- Emboli
- Functional (Hysterical).

CHAPTER 57

Inability to Move a Limb

INTRODUCTION

Inability to move a limb is usually due to pain or paresis. In neonates and infants who are not able to speak, it is difficult to differentiate between the two. It may simply present as not moving the limb. The neonates and young children not moving the limb due to pain is called pseudoparalysis.

In older children, an abscess or swollen joint-like obvious reason is there, it is easy to locate the cause for not moving the limb. However, it is difficult to decide when the patient is present with restricted limb movement without any evident cause.

A clinician should identify some red flags which require urgent attention and prompt action.

Red Flags

- A child presenting with high-grade fever, toxic look, and limp or inability to move the limb, look for septic arthritis or osteomyelitis.
- Nocturnal bone pain is the characteristic of marrow infiltrative disorders like leukemia. Sick look, fever, pallor, petechiae, and lymphadenopathy are other features of leukemia.
- Acute flaccid paralysis may be due to poliomyelitis or Guillain–Barre syndrome (GBS) which may progress rapidly to life-threatening situations like respiratory failure.
- Neonates and infants presenting with restricted limb movement require prompt attention.

PSEUDOPARALYSIS

Inability to move the limb due to severe pain is called pseudoparalysis. It is more common in neonates and young children due to following reasons:
- Congenital syphilis
- Scurvy
- Septic arthritis
- Acute osteomyelitis
- Fractures.

IMPORTANT FEATURES LOCALIZING CAUSE

- Hip pain is often referred to knee or thigh.
- Abdominal conditions like appendicitis and psoas abscess may cause a child to limp
- Characteristic of inability to move the limb due to pain or limp are:
  - Child can make the efforts to move the limb, but restriction is due to pain.
  - Trying to distribute less weight on the affected limb while walking.
  - Severe pain may not allow him to move the limb and with mild to moderate pain child can walk with limp.
- In a case of paresis, child cannot move the limb inspite of his best efforts. The movements of limb are affected as per degree of paresis.
- Children with juvenile idiopathic arthritis (JIA) are less mobile or limp in the mornings and get better over the course of the day with activity. In contrast, mechanical

problems trouble the child after use in the evening.
- Fever indicates inflammatory conditions (may be infective or noninfective) or malignancies.
- Multisystem involvement may be seen in systemic diseases such as systemic lupus erythematosus (SLE), systemic-onset JIA, and dermatomyositis.
- Children with coagulation disorders are prone to suffer from hemarthrosis.
- Sickle cell arthropathy is known.
- Gait may be characteristic:
  - Antalgic gait in painful conditions
  - Waddling gait suggests bilateral hip pathology or proximal muscle weakness
  - High steppage gait is seen with foot drop and peroneal nerve injury
  - Toe walking is seen in children with cerebral palsy.
- Paresis (weakness due to neurological conditions) is mainly due to involvement of peripheral nervous system at various sites like anterior horn cells, peripheral nerves, neuromuscular junction, and muscles. The characteristics of each site will help to decide the cause.
  - *Anterior horn cells:*
    - Loss of power
    - Flaccidity
    - Fasciculation
    - Atrophy
    - Absent deep tendon reflex (DTR)
    - No sensory loss, e.g., poliomyelitis, spinal muscular atrophy (SMA)
  - *Peripheral nerves:*
    - Tingling and numbness
    - Gloves and stocking pattern
    - Difficulty in buttoning and unbuttoning clothes
    - Slippage of slippers
    - Flaccidity
    - Absent reflexes, e.g., Guillain–Barré syndrome (GBS), post-diphtheritic polyneuritis.
  - *Neuromuscular junction:*
    - Fatigability increases over the course of the day, maximum in the evening
    - Diplopia
    - Ptosis
    - Ophthalmoplegia
    - Dysarthria, e.g., myasthenia gravis.
  - *Muscles:*
    - Difficulty in getting up from sitting position and climbing stairs (proximal muscles weakness of lower limbs)
    - Difficulty in combing hair and removing clothes (proximal muscle weakness of upper limbs)
    - DTR are preserved, e.g., Duchenne muscular dystrophy, Becker muscular dystrophy, dermatomyositis, etc.

COMMON CAUSES OF INABILITY TO MOVE THE LIMBS

- *Upper limbs:*
  - Birth trauma:
    - Fracture of clavicle, humerus
    - Brachial plexus injury
    - Erb's palsy
  - Pulled elbow
  - Septic arthritis
  - Congenital syphilis
  - Poliomyelitis
  - GBS
- *Lower limbs:*
  - GBS
  - Poliomyelitis
  - Post-diphtheritic polyneuritis
  - Viral myositis
  - Dermatomyositis
  - Synovitis
  - Osteomyelitis
  - Scurvy
  - Sprains
  - Fractures (femur, tibia)
  - Reactive arthritis
  - Sickle arthropathy
  - Deep vein thrombosis.

Jaundice

INTRODUCTION

- Jaundice is defined as the condition characterized by yellowish discoloration of sclera, skin, and mucous membrane due to increase in the serum bilirubin level. Clinical detection of jaundice indicates serum bilirubin >2 mg/dL in older children and >5 mg/dL in neonates.
- Icterus is another terminology for jaundice. It is derived from "Golden Oriole" (icterus Baltimore) bird who has long yellowish-orange feathers.
- One should look for jaundice only in natural light, the brighter is better as it is very difficult to appreciate jaundice in artificial light, especially fluorescent light. Mild jaundice is easily missed in artificial light.
- Severe pallor can cause yellow halo which is mistaken as jaundice by the parents, which should be clarified.
- Commonly, the patient of jaundice presents with complaints of yellow eyes and urine. Apart from jaundice, dark-colored urine may be due to concentrated urine in a case of dehydration or decreased oral intake of fluids, high fever, etc. Yellow urine can also be due to some drugs like vitamin B complex and rifampicin.
- A lemon yellow color (due to combination of pallor and jaundice) of sclera and skin indicates underlying cause as hemolysis.
- Yellow sclera and dark urine indicate hepatitis. Yellow sclera and normal urine indicate hemolysis. Dark yellow sclera and skin, dark urine, and clay stool with scratch marks are pointers for obstructive jaundice.
- Pruritus in obstructive jaundice is due to deposition of bile acids in the skin, irritating the itch receptors.

MISTAKEN FOR JAUNDICE

Following conditions may be mistaken for jaundice:

- *Carotenemia:* Carotenemia is seen in children with lots of consumption of carrots and mangoes. It can also be seen in hypothyroidism and diabetes mellitus due to impaired conversion of carotene to vitamin A. The yellow pigmentation in carotenemia is mainly seen in the palms, soles, and face. Carotene is fat soluble and hence it is not concentrated in fat poor tissues like sclera.
- *Lycopenemia:* Lycopene is a carotene-like pigment seen in tomatoes, beets, and berries. The child, who eats those things in excess, can develop lycopenemia.
- Drugs like Mepacrine (antimalarial) and Quinacrine hydrochloride (antiparasitic) (previously used for treatment of giardiasis) can cause yellowish discoloration of skin in 30% patients treated with them. They can cause yellow discoloration of eyes also.

RECOGNITION OF JAUNDICE

- Look for jaundice at sclera, palate, and under surface of tongue. Bilirubin in the skin is obscured by melanin. Therefore, it is easier to appreciate jaundice in areas of the skin not commonly exposed to the Sun and is relatively free of melanin, like the skin of the abdomen, palm, and soles.
    In the dark children, jaundice can be best seen in the sclera and under surface of the tongue. There is no difficulty in recognizing jaundice in Indian neonates as increased skin pigmentation appears after 2 weeks of life only.
- In the neonates, it is difficult to examine sclera due to physiological photophobia and one should not try to open the eyes forcibly.
    For assessment of jaundice in neonates, press the skin against a bone surface (sternum) for 5 seconds to blanch the skin and observe the skin color. Due to physiological polycythemia in the newborn, blanching of skin is required to appreciate yellow color of the skin. It can also be examined over forehead and tip of nose.
- In new born, if jaundice is clinically detectable, it means, serum bilirubin is more than 5 mg/dL.
- In neonates, as the intensity of jaundice increases, there is a cephalo-pedal progression. This is due to the relative thickness of the skin at various parts being thinnest over face and thickest in the palms and soles.
- In neonates, conjugated (direct) hyperbilirubinemia is defined as serum direct bilirubin >1 mg/dL if the total serum bilirubin is <5 mg/dL or >20% of total serum bilirubin if total serum bilirubin is >5 mg/dL.
- Conjugated (direct) hyperbilirubinemia at any age in a newborn is pathological and requires evaluation.
- *Uniocular jaundice:* If a person within artificial eye develop hepatitis, he will have uniocular jaundice.

Causes of Neonatal Jaundice

- Unconjugated Hyperbilirubinemia:
  - Physiologic jaundice
  - Hemolytic disease of newborn due to Rh, ABO and minor group incompatibility.
  - Breast milk jaundice.
  - Breast feeding jaundice.
  - Increased extravascular bilirubin load due to cephalhematoma, swallowed maternal blood etc.
  - Upper GI tract obstruction like hypertrophic pyloric stenosis, duodenal atresia etc.
  - Congenital hemolytic anaemias like G-6-P-D deficiency, hereditary spherocytosis etc.
  - Familial jaundice like Crigler-Najjar syndrome and Gilbert syndrome.
  - Hypothyroidism.
- Conjugated hyperbilirubinemia:
  - Hepatocellular jaundice
  - Cholestatic jaundice
  - Stool color chart in cholestasis is used for screening program for biliary atresia. Biliary atresia presents as pale stools by 2 weeks and definitely before 4 weeks. Stool color chart has sensitivity of 77% and specificity of 99% **(Fig. 1)**.

Causes of Cholestatic Jaundice

- Obstructive cholestasis:
  - Biliary atresia
  - Choledocal cyst
  - Inspissated bile syndrome
  - Gall stone
  - Neonatal sclerosing cholangitis.

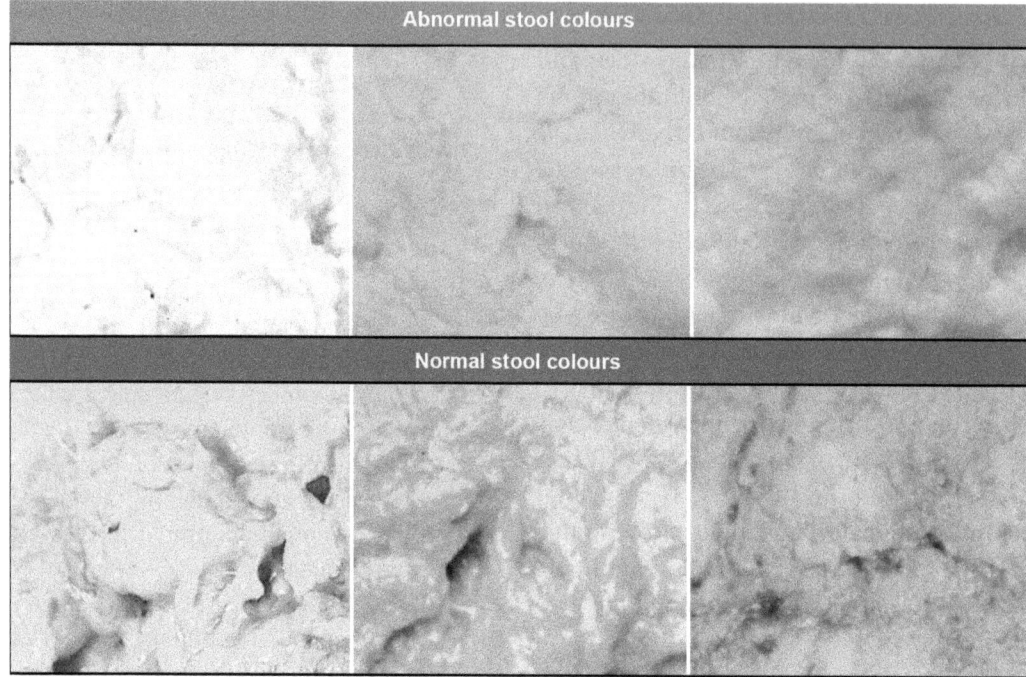

Fig. 1: Check your baby's stool color every day for the first month after birth to screen for biliary atresia.

- Neonatal hepatitis:
  - Viral Infections
    - Herpes simplex
    - Cytomegalovirus.
    - Human Immunodeficiency virus
    - Parvovirus B_{19}
  - Bacterial Infections
    - Sepsis
    - Urinary Tract Infection
    - Congenital syphilis
- Metabolic/Genetic causes:
  - Galactosemia
  - Tyrosinemia
  - Alpha – 1 antitrypsin deficiency
  - Progressive familial intrahepatic cholestasis
  - Alagille syndrome
- Endocrinal disorders:
  - Hypothyroidism
  - Hypopituitarism
- Drugs
- Parenteral nutrition
- Neonatal lupus.

CAUSES OF JAUNDICE IN CHILDREN

Infections

- Viral:
  - Hepatotropic virus A, B, C, D, E.
  - Non hepatotropic viruses like Epstein - Barr virus, mumps, rubella, measles etc.
  - Other viruses like Dengue, Ebola, Lassa fever virus etc.
- Bacterial:
  - Enteric fever.
  - Brucellosis.
  - Disseminated tuberculosis.
  - Septicemia.
  - Weil's disease (leptospirosis).

- Protozoal:
  - Malaria
  - Toxoplasmosis
  - Kala-azar
- Metabolic causes:
  - Wilson's disease
  - Galactosemia
  - Alpha-1-antitrypsin deficiency
  - Cystic fibrosis
  - Tyrosinemia
  - Hereditary fructose intolerance.
- Drugs:
  - Antituberculous drugs like INH, Rifampicin, pyrazinamide etc.
  - NSAIDs
  - Paracetamol
  - Ketoconazole
  - Antipsychotic drugs
- Toxins like Afia toxin.

CHAPTER 59: Lower Gastrointestinal Bleeding

INTRODUCTION

Lower gastrointestinal bleeding (LGIB) means bleeding distal to the ligament of Trietz (duodenojejunal junction), presenting as bleeding per rectum.
- LGIB may be overt (obvious) or occult.
- Overt bleeding can be acute, massive, or chronic intermittent and can present as hematochezia (passage of frank blood per rectum), melena, or streaks of blood. Occult blood is not clinically apparent but becomes manifest by laboratory evidence of iron deficiency anemia or chemical evidence of blood in the stool.

EVALUATION

A meticulous history including details such as bleed is major or minor, chronic, recurrent or acute massive is crucial for further evaluation. Duration of bleeding, number of episodes, frequency, volume, color, presence of clots, mucus, frank blood or mixed with faeces provide lots of information.
- *Site of bleeding:* 10% of upper (gastrointestinal GI) bleeding (UGIB) may present with bleeding per rectum (massive UGIB). Usually, UGIB manifest as hematemesis and melena. Hematochezia (passage of frank blood per rectum) is the manifestation of bleeding from small bowel or colon. Specks (minute quantity) or streaks of bright red blood indicates bleeding from anorectal region.
- Crampy abdominal pain and frequent loose stools mixed with mucus and blood suggest infection (dysentery), inflammation [vasculitis like Henoch–Schonlein purpura (HSP)] or ischemic [necrotizing enterocolitis (NEC), intussusceptions] pathology.
- Painless bleeding is more typical of colonic polyp, Meckel's diverticulum or vascular malformation.
- Passage of painless, large volume, maroon, or bright-red blood, requiring blood transfusion, highly suggest Meckel's diverticulum.
- Painful defection with streaks of blood suggests anal fissure.
- Intermittent severe screaming (due to abdominal pain), vomiting, red currant jelly stool, and presence of mass in abdomen are suggestive of intussusception. There may be recent history of acute gastroenteritis.
- An infant with stool mixed with blood following introduction of bovine milk, one should suspect cow's milk protein allergy.
- An infant of normal weight, on breast milk with blood in the stool may have benign allergic proctocolitis due to transfer of allergen through breast milk (very rare).
- Recent broad-spectrum antibiotics therapy may be followed by passage of blood and mucus in the stools, indicating antibiotic associated colitis or pseudomembraneous colitis. Ampicillin, amoxicillin, clindamycin, and vancomycin are common antibiotics causing pseudomembraneous colitis.
- History of ingestion of beet or coloring agents suggests factitious bleed.

- History of systemic manifestations of bleeding like petechiae, ecchymosis, or epistaxis along with bleeding per rectum may suggest a hematological disorder.
- Abdominal pain, diarrhea, loss of weight, pedal edema (due to hypoproteinemia), and fever suggests inflammatory bowel disease (IBD).
- History of abdominal pain, bleeding per rectum, rashes on gluteal region, legs, and joint pain suggests HSP.
- Per rectal examination is very important. It may reveal polyp, intussusceptions, some mass, etc. Anal fissure is seen on careful inspection of local area.

COMMON CAUSES OF LOWER GASTROINTESTINAL BLEEDING

- *Neonates:*
  - Hemorrhagic disease of new born
  - NEC
  - Malrotation with volvulus
  - Stress ulcer
  - Anal fissure
  - Swallowed maternal blood
- *Older children:*
  - Anal fissure
  - Cow's milk protein allergy
  - Intussusception
  - Pseudomembraneous colitis
  - IBDs (ulcerative colitis, Crohn's disease)
  - HSP
  - Meckel's diverticulum
  - Polyp
  - Vascular malformations
  - Rectal prolapse
  - Hemorrhoids
  - Trauma
  - Foreign body in rectum.

Lymphadenopathy

INTRODUCTION

Lymph nodes are normally small, oval or bean shaped, and located along the course of lymphatic vessels to filter lymph on its way to the blood stream. The primary function of lymph nodes is to filter microorganisms and abnormal cells, collected in lymph fluid.

Palpable lymph nodes are common in children. Lymph node enlargement is caused by proliferation of normal lymphoid elements or by infiltration with phagocytic or malignant cells in response to antigenic, infectious, or neoplastic stimuli.

IS THE MASS A LYMPH NODE?

The following nonlymphoid masses are frequently seen in neck and they should be differentiated with proper physical examination and if indicated by ultrasono study or other necessary investigations:
- Thyroglossal cyst
- Branchial cleft cyst
- Infected sinus
- Goiter
- Thyroid swelling in adolescents
- Thyroiditis
- Thyroid abscess
- Neurofibroma
- Cystic hygroma
- Cervical rib.

IS THE LYMPH NODE ENLARGED?

- Usually, lymph nodes are not palpable in the neonates, if they are palpable, search for the cause. Congenital infections such as rubella, cytomegalovirus (CMV), syphilis, tuberculosis, and toxoplasmosis should be considered as differentials in neonates with lymphadenopathy.
- In older children, cervical and axillary lymph nodes >1 cm and inguinal lymph nodes >1.5 cm in size are considered as significant lymphadenopathy.
- Epitrochlear, supraclavicular, and popliteal lymph nodes of any size should be considered always significant and warrants to decide the cause.

IS THE LYMPHADENOPATHY LOCALIZED OR GENERALIZED?

- Localized (regional) lymphadenopathy indicates infection in the involved node and/or its drainage area.
- Generalized lymphadenopathy is defined as enlargement of lymph nodes of >2 noncontagious regions. It is accompanied by abnormal physical findings in other systems and denotes some systemic disease.

WHAT ARE THE CHARACTERISTICS OF THE LYMPH NODE?

- Acutely infected lymph nodes are tender. Erythema and warmth of the overlying skin are other features of suppurative lymphadenitis. Fever may be there in acute bacterial lymphadenitis.

- With chronic infection, many of these signs are not present.
- Tuberculous lymph nodes are firm in consistency, nontender, and may be matted. It may result in a cold abscess when the caseous material liquefies. Sometimes, the overlying skin gets discolored and spontaneous drainage and sinus formation may develop. Tuberculous cervical lymphadenitis is more common.
  Generalized lymphadenopathy goes against the diagnosis of tuberculosis.
- Presence of fluctuation suggests abscess formation.
- Lymphoma usually presents with painless, rubbery lymphadenopathy, usually involving the cervical or supraclavicular group of lymph nodes. Axillary and inguinal lymph nodes are involved less frequently. Involvement of mediastinal lymph node may be there, manifesting with cough, dyspnea, dysphagia, and voice change. Fever, weight loss, and night sweats are systemic signs in a case of lymphoma.
- Painless, firm, discrete, and shotty glands is the characteristic of syphilitic lymphadenitis.

LOCATION OF LYMPHADENOPATHY SIGNIFIES LIKELY PATHOLOGY

- *Cervical:*
  - Jugulodiagastric: Group A streptococcal
  - Viral infections: Epstein-Barr virus (EBV), CMV
  - Staphylococcal
  - Tuberculosis
  - Diphtheria (bilateral cervical-bull neck)
  - Anterior cervical (single): Kawasaki disease
  - Scalp infection: Pediculosis
  - Seborrheic dermatitis
  - Kikuchi disease
  - PFAPA (periodic fever, aphthous stomatitis, pharyngitis, adenitis) syndrome.
- *Suboccipital and post auricular:* Rubella
- *Supraclavicular:*
  - Malignancy or infection in the mediastinum: Right supraclavicular
  - Metastatic from abdomen (gastric carcinoma): Left supraclavicular
  - Lymphoma
  - Tuberculosis
- *Epitrochlear:*
  - Syphilis
  - Sarcoid
  - EBV
- *Inguinal:*
  - Lower extremities suppurative infection
  - Filariasis
  - Plague
- *Axillary:*
  - Arm and chest infection
  - Malignancy of chest wall
  - Bacillus Calmette–Guerin (BCG) adenitis (left axillary).

CAUSES OF GENERALIZED LYMPHADENOPATHY

- Viral infections: EBV, human immunodeficiency virus (HIV), CMV
- Leukemias [acute lymphocytic leukemia (ALL)]
- Lymphomas
- Histiocytic disorders
- SLE
- Juvenile idiopathic arthritis (JIA)
- Brucellosis
- Sarcoidosis
- Syphilis
- Plague
- Histoplasmosis
- Fungal infections
- Kala-azar
- Chronic granulomatous
- Drug reaction: Phenytoin, carbamazepine, hydralazine, cephalosporins, sulfonamides, captopril, allopurinol.

CHAPTER 61

Macrocephaly

INTRODUCTION

Large head (macrocephaly) is not an uncommon complaint put forward by parents in our daily outdoor practice.
- Occipitofrontal circumference (OFC) should be measured by fiberglass measure tape and not by plastic (tailor) measure tape.
- *Normal head circumference growth velocity:*
  - <3 months: 2 cm/month
  - 3–6 months: 1 cm/month
  - 6–12 months: 0.5 cm/month
  - 1–3 years: 1 cm/6 months
  - 3–5 years: 1 cm/year
- Adult head size is achieved by 5–6 years.
- Serial head circumference should be measured monthly for first year, 3 monthly for second year, and 6 monthly for 3–5 years.
- Macrocephaly is defined as a head circumference (OFC) that is >2 standard deviation above the mean for age, sex, race, and gestation. It is not a disease, but a syndrome of diverse causes.
- Serial measurements of head circumference and plotting the readings on growth chart is an important step to detect macrocephaly.
- Evaluation of a child is necessary whenever a single-head circumference measurement is above the range of normal, or when graphing the serial measurements document a progressive, relative enlargement of head as evidence by the crossing of one or more percentile lines.
- *Important points on history taking:*
  - What is the age of the child? *(congenital/acquired)*
  - Any congenital defect like meningocele or talipes? *(associated hydrocephalus)*
  - Was the patient abnormal from birth or was there a period of normal growth and development before deterioration set in? *(congenital/acquired/neurodegenerative)*
  - Is there a history of (H/o) central nervous system (CNS) infection, trauma, or intracranial hemorrhage? [*bacterial meningitis, hemolytic disease of the newborn (HDN), H/o fall, etc.*]
  - Is there H/o irritability/headache, projectile vomiting, seizures? [*suggesting raised intracranial pressure (ICP)*]
  - Is there a family H/o neurologic or cutaneous abnormalities?
- *Large head may result due to:*
  - Familial macrocephaly (common, not pathological)
  - Increased cerebrospinal fluid (CSF) space (hydrocephalus)
  - Subdural fluid (subdural hematoma, empyema, and hygroma)
  - Thick skull due to skeletal abnormalities (hemolytic anemia, rickets, achondroplasia, and osteopetrosis)

- Increased brain volume (megalencephaly)
- Abnormal brain storage (gray matter/white matter abnormalities).

■ Examination of anterior fontanelle (AF) is important. Delayed closure of AF, wide open and tense pulsatile AF suggest hydrocephalus or raised ICP.
■ In infants, transillumination of skull may be positive in subdural effusion, porencephalic cysts, hydranencephaly, etc. It should be confirmed by ultrasonography (USG) cranium.
■ Auscultation of skull may reveal intracranial bruits (vein of Galen malformation).
■ Eye examination (including fundus examination) is essential for evaluating large head. It may show papilledema (hydrocephalus, raised ICP), macular degeneration (lipid metabolic disorders), chorioretinitis, and cataracts (intrauterine infections).
■ The patient and family should be examined for cutaneous lesions such as angiomas, cafe-au-lait spots, shagreen patches, telangiectasia, and subcutaneous nodules. (neurocutaneous disorders).

COMMON CAUSES OF MACROCEPHALY

■ *Congenital:*
  - Benign/familial
  - Hydrocephalus
  - Cranio-skeletal dysplasia
  - Achondroplasia
  - Porencephaly
  - Megalencephaly
■ *Infections:*
  - Intrauterine infections (toxoplasmosis causing hydrocephalus)
  - Hydrocephalus [complications of acute bacterial meningitis (ABM) and tuberculous meningitis (TBM)]
  - Subdural effusion/empyema (ABM)
■ *Degenerative:*
  - Alexander disease
  - Canavan disease
■ *Metabolic:*
  - Mucopolysaccharidosis
  - Gangliosidosis
  - Hypoparathyroidism
■ *Space-occupying lesions:*
  - Tumors
  - Subdural hematoma
■ *Neurocutaneous disorders:*
  - Tuberous sclerosis
  - Neurofibroma.

Common Causes of Hydrocephalus

■ Bacterial meningitis
■ Tuberculous meningitis
■ Congenital hydrocephalus
■ Intracranial hemorrhage
■ Aqueductal stenosis
■ Arnold–Chiari malformation
■ Dandy–Walker syndrome
■ Space-occupying lesions (tumors)
■ Achondroplasia.

Common Causes of Megalencephaly

■ Idiopathic
■ *Gray matter disorders:*
  - Tay-Sachs disease
  - Mucopolysaccharidosis
■ *White matter disorders:*
  - Canavan disease
  - Alexander disease
  - Metachromatic leukodystrophy
■ Neurofibroma and tuberous sclerosis
■ Soto's syndrome (pituitary gigantism).

Macroglossia

INTRODUCTION

Macroglossia is an abnormal enlargement of tongue and is a very significant finding in children of different age groups.

COMMON CAUSES OF MACROGLOSSIA

- *Syndromic conditions:*
  - Down syndrome
  - Beckwith-Wiedemann syndrome (hypoglycemia, macroglossia, macrosomia, unusual ear creases, abdominal wall defects, renal anomalies, etc.)
- Hypothyroidism
- *Storage disorders:*
  - Mucopolysaccharidosis
  - Pompe disease
  - Gangliosidosis
  - Mucolipidosis
- *Benign tumors:*
  - Hemangioma
  - Lymphangioma
  - Hemangiolymphangioma
  - Neurofibroma
  - Rhabdomyoma
- *Miscellaneous:*
  - Angioneurotic edema
  - Infection
  - Trauma (hematoma)
- Idiopathic.

Microcephaly

INTRODUCTION

Microcephaly describes a small head, and a small head generally denotes a small brain because it is brain growth that produces head enlargement, except microcephaly secondary to craniosynostosis. Serial measurements of head circumference and their plotting on growth chart catches microcephaly at the earliest. Methodological evaluation is essential for early diagnostic and therapeutic interventions to prevent irreversible damage to brain.

DEFINITION

Microcephaly is defined as head circumference that measures >3 standard deviation (SD) below the mean for age and sex.
- It is relatively common in pediatric practice, especially among developmentally delayed children.
- Microcephaly is a physical sign associated with neurological and non-neurological conditions such as cerebral palsy, neurodegenerative diseases, and malnutrition.
- It is not a single malformation but a product of arrested proliferation of neurons due to various reasons. It may be accompanied by any of the disorders of neuronal migration. It may not be purely congenital, and can also occur due to poor brain development during first 2 years of life.
- Microcephaly can be microcephaly vera (MV) which is purely due to nonproliferation of the germinal neuroblasts or microcephaly with simplified gyral pattern (MSG) in which hypoplasia is coupled with disordered migration.
- Microcephaly vera is characterized by thin cortex and scarcity of neurons in layers II and III of the cortex. The children have underlying degree of mental retardation but seizures are rare.
- MSG is associated with lissencephaly and has a worse prognosis. Severe mental retardation is accompanied by intractable seizures, developing in the neonatal period along with diffuse spasticity.
- *Serial measurements of head circumference and plotting them on growth chart:*
  - Head circumference (occipitofrontal circumference) should be measured after 24 hours of birth of the baby, meanwhile caput succedaneum disappears.
  - A flexible, nonstretchable measuring tape (made of fiber glass and not plastic) must be used with 1 cm increments.
  - The tape is positioned at supraorbital ridges in front and external occipital protuberance at posterior.
  - Serial head circumference measurements are more meaningful than a single reading.
  - The head circumference of each parent and sibling should be recorded and taken into consideration.

- Following birth asphyxia, central nervous system (CNS) infections, kernicterus, or any brain insult in first 2 years of life should be followed up with serial head circumference measurements and plotting them on growth chart to detect the microcephaly earliest.
- *Head circumference in relation with other growth parameters:*
  - Head, length, and weight all at same percentile: Syndromic microcephaly
  - Head is small but length and weight percentile are even lower: Malnutrition and chronic disease
  - Head small but length and weight percentile normal: Primary microcephaly
- Microcephaly can be subdivided into two main groups: Primary (genetic) microcephaly and secondary (nongenetic) microcephaly.
- *Primary microcephaly:*
  - Usually, have no associated malformations
  - Follow Mendielian pattern of inheritance
  - Associated with a specific genetic syndrome (MV)
  - Affected infants are usually identified at birth because of a small head circumference.
  - The more common types include familial and autosomal dominant microcephaly and a series of chromosomal syndromes.
  - It is also associated with seven gene loci and at least seven single etiologic genes have been identified, autosomal recessive inheritance.
  - Many X-linked causes of microcephaly are caused by gene mutations that lead to severe structural malformations, such as lissencephaly, holoprosencephaly, and polymicrogyria. These findings are seen in MRI of brain.
- *Secondary microcephaly:*
  - The brain has formed normally, but disease process impairs further growth.
  - Large number of noxious agents that can affect a fetus in utero or an infant during periods of rapid brain growth, particularly first 2 years of life.
- *Acquired microcephaly:* It can be seen in conditions such as Rett, Seckel, and Angelman syndromes, encephalopathy associated with human immunodeficiency virus (HIV), and severe seizure disorders.
- Primary disorder of skull bones like craniosynostosis can cause microcephaly, but they are associated with abnormal shape of skull and signs of raised intracranial pressure, e.g., Carpenter syndrome, Apert syndrome, Crouzon syndrome, etc.

COMMON CAUSES OF MICROCEPHALY

- *Primary (genetic) microcephaly:*
  - Familial (autosomal recessive)
  - Autosomal dominant
  - Syndromes:
    - Down syndrome (trisomy 21)
    - Edward syndrome (trisomy 18)
    - Cri-du-chat syndrome (5p deletion)
    - Cornelia de Lange syndrome
    - Rubinstein–Taybi syndrome
- *Secondary (nongenetic) microcephaly:*
  - Congenital infections:
    - Cytomegalovirus (CMV)
    - Zika
    - Rubella
    - Toxoplasmosis
  - Hypoxic encephalopathy (birth asphyxia)
  - Meningitis/encephalitis
  - Malnutrition
  - Metabolic (hypoglycemia)
  - Radiation
  - Drugs (fetal alcohol and fetal hydantoin).

Movement Disorders

INTRODUCTION

- Movement disorders are characterized by abnormal or excessive involuntary movements that may result in abnormalities in posture, tone, balance, or motor control.
- Basically movement disorders are classified as akinetic syndrome and hyperkinetic or dyskinetic syndrome.
    In akinetic syndrome, there is slowness or paucity of movement, for example, parkinsonism, which is rare in children.
    In dyskinetic syndrome, there are excessive movements, e.g., chorea, athetosis, ballismus, tremor, dystonia, tics, and stereotype behavior.
- Movement disorders can be grouped according to the speed of movement. Fastest being myoclonus, slightly slower ballismus, then chorea, athetosis, and slowest dystonia.
- *Import points in history for evaluation of movement disorders:*
    - Distribution: Orofacial chorea
    - Unilateral or generalized: Hemidystonia associated with structural lesion
    - Speed of movement: Hyperkinetic or hypokinetic
    - Rhythmic or jerky: Rhythmic—tremor, palatal myoclonus
    - Rest tremor in parkinsonism
    - Action tremor
    - Tics can be suppressed by the person.
    - Tics are usually associated with urge.
    - Most movements disappear during sleep except ballismus.
    - Episodic: Paroxysmal dyskinesia should be differentiated from seizures.
    - Movement disorders and seizures can be differentiated by the preservation of consciousness.
    - Association with functional motor impairment
    - Aggravating or alleviating factors
- If clinician has not observed movement disorder, following are the ways to collect information:
    - Video recording by parents
    - Ask the parents to demonstrate what they have observed.
    - Clinician can show different movements for identification by parents.
    - Classic recording of various movement disorders can be shown to parents to identify one which is observed in their child.

CAUSES OF MOVEMENT DISORDERS

- *Chorea:*
    - Rheumatic
    - Systemic lupus erythematosus (SLE)
    - Thyrotoxicosis
    - Hypoparathyroidism
    - Drugs
    - Basal ganglia infarct

- *Athetosis:*
  - Perinatal hypoxia/trauma
  - Kernicterus
- *Dystonia:*
  - Perinatal hypoxia/trauma
  - Encephalitis (Japanese)
  - Wilson disease
  - Basal ganglia stroke
  - Drugs
- *Myoclonus:*
  - Epileptic
  - Mitochondrial
  - Gangliosidosis
  - Biotinidase deficiency
  - Hepatic failure
  - Renal failure
  - Subacute sclerosing panencephalitis (SSPE)
  - Opsoclonus myoclonus syndrome
  - Post hypoxia
  - Drugs
- *Tremor:*
  - Hypoglycemia
  - Hypocalcemia
  - Hyperthyroidism
- *Bradykinesia:*
  - Parkinson's disease
  - Wilson's disease
  - Drugs
- *Drugs causing movement disorders:*
  - Phenytoin
  - Carbamazepine
  - Valproic acid
  - Metoclopramide (dystonia)
  - Domperidone (dystonia)
  - Salbutamol (tremors)
  - Terbutaline (tremors)
  - Lamotrigine (tics)
  - Antipsychotics
  - Steroids.

CHARACTERISTICS AND SITE OF LESION OF MOVEMENT DISORDERS

Movement disorder	Characteristics	Site of lesion
Chorea	Involuntary, purposeless/quasi purposive, movements of jerky, dance-like proximal more than distal muscles	Caudate nucleus
Athetosis	Slower, writhing, irregular movements, predominantly in hands and wrist	Putamen nucleus

Dystonia	Contraction of agonist and antagonist muscles which lead to intermittent or persistent abnormal posture or twisting
	• *Focal:*
	  – Ocular muscles: Blepharospasm
	  – Tongue: Lingual dystonia
	  – Vocal cord: Dystonic dysphonia
	  – Mouth: Oromandibular dystonia
	  – Neck: Torticollis
	  – Hand: Writer's cramp
	• Segmental
	• Generalized
		Putamen nucleus

Hemiballismus	Violent, flinging movements which are irregular, usually affecting one side	Subthalamic nucleus
Dyskinesia (orofacial dyskinesia)	Commonly denotes movements of mouth and face, usually drug-induced	

Contd...

Contd...

Movement disorder	Characteristics	Site of lesion
Myoclonus	Sudden, shock-like contraction of a muscle or a group of muscles leading to involuntary purposeless jerk of the affected limb	
Ataxia	Inability to control balance, typically is caused by cerebellar dysfunction	• Cerebellum • Proprioception
Tremor	Tics are rapid, complex, involuntary, repetitive, segmental movements	
Tourette syndrome	There are motor ticks and vocalization lasting longer than 12 months, start between 2 and 10 years of age, may fluctuate in severity over time.	
Stereotype	Repetitive, patterned involuntary movements that have no apparent function	

ALGORITHM OF MOVEMENT DISORDERS

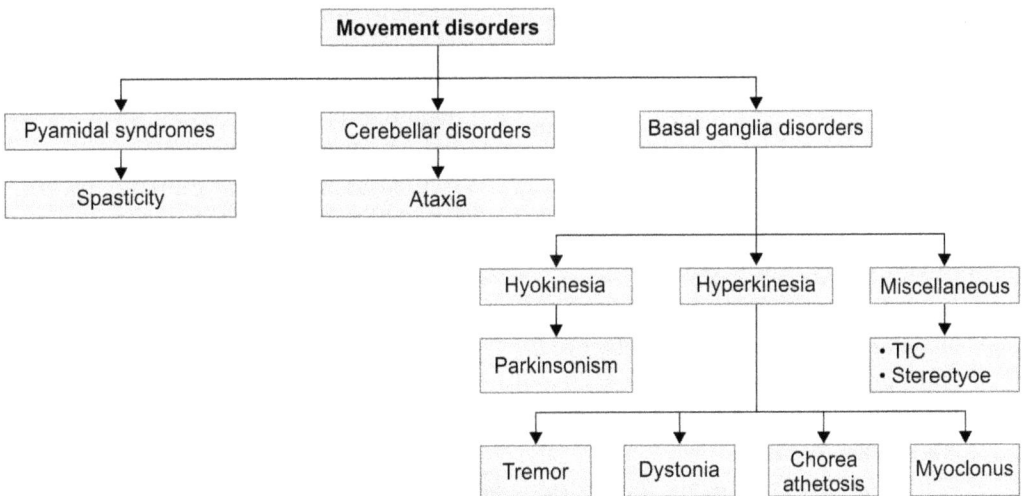

65 Neck Masses

INTRODUCTION

Neck masses are very common in infants and children. A neck mass is a lump or swelling in the neck that can be large and visible or very small. Some neck masses are present since birth (congenital neck masses) and can be due to abnormal embryonic development. Many neck masses become visible when the child has upper respiratory infection. Some are not found until they become enlarged and painful from infection. Neck masses in children are usually benign, but rarely they can be malignant.

CAUSES OF NECK MASSES

- *Lymphadenopathy:*
  - Jugulodigastric (Group A streptococcal infection)
  - Anterior cervical—single lymph node (Kawasaki disease)
  - Viral infections [Epstein-Barr virus (EBV), cytomegalovirus (CMV), and human immunodeficiency virus (HIV)]
  - Staphylococcal
  - Tuberculosis
  - Atypical mycobacterium
  - Sarcoidosis
  - Diphtheria (bilateral cervical—bull neck)
  - Scalp infection (pediculosis)
  - Seborrheic dermatitis
  - Leukemia
  - Lymphoma
  - Histiocytosis
  - Kikuchi–Fujimoto disease
  - PFAPA (periodic fever, aphthous stomatitis, pharyngitis, cervical adenitis) syndrome
- Deep neck abscesses or cellulitis (bacterial, tuberculosis, and cat scratch disease).
- *Thyroglossal duct cyst:* Most common congenital midline swelling, moving with deglutition **(Fig. 1)**.
- *Branchial cleft cyst:* It develops following failure of branchial cleft to develop normally. This may appear as an open space called cleft sinus, which may be unilateral or bilateral. The cyst or sinus can be infected **(Figs. 2A and B)**.
- *Dermoid cyst:* A dermoid cyst is a pocket or cavity under the skin that contains tissues

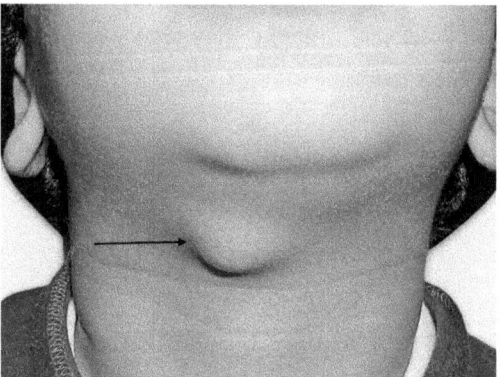

Fig. 1: Thyroglossal cleft cyst.

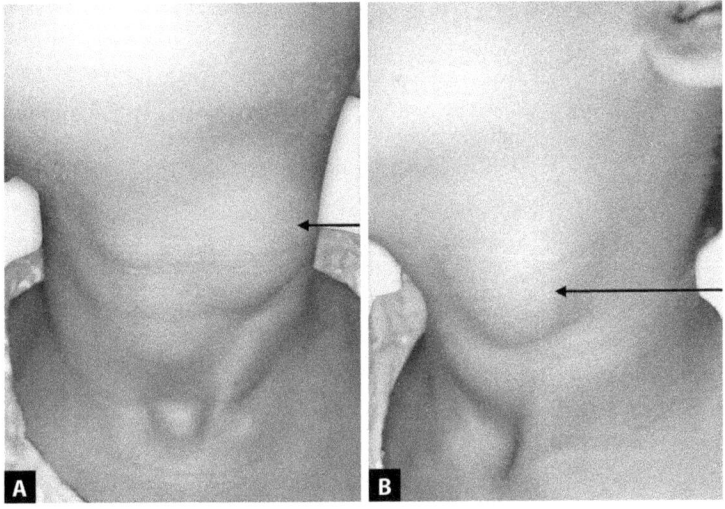

Figs. 2A and B: Branchail cleft cyst.

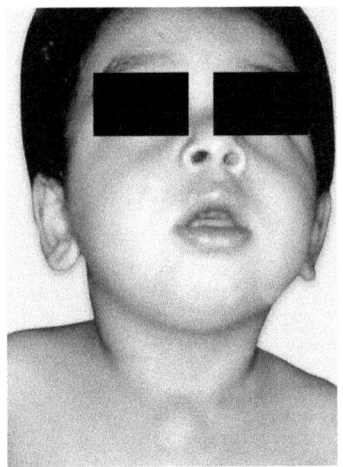

Fig. 3: Dermoid cyst.

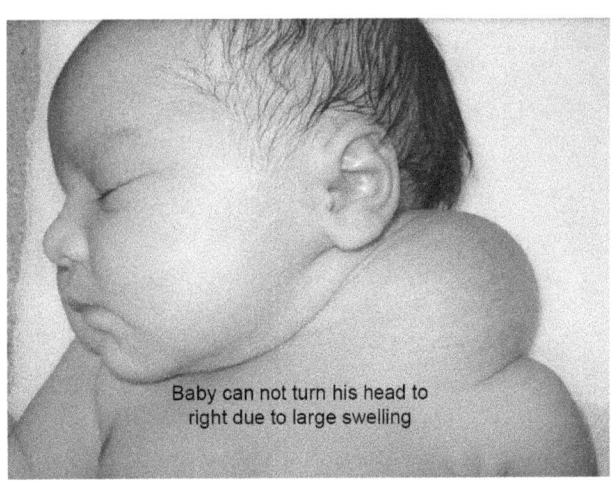

Baby can not turn his head to right due to large swelling

Fig. 4: Cystic hygroma.

normally present in the outer layers of the skin. Dermoid cyst is a midline neck swelling. It may be visible at birth or in early infancy but often is not seen until years later **(Fig. 3)**.
- *Vascular malformations:*
  - Lymphangioma
  - Cystic hygroma **(Fig. 4)**
  - Hemangioma
  - Venous malformations
- Sternocleidomastoid tumor
- Ranula
- Thyroid mass (goiter, ectopic thyroid)
- Teratoma
- Lipoma
- Thymic cyst, ectopic thymus, and thymoma
- Salivary gland infection, salivary gland tumors
- Parathyroid mass.

ANATOMICAL LOCATION AND ETIOLOGY

Location/etiology	Congenital	Inflammatory	Neoplastic
Anterior sternocleidomastoid	• Branchial cleft cyst • Vascular malformations	• Lymphadenitis • Sternocleidomastoid tumor of infancy	• Lymphoma • Rhabdomyosarcoma
Midline	• Thyroglossal duct cyst • Dermoid cyst		• Thyroid tumor • Teratoma
Occipital	• Vascular malformation • Hemangioma	Lymphadenitis	• Metastasis • Neuroblastoma
Temporal	• Hemangioma • Vascular malformations	• Lymphadenitis • Sialadenitis	Salivary gland tumor
Pre auricular	• Branchial cleft cyst • Preauricular cyst		
Submandibular	• Branchial cleft cyst • Vascular malformations	• Lymphadenitis • Sialadenitis	• Salivary gland tumor
Submental	• Thyroglossal duct cyst • Dermoid cyst	• Lymphadenitis • Sialadenitis	
Supraclavicular	• Vascular malformation		• Lymphoma • Metastasis

Nuchal Rigidity

INTRODUCTION

Nuchal rigidity (stiff neck) is an alarming complaint. The cause may be simple like drug-induced dyskinesia, cervical lymphadenitis, and viral myalgia to serious conditions like meningitis.

ONSET OF COMPLAINT

- Acute history may suggest meningitis, drug-induced dyskinesia, trauma, viral-induced myalgia, etc.
- Hyperacute onset is the characteristic of subarachnoid hemorrhage.
- Longer duration and noticed since infancy may be due to sternomastoid tumor or cervical vertebral anomalies.
- History of (H/o) trauma, fever, sore throat, and convulsions will help to decide the cause.
- History of drugs, especially phenothiazine derivatives, antiemetics like metoclopramide, etc. suggests drug-induced dyskinesia.
- It may be meningism due to right upper lobe pneumonia.
- Nuchal rigidity with signs of raised intracranial pressure may be due to space-occupying lesion (SOL) or hydrocephalus.
- Presence of dysmorphism or other congenital malformations may suggest vertebral anomalies.

- *Associated symptoms:*
  - Fever, headache, vomiting, altered sensorium and/or convulsions suggest meningitis.
  - Fever, enlarged cervical lymph nodes, and stiffness of neck suggest acute bacterial cervical lymphadenitis.
  - Acute otitis media may be associated with nuchal rigidity.
  - Fever, cough, and breathlessness suggest pneumonia and stiffness of neck may be due to meningism.
  - Stiffness of neck associated with features of Kawasaki disease suggests aseptic meningitis.

CAUSES OF NUCHAL RIGIDITY (STIFF NECK) IN CHILDREN

- *Infections:*
  - Meningitis: Inflamed meanings are irritated, causing spasms of neck muscles, resulting in nuchal rigidity (stiff neck).
    Meningitis may be due to bacterial, viral, tuberculous, rickettsial, or fungal infections.
  - The neck stiffness resulting from subarachnoid hemorrhage is called meningism.
  - Right upper lobe pneumonia causing neck stiffness is called meningismus.

- Cervical lymphadenitis: Acute posterior cervical lymphadenitis may cause nuchal rigidity due to tender swelling.
- Poliomyelitis and Guillain-Barré syndrome may cause nuchal pain and rigidity during preparalytic stage.
- Retropharyngeal abscess: The classical presentation of retropharyngeal abscess in younger child less than 3-4 years of age, fever, irritability, dysphagia, drooling, muffled voice, torticollis, and refusal to extend the neck. The neck is kept flexed only. It is also called as Bolte sign.
- Cervical spine osteomyelitis can present with fever, pain, and restricted movement of neck.
- Other causes:
  - Tetanus
  - Otitis media
  - Brain abscess
  - Dental abscess
- *Vascular causes:*
  - Subarachnoid hemorrhage
  - Cerebral aneurysm
  - Intracranial venous thrombosis
- *Neoplasms:*
  - Brain abscess
  - Meningeal leukemia
  - Posterior fossa tumors
- *Skeleton muscular disorders:*
  - Subluxations, dislocations, and fractures of cervical vertebrae
  - Vertebral anomalies like Klippel-Feil syndrome
  - Juvenile rheumatoid arthritis
  - Kawasaki disease
- *Drug-induced dyskinesia/dystonia:*
  - Phenothiazines
  - Metoclopramide
  - Hypervitaminosis A.

Nystagmus

INTRODUCTION

Nystagmus is defined as an involuntary, rhythmic, oscillatory movements of the eyes. The searching movements of eyes associated with severe visual impairment or blindness should not be mistaken as nystagmus. Opsoclonus should be differentiated from nystagmus. Opsoclonus is a condition characterized by nonrhythmic, chaotic, rapid eye movements that often occurs in bursts. It is commonly associated with neuroblastoma in young children.

The most common causes of nystagmus include disorders affecting central vision, drugs, hereditary conditions, and disorders affecting the vestibular apparatus of the ear. Neoplasms involving brain stem must always be considered in the differential diagnosis.

COMMON CAUSES OF NYSTAGMUS

- *Physiological causes:*
  - End position nystagmus (on extreme lateral gaze)
  - Optokinetic nystagmus: It is induced when a series of objects are followed across the field of vision; e.g., to see the trees while travelling in the train.
  - Evoked vestibular nystagmus: Rotation of the body or irrigation of the ear with cold or warm water can induce this type of nystagmus.
- *Congenital nystagmus:* Generally, presents in the first 6 months of life.
  - Ocular causes:
    - Poor central vision: If a child is born blind or becomes blind before the age of 2–3 years, nystagmus usually follows. The eye movements are random and not rhythmic, and called searching movements. Some children may develop nystagmus after visual loss up to age of 5 years. Defective vision acquired in older children and adults is not associated with nystagmus.
    - Structural anomalies of globe and opacities affecting transmission of images
    - Retinal abnormalities
    - Abnormalities of the afferent visual pathways
    - Down syndrome
    - Congenital cataracts
    - Clouding of cornea
    - Chorioretinitis
    - Albinism
    - Congenital optic atrophy
    - Coloboma
    - Retinal detachment
    - Retinal infections [toxoplasmosis, cytomegalovirus (CMV)]
    - Vitreous hemorrhage
    - Cortical blindness
    - Hereditary nystagmus

- Maternal drugs like hydantoin, alcohol, etc.
- Hypothyroidism
- Hyperbilirubinemia
- *Acquired nystagmus:*
  - Drugs:
    - Anticonvulsants (phenobarbitone and hydantoin)
    - Antihistaminic
    - Codeine
    - Alcohol
    - Lead poisoning
    - Quinine
    - Nicotine
  - Spasmus nutans: This disorder has onset between 4 and 18 months of age. It is characterized by nystagmus, head nodding, and torticollis. One should look for other neurologic signs suggestive of an intracranial neoplasm.
  - Disorders affecting vestibular system:
    - Tumors of brain stem or upper spinal cord may involve vestibular nuclei and associated tracts, causing nystagmus.
    - Trauma: Head injury causing fracture of petrous portion of temporal bone; vertigo is a common accompanying symptom
    - Labyrinthitis following middle ear infection
    - Benign paroxysmal vertigo
  - Arnold–Chiari malformation
  - Basilar impression: In this skeletal malformation, it causes pressure on medulla and upper cervical spinal cord. It manifests with neck stiffness, progressive lower limb weakness, head tilt, and short neck. It may be associated with nystagmus.
  - Neurological disorders:
    - Acute cerebellar ataxia
    - Brain tumors
    - Encephalitis
    - Tuberculous meningitis
    - Ataxic cerebral palsy
    - Demyelinating disorders
    - Degenerative diseases
    - Cerebellar abscess
    - Extradural hematoma
- *Opsoclonus:* Opsoclonus is a condition characterized by nonrhythmic, chaotic, rapid eye movements. It often occurs in bursts. It is most commonly associated with neuroblastoma in young children. Polymyoclonus (dancing eyes, dancing feet) may be present in neuroblastoma. It may be due to post infectious encephalopathy in older children and adults.
- *Miscellaneous causes:*
  - Maple syrup urine disease
  - Hypervalinemia
  - Trembling chin syndrome
  - Scorpion bite.

Obesity

INTRODUCTION

Childhood obesity is a major public health problem of the modern world which has shown increasing trends globally in the recent years. The World Health Organization (WHO) has declared obesity as the most neglected epidemic of modern times with significant health consequences. Obesity is quite on the rise in Indian children.

DEFINITION

Body mass index (BMI) is the most commonly used parameter to define and classify the severity of obesity. Every child should have his/her BMI calculated every year and get it plotted on BMI charts **(Figs. 1 and 2)**.

- Calculation of BMI:

$$BMI = \frac{\text{Weight in Kg}}{\text{Height in m}^2} \text{ kg/m}^2$$

- BMI >85th percentile for age and sex is overweight.
- BMI >95th percentile for age and sex is defined as obesity.
- Other parameters to define obesity:
  - Skin-fold thickness
  - Waist circumference
  - Total body fat
  - Fat mass index.

BMI remains the most widely accepted and used parameter for defining obesity in children.

HISTORY

- History of maternal gestational diabetes mellitus (DM) or any other complication of pregnancy like gestational hypertension and intrauterine growth restriction (IUGR)
- Birth weight
- Weight gain during infancy, toddler, and adolescent age
- Dietary history in details like number of meals, frequency of junk food, night meals, and cold drinks
- Detailed history of sleep pattern including daytime somnolence
- Screen time (TV, computer, mobile, videogames, etc.)
- Details of physical activity
- Developmental assessment
- Menstrual history in girls: Age of menarche, menstrual irregularities
- Family history of obesity; DM in grandparents, parents, and siblings; history of coronary artery disease in family
- History of medications by the child, especially steroids and psychotropic medicines.

PHYSICAL EXAMINATION

Apart from routine, general, and systemic physical examination, the following points should be recorded in all children with overweight and obesity:

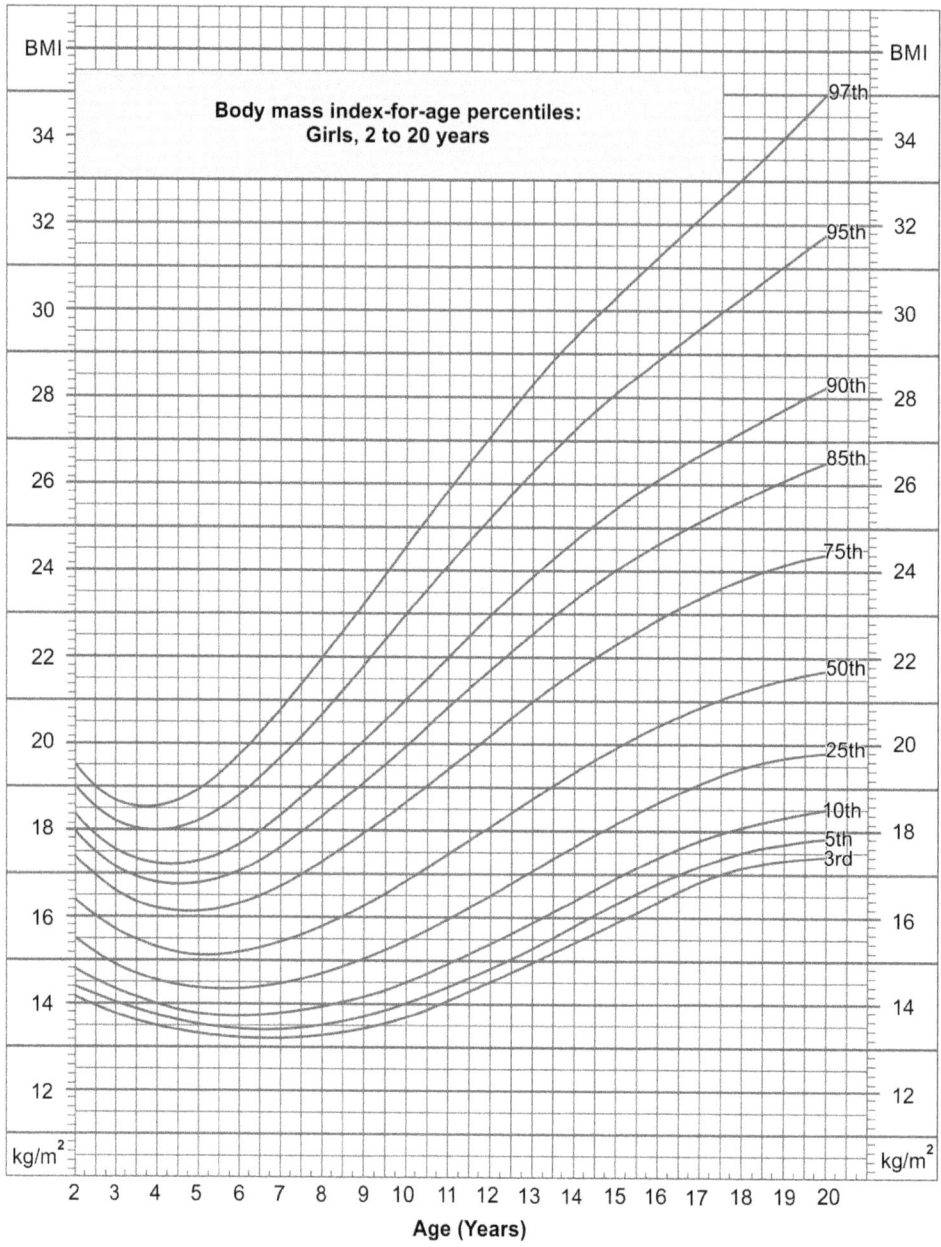

Fig. 1: Body mass index (BMI) chart for girls.

- Anthropometric measurements: Weight, height, BMI, and waist and hip circumference
- Vitals:
  - Bradycardia: Hypothyroidism.
- Blood pressure (Hypertension): Cushing syndrome
- Body fat distribution
- Signs of insulin resistance: Acanthosis nigricans, skin tags

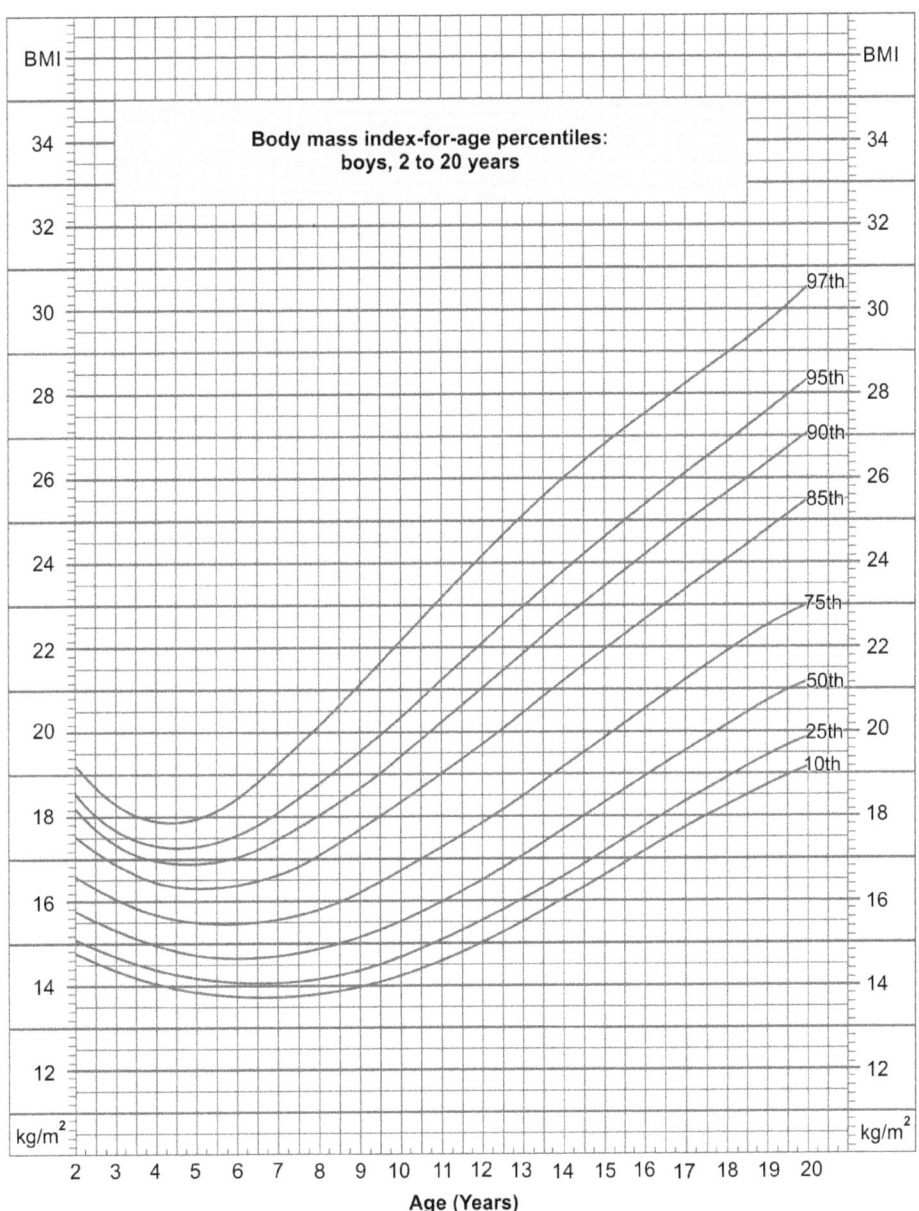

Fig. 2: Body mass index (BMI) chart for boys.

- Sign of hyperandrogenism in girls: Acne, hirsutism, increased hair fall
- Stretch marks, striae of Cushing's syndrome
- Fundus examination: Papilledema (pseudotumor cerebri)
- Neck: Goiter
- Any dysmorphic features which may suggest syndromic (Down syndrome, Laurence-Moon-Biedl syndrome, Prader-Willi syndrome) or secondary cause of obesity
- Pubertal status
- Psychiatric evaluation.

RISK FACTORS OF CHILDHOOD OBESITY

- Prenatal factors: IUGR (Barker's hypothesis on fetal origin of adult diseases)
- Early feeding practice: Lack of breastfeeding (BF), increased formula feed, and early introduction of complementary feeds
- Dietary: Increased consumption of junk food, sweetened beverages, and less fiber in diet
- Lifestyle: Increased screen time, lack of physical activities, and irregular sleep
- Family history of obesity
- Medications: Antipsychotics, antiepileptics, and steroids

COMORBIDITIES LINKED WITH OBESITY IN CHILDREN AND ADOLESCENTS

- *Metabolic:* Metabolic syndrome, type II DM
- *Cardiovascular:* Hypertension, atherosclerosis, left ventricular hypertrophy
- *Respiratory:* Sleep abnormalities, obstructive sleep apnea syndrome
- Gastrointestinal: GERD, Fatty liver, cholelithiasis, and hernia
- *Endocrinal:* Type II DM, polycystic ovarian disease
- *Musculoskeletal:* Osteopenia
- *Psychosocial:* Low self-esteem, depression, anxiety, social isolation
- *Dermatological:* Striae, intertrigo, acanthosis nigricans, carbuncle, and cellulitis
- *Miscellaneous:* Pseudotumor cerebri, proteinuria, etc.

CAUSES OF CHILDHOOD OBESITY

Primary (Constitutional) Obesity

- Most common (>95% cases)
- Genetic disorder
- Imbalance between energy intake and energy expenditure
- Increased intake of junk foods and sweetened beverages
- Decreased intake of fibers
- Decreased physical activity
- Increased screen time
- Ignorance of seriousness of the condition.

Secondary Obesity

- Monogenic and polygenic
- Syndromic:
  - Prader–Willi syndrome
  - Laurence–Moon–Biedl syndrome
  - Down syndrome
  - Fragile X syndrome
  - McCune–Albright syndrome
- Endocrinal:
  - Cushing syndrome
  - Hypothyroidism
  - Pseudohypoparathyroidism
- Hypothalamic:
  - Tumors like craniopharyngioma
  - Tuberculosis, sarcoidosis, viral encephalitis
  - Pituitary surgery
  - Head trauma
  - Cranial radiotherapy
  - Antipsychotic and antidepressant drugs.

Odynophagia

INTRODUCTION

Odynophagia is a disorder in which swallowing is painful. A person may feel pain in mouth, throat, or esophagus when swallowing food, liquid, or saliva. It should be differentiated from dysphagia when a person finds difficulty in swallowing which may be painful or without pain. Dysphagia may occur alongside odynophagia, but the two conditions can also occur separately. When dysphagia and odynophagia occur together, it means that swallowing is both difficult and painful.

COMMON CAUSES OF ODYNOPHAGIA

- *Infectious:*
  - Tonsillitis
  - Pharyngitis
  - Esophagitis
  - Oral ulcers
  - Candidiasis (oral thrush)
  - Herpes infection
  - Human immunodeficiency virus (HIV)
- Gastroesophageal reflux disease (GERD)—retrosternal heart burn due to reflux esophagitis
- HIV
- Candidiasis of esophagus
- Trauma in mouth, throat, or esophagus
- Drinking very hot or cold drinks
- Esophageal malignancy (in adults).

Oral Ulcers

INTRODUCTION

Oral ulcers in children is a common problem in pediatric practice. The causes for oral ulcers can range from simple trauma, infections, and nutritional deficiencies to drug-induced systemic diseases like autoinflammatory and collagen disorders.

Geographic tongue should not be mistaken for oral ulcers **(Fig. 1)**
- An ulcer is defined as complete breach of the epithelium, which becomes covered with a fibrin slough and appears as a white lesion surrounded by erythema.
- If a mucosal lesion lasts over 14 days, it is considered as chronic; otherwise, it is regarded as an acute ulcer.
- Recurrent ulcers are defined as similar episodes with intermittent healing and are described as recurrent aphthous stomatitis.
- Oral ulcers can be solitary or multiple ulcers.

CLASSIFICATION

Acute Ulcers
- Single ulcer:
  - Traumatic ulcer (bite injury)
  - Thermal injury
  - Mechanical irritation
- Multiple ulcers:
  - Herpetic gingivostomatitis
  - Herpangina
  - Hand, foot, mouth disease (HFMD)
  - Infectious mononucleosis
  - Candidiasis
  - Chemical/toxic/drug induced
  - Diphtheria
  - Erythema multiforme
  - Stevens–Johnson syndrome
  - Chemotherapy
  - Radiation therapy
  - Graft-versus-host disease (GvHD).

Chronic Ulcers (>14 days)
- Single ulcers:
  - Traumatic ulcer
  - Tuberculous ulcer
  - Syphilitic ulcer

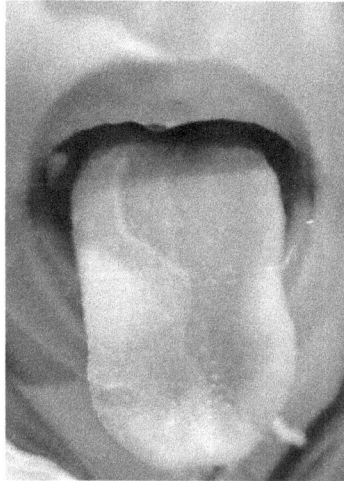

Fig. 1: Geographic tongue.

- Fungal ulceration (mucormycosis, histoplasmosis, blastomycosis)
- Cytomegalovirus (CMV) infection
- Sarcoidosis
- Multiple ulcers:
  - Necrotizing ulcerative gingivitis
  - Pemphigus vulgaris
  - Lichen planus
  - Granulomatosis.

Recurrent Ulcers

- Single ulcers:
  - Celiac disease
  - Crohn's disease
  - Behcet's disease
- Multiple ulcers:
  - Nutritional (deficiency of vitamins B_2, B_6, B_{12}, folic acid, zinc, etc.)
  - Recurrent herpetic stomatitis
  - PFAPA (periodic fever, aphthous stomatitis, pharyngitis, adenitis) syndrome
  - Systemic lupus erythematosus (SLE)
  - Sjogren's syndrome
  - Pyoderma gangrenosum
  - Cyclic neutropenia
  - Hyperimmunoglobulin D
  - Familial Mediterranean fever.

Traumatic Oral Ulcers

- They may be traumatic, thermal, chemical, or mechanical.
- Repetitive local traumatic ulcers can be due to aggressive tooth brushing or ill-fitting dental braces.
- Cerebral palsy, bruxism, and autism spectrum disorder (ASD) are other causes.

INFECTIONS

- Herpetic gingivostomatitis is a manifestation of herpes simplex virus type 1 (HSV-1). It is the most common viral cause of oral ulcers and occurs in children from 6 months to 5 years of age.

  The initial sign is hyperemia of the oral and perioral mucosa, fever, and widespread superficial fluid-filled vesicles which rapidly break down to form a cluster of small ulcers. Along with it, recurrent episodes of herpes labialis are known to occur.
- Herpangina:
  - <5 years of age
  - Sudden pharyngeal pain, fever, and multiple ulcers in the posterior pharyngeal wall
  - It is caused by enteroviruses, particularly coxsackievirus.
- HFMD:
  - HFMD is also caused by enteroviruses, most commonly coxsackievirus A16.
  - It presents with multiple oral blisters and a prodromal phase of fever and sore throat.
  - Whilst herpangina lesions are typically only found in the back of mouth (palatine arch, soft palate, uvula, and tonsils), HFMD blisters occur in the front of the mouth along with lesions on soles of feet and palms.
- Epstein–Barr virus (EBV):
  - Fever, pharyngitis, lymphadenopathy, and fatigue are characteristic features.
  - Hepatosplenomegaly and atypical lymphocyte on peripheral smear examination
  - Oral hairy leukoplakia is a benign, asymptomatic, white hyperkeratosis lesion on lateral borders of the tongue.
- CMV:
  - Asymptomatic in healthy, immunocompetent children
  - Fever, myalgia, cervical lymphadenopathy, and mild hepatitis are other clinical features.

- It can cause shallow oral ulceration with rolled margins and yellow slough or pseudomembrane—most prevalent on the hand and soft palate.
- Commonly associated with human immunodeficiency virus (HIV)
- Tuberculosis: Primary oral tuberculous lesions are rare, but do occur in children, affecting gingival and mucobuccal folds, usually presenting with a single lesion associated with enlarged submandibular lymph-nodes.
- Syphilis:
  - Syphilitic lesions are rare, but known to occur. These lesions are painless.
  - Necrotizing ulcerative gingivitis occurs due to poor oral hygiene and malnutrition.
  - Candidiasis infection is common to cause oral thrush and ulceration. Mucormycosis occurs in immunocompromised individuals.
  - Oral thrush is common in newborns, HIV, and immunodeficiency disorders with T-cell dysfunction.
- *Nutritional deficiencies:* Vitamin B_2, vitamin B_6, vitamin B_{12}, folic acid, iron, and zinc deficiencies are known to cause recurrent aphthous stomatitis.
- *Gastrointestinal (GI) diseases:*
  - Celiac disease
  - Crohn's disease
  - Ulcerative colitis
- *Autoinflammatory conditions:*
  - Erythema multiforme (may be secondary to HSV-1, mycoplasma, etc.)
- Pemphigus vulgaris
- Behcet's disease:
  - Fever, mucocutaneous lesions, involvement of joints, eyes, vascular, neurologic, and GI tract common.
  - Oral manifestations are discrete, round ulcers with a yellow-gray pseudomembranous base and a red halo, affecting lips, tongue, cheeks, and palate, disappearing without scarring.
  - Genital ulcers, skin lesions, and ocular lesions are common.
- SLE:
  - Multisystem disease [GI, renal, hematologic, cyclic vomiting syndrome, pulmonary, musculoskeletal, cutaneous]
  - Oral or nasopharyngeal ulcers are painless.
- PFAPA syndrome:
  - <5 years of age
  - Periodic fever, aphthous stomatitis, pharyngitis, adenitis (PFAPA) syndrome.
- Sjogren's syndrome
- Cyclic neutropenia
- Hyperimmunoglobulin D.

DRUGS

- Diphenyl hydantoin
- Sulfas
- Methotrexate
- Tetracyclines
- Gold salts
- Chemotherapy and radiotherapy.

71 Other Clinical Signs

INTRODUCTION

Thorough and repeated physical examination is rewarding in clinical medicine. Each clinical sign, may be minute, should be noted. On analysis of the case, small finding on physical examination, may turned out to be a pathognomonic sign for some condition. Sign of dysmorphism, skin lesions and important findings on eye examination are included in this chapter. The description of appearance of the signs, their importance & their association with clinical conditions are described in this chapter.

HYPERTELORISM

Hypertelorism means increased distance between two bodily parts or organs, e.g., eyes, kidneys, nipple, etc. Hypertelorism is commonly used for eyes (orbital hypertelorism).

Orbital hypertelorism **(Figs. 1 and 2)**:
- The distance between two medical canthi measured at the level of posterior lacrimal crest is known as inner canthal distance (ICD).
- The outer canthal distance (OCD) is between two lateral canthi.
- The distance between two mid-pupillary regions in the front gaze is called interpupillary distance (IPD).
- The palpebral fissure length (PFL) is the distance between the medial and lateral canthi.
- Orbital hypertelorism: Increased ICD, OCD, and IPD; normal PFL.

Causes of Hypertelorism
- Racial
- Down syndrome
- Trisomy 18
- Congenital hypothyroidism
- Noonan syndrome
- Turner syndrome
- Williams syndrome

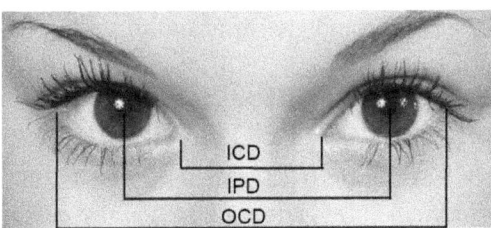

Fig. 1: Measurement of inner canthal distance (ICD), interpupillary distance (IPD), and outer canthal distance (OCD).

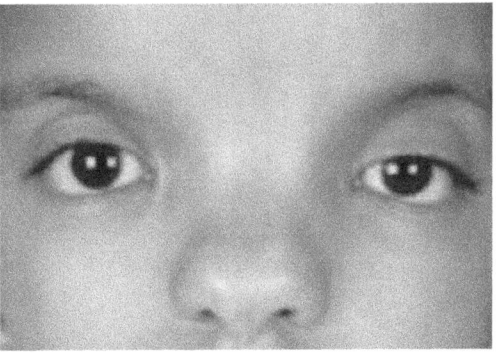

Fig. 2: Hypertelorism.

- Apert syndrome
- Rubinstein–Taybi syndrome
- Sotos syndrome
- Larsen syndrome
- LEOPARD syndrome
- Sjögren–Larsson syndrome
- DiGeorge syndrome
- Thalassemia major
- Ehlers–Danlos syndrome
- Waardenburg syndrome.

HYPOTELORISM

Hypotelorism is detected during antenatal ultrasonography as a part of anomaly scan. Hypotelorism is defined as decreased interorbital (medial aspects of orbital walls) distance <5th percentile.

Causes of Hypotelorism

- Holoprosencephaly
- Trigonocephaly
- Trisomy 13
- Oculodentodigital syndrome.

TELECANTHUS (PSEUDOHYPERTELORISM)

There is increased ICD, but normal OCD, IPD, and small PFD in telecanthus. It is also called as pseudohypertelorism **(Fig. 3)**.

Causes of Telecanthus

- Down syndrome

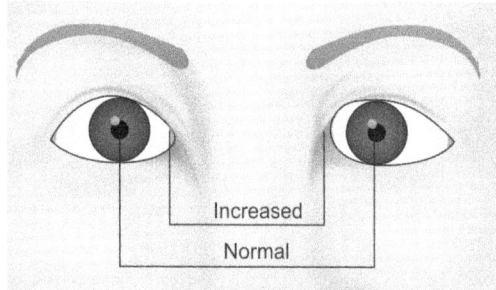

Fig. 3: Telecanthus.

- Fetal alcohol syndrome
- Cri-du-chat syndrome
- Klinefelter syndrome
- Turner syndrome
- Ehlers–Danlos syndrome
- Waardenburg syndrome.

EPICANTHAL FOLD

A skin fold of the upper eyelid covering the inner corner of the eye is called as epicanthal fold. Epicanthal folds may be normal for people of Asiatic descent. Epicanthal folds also may be seen in young children before the bridge of nose begins to rise **(Fig. 4)**.

Causes of Epicanthal Folds

- Down syndrome
- Fetal alcohol syndrome
- Turner syndrome
- Phenylketonuria
- Williams syndrome

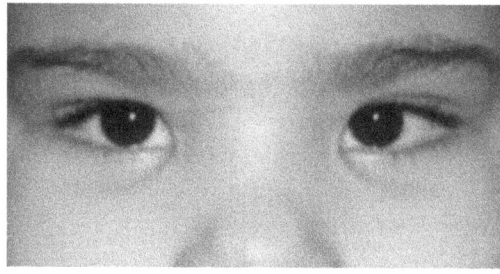

Fig. 4: Epicanthal fold.

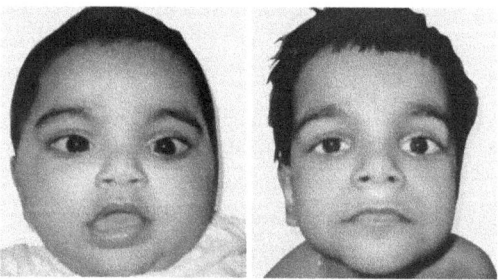

Fig. 5: Long philtrum.

- Noonan syndrome
- Rubinstein-Taybi syndrome.

LONG PHILTRUM

The philtrum or median cleft is a vertical indentation in the middle area of the lip, extending from the nasal septum to the tubercle of the upper lip.

Long philtrum is defined as the distance between the nasal base and midline upper lip vermilion border >2 standard deviation (SD) above the mean **(Fig. 5)**. Length or philtrum >13 mm in a female and >15 mm in a male is considered as long philtrum. Long philtrum is associated with several syndromes.

SHORT PHILTRUM

Short philtrum is associated with cleft lip, cri-du-chat syndrome, alagille syndrome, cranio-fascio-skeletal syndrome, DiGeorge syndrome, holoprosencephaly, etc.

SLANTING OF THE EYES

A line drawn from the inner corners to the outer corners determines the slant of eyes.
- Upward slanting of eyes **(Fig. 6)**: It is upward and lateral slant. It is also called as mongoloid slanting of eyes.
  - Racial
  - Down syndrome
  - Prader-Willi syndrome
  - Ectodermal dysplasia
- Downward slanting of eyes is seen in Sotos syndrome.

LOW SET EARS

The ear is set when the helix of the ear meet the cranium at the level below that of a horizontal plane through both inner canthi, is called low set ears **(Fig. 7)**.

Conditions Associated with Low Set Ears

- Down syndrome—(Trisomy 21)
- Turner syndrome
- Noonan syndrome
- Patau syndrome—(Trisomy 13)
- DiGeorge syndrome
- Cri-du-chat syndrome
- Edwards syndrome—(Trisomy 18)
- Fragile X syndrome
- Beckwith-Wiedemann syndrome
- Potter syndrome
- Trencher-Collins syndrome.

CRANIOTABES

Craniotabes is softening and thinning of skull bones which can be indented like a ping-pong ball **(Fig. 8)**. The sign should be elicited away from the suture line. It is found normally

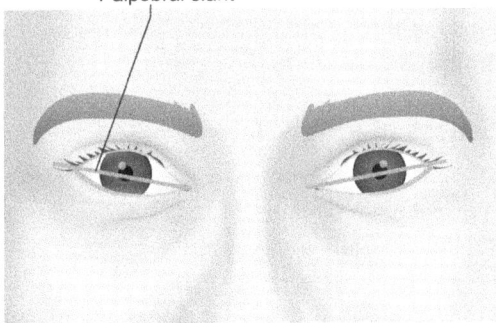

Fig. 6: Upward slanting of eyes.

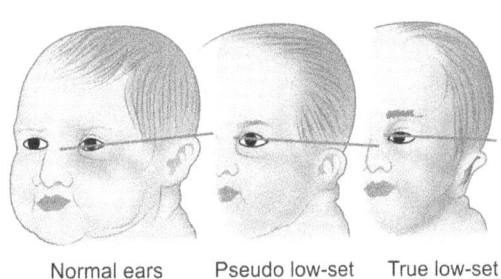

Fig. 7: Low set ears.

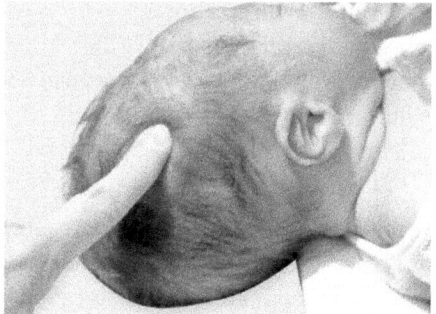

Fig. 8: Craniotabes.

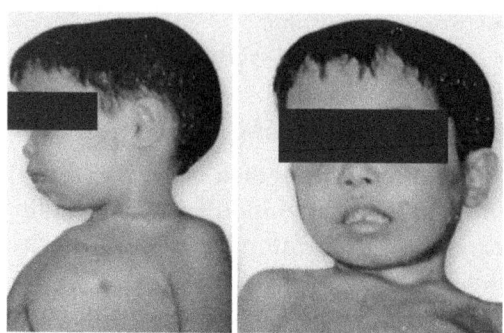

Fig. 9: Frontal bossing.

in preterm babies. It is seen mostly in the occipital and parietal bones.

Causes of Craniotabes

- Physiological
- Rickets (sign of active rickets)
- Congenital syphilis
- Hydrocephalus
- Osteogenesis imperfecta
- Lacunar skull
- Hypervitaminosis A.

BOSSING OF SKULL

Protuberance of the skull is called as bossing of skull, most often in the frontal bones of the forehead (frontal bossing) **(Fig. 9)**.

Conditions Associated with Frontal Bossing

- Rickets
- Thalassemia major
- Congenital syphilis
- Achondroplasia
- Acromegaly
- Cleidocranial dysostosis
- Crouzon syndrome
- Extramedullary hematopoiesis (chronic hemolytic anemia, chronic iron deficiency, anemia)
- Hurler syndrome
- Ectodermal dysplasia
- Pyknodysostosis
- Ehlers–Danlos syndrome.

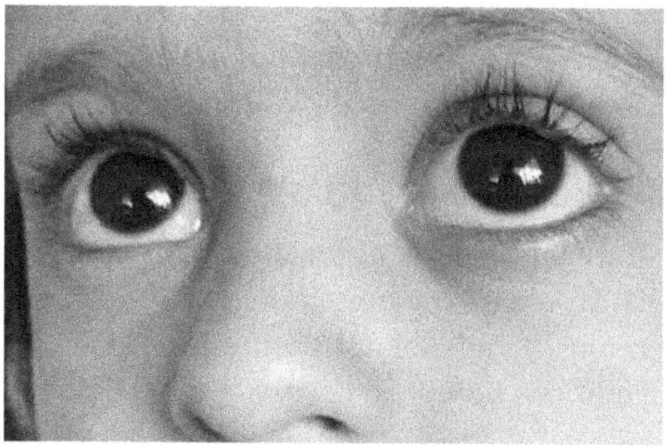

Fig. 10: Blue Sclera.

BLUE SCLERA

The blue color of the sclera is caused by thinness and transparency of the collagen fibers of the sclera, allowing the veins in the underlying tissues to show through **(Fig. 10)**.

Causes of Blue Sclera

- Normal in newborns, especially preterm
- Osteogenesis imperfecta
- Ehlers–Danlos syndrome
- Marfan syndrome
- Severe, chronic iron deficiency anemia
- Diamond-Blackfan syndrome.

Other Clinical Signs

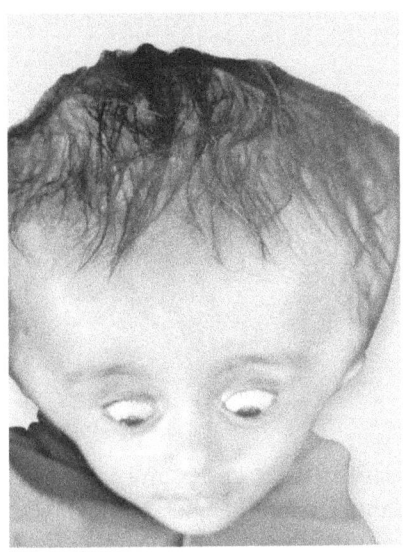

Fig. 11: Setting sun sign.

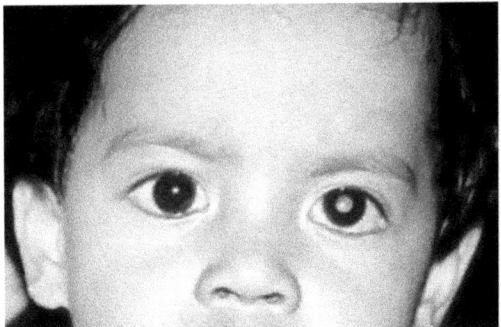

Fig. 12: Cat's eye in retinoblastoma on left side.

SETTING SUN SIGN

The eyes are rolled downward, iris is completely covered by the eyelids and upward sclera is visible. It occurs due to involvement of center of upward gaze which is located in the pretectal area of brainstem **(Fig. 11)**.

Conditions with Setting Sun Sign
- Hydrocephalus
- Kernicterus
- Parinaud syndrome
- Preterm infants (due to immaturity of reflexes)
- Laron dwarfism.

CAT'S EYE

Normally, when the light shines through the pupil, red reflex is seen. In cat's eye, it appears white, instead of normal red **(Fig. 12)**.

Causes of Cat's Eye
- Cataract
- Retinoblastoma
- Retinal detachment

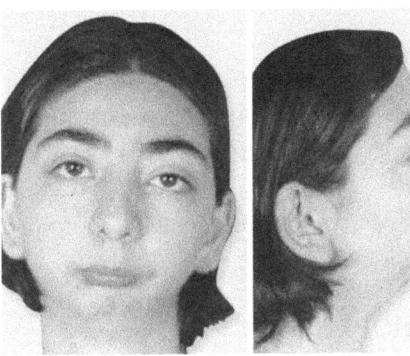

Fig. 13: Micrognathia.

- Retinopathy of prematurity
- Organized vitreous hemorrhage.

MICROGNATHIA (HYPOPLASIA OF MANDIBLE) (FIG. 13)

Causes of Micrognathia
- Pierre–Robin syndrome
- Trisomy 13 (Patau syndrome)
- Trisomy 18 (Edward syndrome)
- Cri-du-chat syndrome
- Fetal alcohol syndrome
- Trencher-Collin syndrome
- Progeria.

TRISMUS (LOCK JAW)

There is inability to open the mouth.
- Tetanus
- Temporomandibular joint arthritis

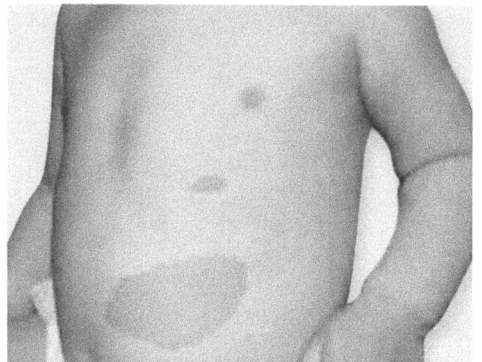

Fig. 14: Café-au-lait lesions.

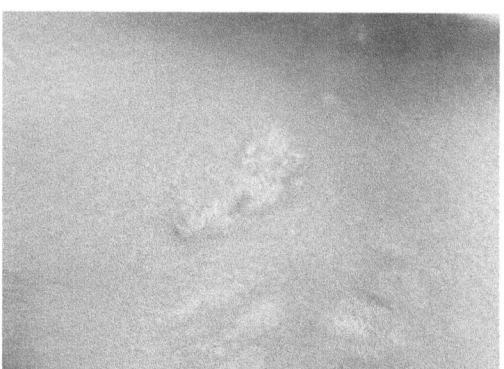

Fig. 15: Shagreen patch.

- Encephalitis
- Strychnine poisoning
- Tumor of the jaw (rhabdomyosarcoma)
- Infantile Gaucher disease
- Trauma
- Drugs: Phenothiazines, metoclopramide
- Functional.

MICROPENIS

Stretched penile length <2.5 cm in infants is diagnosed as micropenis.
- Prader–Willi syndrome
- Hypopituitarism
- Down syndrome
- Klinefelter syndrome.

CAFÉ-AU-LAIT LESIONS

Café-au-lait name is derived from French language, meaning coffee with milk, (brown coffee spots in white milk) **(Fig. 14)**.
- Café-au-lait lesions are hyperpigmented, flat macules, and light brown to dark brown.
- Café-au-lait spots with smooth borders (coast of California) are seen in neurofibromatosis.
- Café-au-lait spots with rough borders (coast of Maine) are characteristics of McCune–Albright syndrome.
- Café-au-lait spots may be earliest manifestations of neurofibromatosis.
- Pre pubertal >5 mm in size and five in numbers, while post pubertal >15 mm in size and six in numbers are considered as significant.

Conditions with Café-au-lait Lesions

- Neurofibromatosis (almost 100%)
- McCune–Albright syndrome
- Noonan syndrome
- Tuberous sclerosis
- Ataxia-telangiectasia
- Chediak–Higashi syndrome
- Fanconi disease
- Gaucher disease
- Bloom syndrome.

SHAGREEN PATCH

Shagreen patch is a plaque representing connective-tissue nevus **(Fig. 15)**. Connective-tissue nevi are uncommon skin lesions that occur when the deeper layers of the skin do not develop correctly or the components of these layers occur in the wrong proportion. Shagreen patch are oval shaped and nevoid, skin colored or occasionally pigmented, and smooth or crinkled. The word shagreen refers to a type of roughened untanned leather. Shagreen patch is the feature of tuberous sclerosis.

Other Clinical Signs

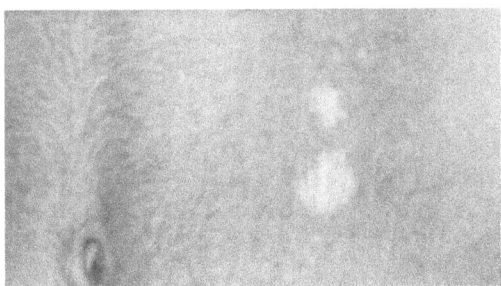

Fig. 16: Ash leaf.

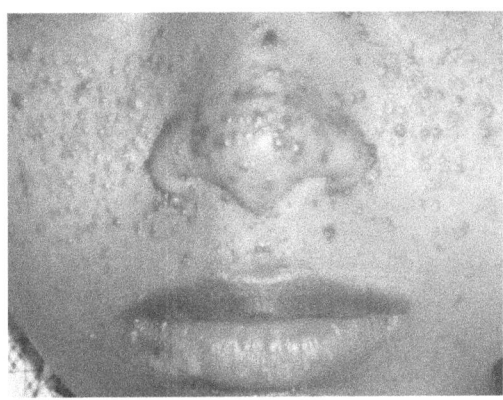

Fig. 17: Adenoma sebaceum.

ASH LEAF

This is hypomelanotic macule which is most easily visualized with a wood's light. Ash-leaf spots are found at birth or in early infancy in 87% of patients with tuberous sclerosis. The ash-leaf spot is the earliest skin lesion in tuberous sclerosis **(Fig. 16)**.

ADENOMA SEBACEUM

The typical lesions of adenoma sebaceum appear as small erythematous nodules about the center of the face, and there may be other nevoid lesions, such as pigmented spots, fibromatous nevi, and papillomas. The syndrome of epilolia includes adenoma sebaceum, and tuberous sclerosis with mental deficiency and epilepsy **(Fig. 17)**.

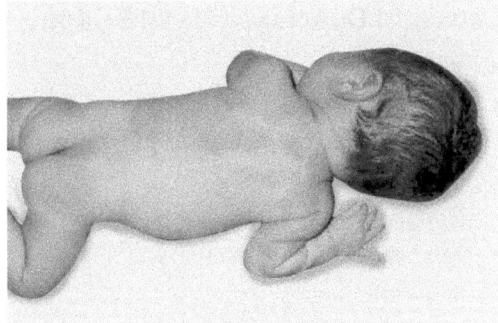

Fig. 18: Mongolian Spots.

MONGOLIAN SPOTS (MS)

New term of MS is congenital Dermal Melanocytosis. They are considered due to accumulation of melanocytes within dermis. They are bluish or slate gray macular lesions of variable size, commonly seen over lumbosacral area and buttocks. These lesions are usually benign and they disappear gradually. Persistent MS and unusual sites like shoulders and face have been found associated with GM1 gnagliosidosis, Hurler's disease, Hunter's syndrome, mucolipidosis, Niemann – Pick disease etc. **(Fig. 18)**.

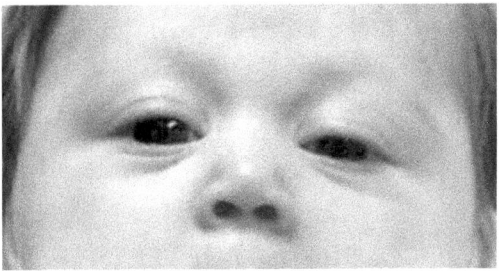

Fig. 19: Depressed nasal bridge.

DEPRESSED NASAL BRIDGE

Nasal bridge is the bony area at the top of the nose. If it is low nasal bridge, the area is flat and does not protrude. The degree of flatness can vary depending on the person **(Fig. 19)**.

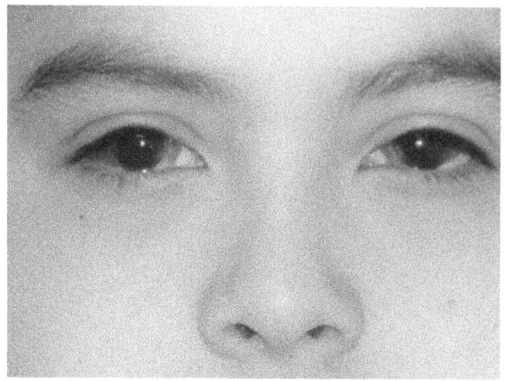

Fig. 20: Subconjunctival hemorrhage.

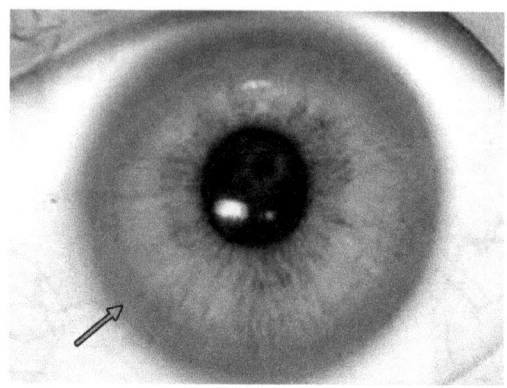

Fig. 21: Kayser–Fleischer ring.

Causes of Depressed Nasal Bridge

- Racial (Asians)
- Down syndrome
- Congenital hypothyroidism (cretinism)
- Thalassemia major
- Congenital syphilis
- Mucopolysaccharidosis (Hurler syndrome).

SUBCONJUNCTIVAL HEMORRHAGE (FIG. 20)

- Whooping cough (pertussis)
- Severe cough
- Leukemia
- Immune thrombocytopenia purpura (ITP)
- Trauma (birth or mechanical injury).

DISCOLORATION OF TEETH

- Poor orodental hygiene
- Caries
- Fluorosis
- Oral iron therapy
- Tetracycline therapy
- Porphyria
- Lead poisoning.

KAYSER–FLEISCHER (K–F) RING

Kayser-Fleischer rings are dark rings that appear to encircle the cornea of the eye **(Fig. 21)**. They are due to copper deposition in the Descemet's membrane as a result of liver diseases. Though K-F ring is pathognomonic of Wilson disease, it is also seen in various other hepatic conditions. It is seen at the sclerocorneal junction mostly as golden-brown/greenish-yellow in color. Detection of the K-F rings in asymptomatic cases can help in clinching early diagnosis and starting early treatment. K-F ring is correlated with disease severity, disappears on treatment, and reappears on discontinuation of the treatment. K-F ring is initially evident at superior and then inferior corneal poles and becomes circumferential later. Slit lamp examination is considered the best for detection of the K-F rings, but it may be detected with torchlight in later stages.

Causes of Kayser–Fleischer Rings

- Wilson disease
- Cryptogenic cirrhosis of liver
- Partial biliary atresia
- Autoimmune hepatitis.

CHERRY-RED SPOT

Due to the special features of the macula, certain diseases affecting the retina produce a visible sign on ophthalmoscopic examination of eye are called as cherry-red spot **(Fig. 22)**. It is a bright-red spot at the center of the macular surrounded and accentuated by grayish-white or yellow halo. The halo is a result of a loss of transparency of the retinal ganglion cell layer secondary to deposition of lipid substance. Because ganglion cells are not present in the fovea, the retina surrounding the fovea is opacified, but the fovea transmits the normal underlying choroidal red color, giving rise to cherry-red spot.

Cherry-red spot may develop as a result of ischemia secondary to central retinal artery occlusion or orbital contusion.

It should be appreciated that cherry-red spot is not a disease, but an ophthalmoscopic evidence of a pathology that may involve the peripheral layers of the retina and multiple systems of the body.

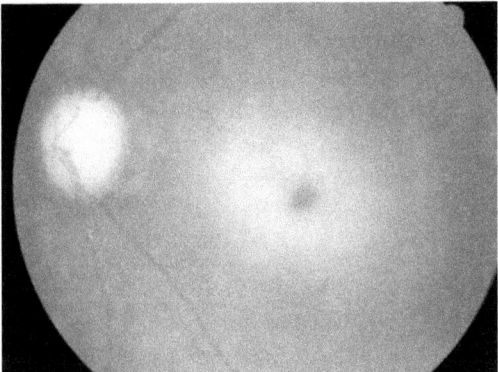

Fig. 22: Cherry-red spot.

Causes of Cherry-Red Spot

- Tay-Sachs disease
- Sandhoff disease
- GM2 gangliosidosis
- Metachromatic leukodystrophy
- Niemann-Pick disease
- Farber's disease
- Goldberg's syndrome
- Gaucher disease
- Hurler syndrome
- Spranger's disease
- Wolman disease
- Dapsone poisoning.

CHAPTER 72: Otorrhea (Ear Discharge)

INTRODUCTION

Otorrhea often arises from the external ear, in the setting of nonintact tympanic membrane, the middle and even inner ear may be source as well. Suctioning the ear discharge out of the canal to visualize the tympanic membrane is both therapeutically and diagnostically useful.

CAUSES OF OTORRHEA

- Cerumen (often brownish color, may be associated with otalgia or pruritus)
- Otitis externa
- Acute otitis media with tympanic membrane perforation
- Chronic perforation drainage
- Chronic suppurative otitis media (CSOM) —chronic middle ear and/or mastoid infection with perforated tympanic membrane; it is known to cause following complications in children:
  - Acute bacterial meningitis
  - Tuberculous meningitis
  - Tetanus
  - Mastoid abscess
  - Brain abscess
  - Cholesteatoma
- Tympanostomy tube drainage
- Cholesteatoma
- Myringitis
- Foreign body
- Eczema.

73 — Pallor (Anemia)

INTRODUCTION

Pallor is a very common symptom and sign in pediatric practice. The most common cause for pallor in children is anemia. But pale appearance may be seen in some other conditions as well, which should be kept in mind.

CAUSES OF PALLOR

- Anemia
- Poor perfusion (shock): Due to peripheral vasoconstriction
- Nephrotic syndrome (due to edema)
- Congestive heart failure (decreased perfusion)
- Vasovagal syncope
- Hypothyroidism.

ANEMIA

Definition

Anemia is defined as reduction in the oxygen-carrying capacity of blood, due to reduced hemoglobin (Hb) concentration and red cell mass [hematocrit (HCT)], leading to tissue hypoxia.

World Health Organization (WHO) cutoff values for diagnosis of anemia

Age/Sex	Hb (g/dL)
• New born	<14
• At 3 months	<9

Contd...

Contd...

Age/Sex	Hb (g/dL)
• 6 months to 6 years	<11
• 6–14 years	<12
• Adult males	<13
• Adult females	<12
• Pregnant women	<11

Grades of Anemia

- Mild: Hb <10 g/dL
- Moderate: Hb 7–10 g/dL
- Severe: Hb 7–5 g/dL
- Very severe: Hb <5 g/dL.

Clinical Features

- Pallor
- Tiredness
- Lassitude
- Easy fatigability
- Weakness
- Behavioral changes
- Decreased cognition
- Decreased scholastic performance
- Poor academic achievement
- Irritability
- Excessive crying
- Breath-holding spell (BHS)
- Temper tantrums
- Shortness of breath (exercise intolerance)
- Growth retardation.

CAUSES OF ANEMIA

- *Decreased (inadequate) red blood cells (RBCs) production:*
  - Bone marrow pathology (hypoplastic or infiltrative disorders)
  - Deficiency of hematopoietic factors (nutritional) (iron, vitamin B_{12}, folic acid, etc.)
- *Blood loss:*
  - Hemorrhage (trauma)
  - Gastrointestinal (GI) tract bleeding (overt or occult)
  - Worms infestations (hook worms)
- *Increased destruction of RBCs (hemolytic anemia):*
  - Congenital:
    - Hemoglobinopathy (thalassemia, sickle cell disease)
    - RBC cell wall (membrane) defect (hereditary spherocytosis)
    - Enzymatic defects (G6PD deficiency, pyruvate kinase deficiency)
    - Autoimmune hemolytic anemia
  - Acquired:
    - Malaria
    - Hemolytic uremic syndrome (HUS).

TIME TAKEN TO DEVELOP ANEMIA

Symptoms depend upon not only on severity but also on time taken to develop anemia (rate of drop of Hb).

Acute Anemia

- Hemorrhage (external or internal)
- *Hemolysis:*
- Enzyme deficiency (G6PD deficiency)
- Immune mechanism (autoimmune hemolytic anemia)
- Severe complicated malaria
- Presence of icterus suggests hemolysis or internal hemorrhage
- Child may present with signs of congestive cardiac failure, breathlessness, and restlessness.

Chronic Anemia

- Chronic blood loss can be either obvious (recurrent hematemesis) or occult (occult blood loss in stools).
- Chronic hemolysis can be due to recurrent malaria in endemic areas.
- Children may remain asymptomatic for long duration if the onset of anemia is insidious (may be brought walking with minimal symptoms even though Hb is as low as 3–5 g/dL).

HISTORY TAKING

Age

- *Neonates:*
  - Blood loss (fetomaternal hemorrhage, hemorrhagic disease of newborn)
  - Hemolytic disorders (Rh incompatibility, ABO incompatibility, G6PD deficiency, malaria, hereditary spherocytosis)
- *Anemia in childhood:*
  - Nutritional anemia (most common) (6 months to 3 years)
  - Beta thalassemia (most cases present at 6 months)
  - Alpha thalassemia (anemia or hydrops fetalis just after birth)
  - Congenital bone marrow aplasia (soon after birth) (Diamond-Blackfan syndrome).

Family History

- G6PD deficiency is more common in Parsis and Sindhis.
- Thalassemia is more common in Punjabis, Lohanas, Kutchhis, Khatris, and Mahars.

- Sickle cell disease is more common in tribal community.
- History of (H/o) beta-thalassemia (BT) indicates an inherited cause such as thalassemia, G6PD deficiency, and hereditary spherocytosis.
- Repeated history of blood transfusions usually indicates non-nutritional anemia such as hemoglobinopathy and bone marrow hypofunction.
- Pedigree chart including expired members should be charted meticulously including two generations on each side:
  - X-linked disorder (G6PD deficiency)
  - Autosomal recessive (thalassemia)
  - Autosomal dominant (hereditary spherocytosis)
- H/o consanguineous marriage is helpful to recessive conditions.
- A family history of neonatal hyperbilirubinemia, jaundice, splenomegaly, splenectomy, and gall stones should be asked. It suggests hemolytic anemia like hereditary spherocytosis.

Dietary History
- Predominantly milk-based diet with minimal or no complementary feeding is more likely to suffer from nutritional anemia. It is common in infants and toddlers.
- H/o pica suggests worm infestations and iron deficiency anemia.
- A child on goat's milk is predisposed to folic acid deficiency and megaloblastic anemia.
- Cow's milk allergy has been reported in children who are on cow's milk and on breastfed infants whose mother is consuming cow's milk.
- Exclusively breastfed infants are less likely to develop iron deficiency anemia in spite of poor source of iron in breast milk due to its good bioavailability.
- Megaloblastic anemia is found in vegetarians due to less availability of vitamin B_{12}.
- Megaloblastic anemia develops in nonvegetarians due to lack of green vegetables in their food, resulting in folic acid deficiency.

History of bleeding
- H/o skin bleeds (petechiae or ecchymosis) or bleeding from any other sites suggests platelets or hepatic involvement and chronic liver disorder.
- Skin bleeds associated with anemia and fever may be due to hypoplastic or infiltrative bone marrow disorders.
- Stool examination for consecutive 3 days for occult blood is very important. It may be due to drugs like aspirin, cow's milk allergy, Crohn's disease, ulcerative colitis, etc.
- Painless, massive bleeding per rectum may be in a case of polyp or Meckel's diverticulum.

History of Drug Ingestion
- Chloramphenicol, non-steroidal anti-inflammatory drugs (NSAIDs), and sulfas can cause bone marrow hypoplasia.
- Cephalosporin and alpha-methyldopa can cause hemolysis
- Primaquine, nitrofurantoin, sulfas, furazolidone, etc., can cause hemolysis in children with G6PD deficiency.
- Pyrimethamine (antifolate) and phenytoin are known to cause megaloblastic anemia.

History of Infections
- Malaria
- Chronic bacterial infections
- Kala-azar.

PHYSICAL EXAMINATION
- Pulse, respiratory rate, and blood pressure (BP) indicate severity of anemia.

- Look for pallor, puffiness of face, edema of feet, jugular venous pressure (JVP), and tenderness of liver to diagnose congestive heart failure.
- Hypertension in a case of anemia may be due to renal disease or collagen disease like systemic lupus erythematosus (SLE).
- *Facies:*
  - Hemolytic facies: Frontal and parietal bossing, large head, depressed nasal bridge, malar prominence, sallow complexion, malocclusion of teeth
  - Cretin facies in hypothyroidism
  - Diamond–Blackfan is characterized by box-like face, high arched palate, and triphalangeal thumb.
- *Eyes:*
  - Microcornea (Fanconi anemia)
  - Conjunctival vessels tortuosity (sickle cell disease)
  - Mild jaundice without high-colored urine indicates hemolytic anemia
  - Blindness in osteopetrosis
- *Nail changes:*
  - Platynychia, kolionychia, and brittle nails are suggestive of iron deficiency.
  - Dyskeratotic nails in dyskeratosis congenita
  - Anemia and clubbing:
    - Celiac disease
    - Crohn's disease
    - Ulcerative colitis
    - Bacterial endocarditis
    - Arteriovenous malformations
- *Lymphadenopathy:*
  - Leukemia
  - Lymphoma
  - Human immunodeficiency virus (HIV)
  - Tuberculosis
  - Epstein–Barr virus (EBV)
- *Hepatosplenomegaly:*
  - Malaria
  - Hemolytic anemia
  - Thalassemia
  - Leukemia, lymphoma, chronic myeloid leukemia (CML)
  - Portal hypertension
  - HIV
  - Kala-azar
  - Tropical splenomegaly
- *Bleeding manifestations:*
  - Hypoplastic/aplastic bone marrow
  - Malignancy
- *Mucosal changes:*
  - Glossitis, angular cheilosis, bald tongue in iron, vitamin B_{12}, and folic acid deficiency.
- *Skeletal changes:*
  - Anemia, thrombocytopenia and absent radius [thrombocytopenia-absent radius (TAR) syndrome].
  - Bifid thumb, triphalangeal thumb, polydactyly, syndactyly, short stature, microcephaly, etc., may be seen in Diamond–Blackfan syndrome, Fanconi anemia, dyskeratosis congenita, etc.
- *Skin changes:*
  - Pallor
  - Multiple nutrients deficiency
  - Hyperpigmented knuckles (vitamin B_{12} and folic acid deficiency)
  - Generalized hyperpigmentation (Fanconi anemia)
  - Nonhealing ulcer over lower limb (chronic hemolytic anaemia especially sickle cell disease)
  - Hemangioma (Kasabach–Merrit syndrome)
- *Palmar pallor:*
  - No pallor (no anemia)
  - Palmar pallor (some anemia)
  - Palmar creases pallor (severe anemia)

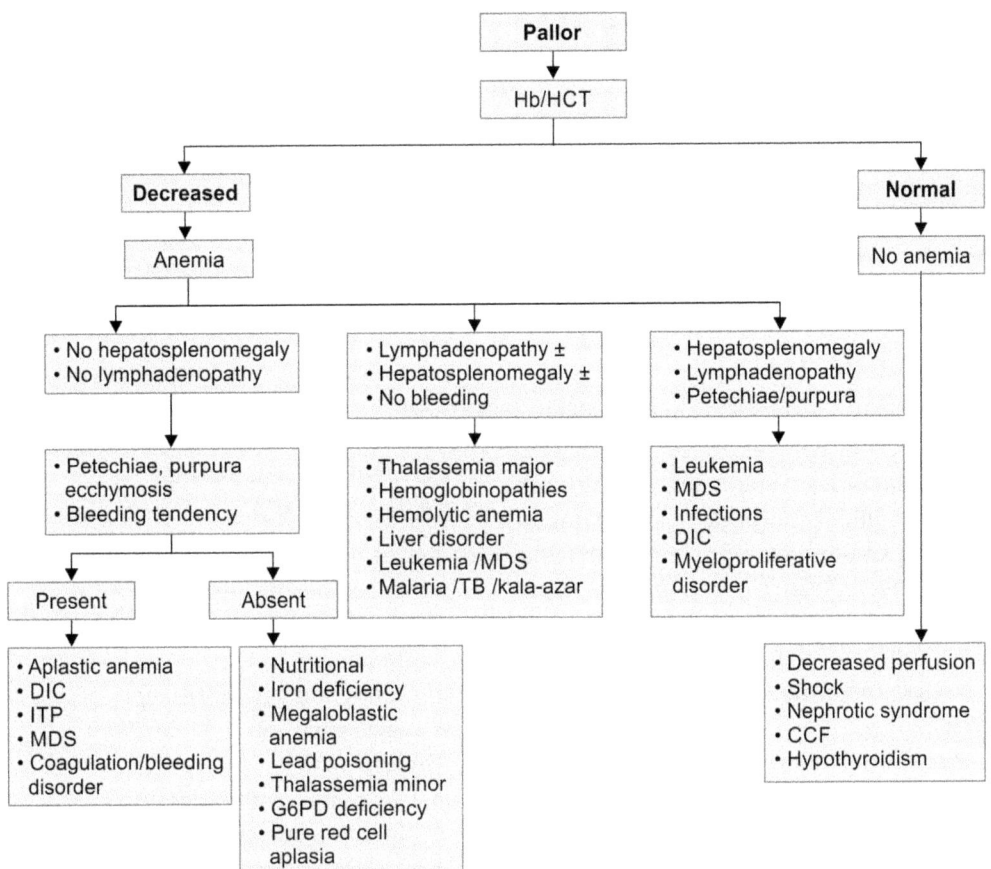

(CCF: congestive cardiac failure; DIC: disseminated intravascular coagulation; Hb: hemoglobin; HCT: hematocrit; ITP: immune thrombocytopenia; MDS: myelodysplastic syndrome; TB: tuberculosis)

Papilledema

INTRODUCTION

The ophthalmic examination of the eyes is an integral part of clinical examination. Every clinician should learn ophthalmic examination of eyes. Papilledema (optic disc swelling or edema) is an ominous sign. In papilledema, the optic nerve head is hyperemic, the cup is full, margins blurred with peripapillary retinal edema and hemorrhages, and the retinal veins at the disk are tortuous and dilated **(Figs. 1A and B)**.

Papilledema may be asymmetric, unilateral, or bilateral. In acute papilledema, acuity of vision, color vision, and pupillary reflexes may be normal, but the field of vision is affected. Chronic papilledema leads to loss of vision and loss of visual fields. Papilledema is most commonly due to raised intracranial pressure.

COMMON CAUSES OF PAPILLEDEMA

- *Raised intracranial pressure:*
  - Space-occupying lesions
  - Hydrocephalus
  - Meningitis
  - Intracranial hemorrhage
  - Hypertension
- *Optic neuritis:*
  - Post-viral syndromes
  - Meningoencephalitis
  - Loss of vision or pain on eye movements
  - Vision usually improves within a few weeks

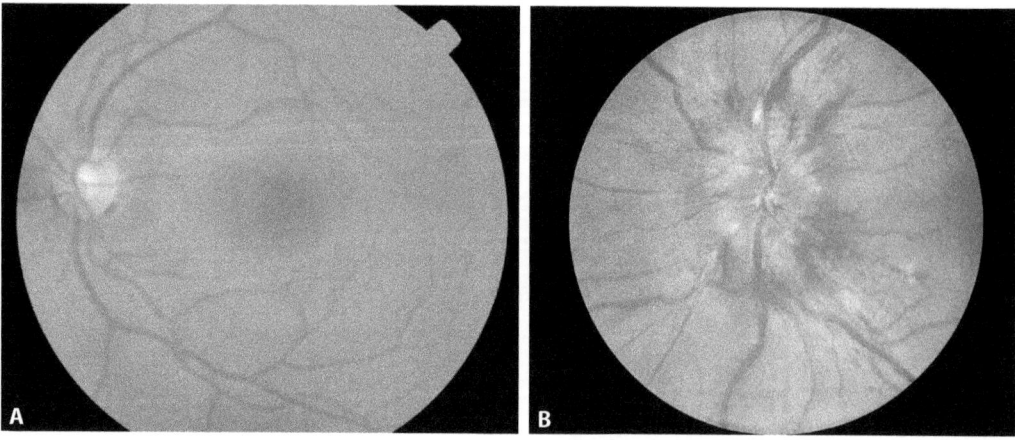

Figs. 1A and B: A. Normal fundus examination; B. Signs of papilledema.

- *Optic neuropathy:*
  - Compressive (neurofibromatosis, optic nerve glioma)
  - Infiltrative diseases [leukemia, lymphoma, tuberculosis, sarcoidosis, toxoplasmosis, and cytomegalovirus (CMV) infection]
  - Toxic/nutritional optic neuropathy (thiamine, vitamin B_{12}, tobacco, and alcohol)
- Retinal hemorrhage and loss of vision
- Malignant hypertension

- *Pseudotumor cerebri (benign raised intracranial pressure):*
  - Nausea, head, vomiting, diplopia, and transient impairment of vision are manifestations.
  - Normal cerebrospinal fluid (CSF)
  - Normal radioimaging
  - More common in obese persons. Drugs such as nalidixic acid, vitamin A, vitamin D, and steroids are known to cause pseudotumor cerebri.

Parotid Gland Swelling

INTRODUCTION

The normal parotid gland is not palpable. Mumps is the most common cause of parotid gland swelling. In some cases, swelling of the parotid gland is recurrent which requires methodological evaluation. Lymphadenopathy and masseter muscle hypertrophy may mimic parotid swelling, which should be differentiated.

The common causes of parotid gland swelling are as follows:
- *Infections:*
  - Viral infections:
    - Mumps
    - Parainfluenza types 1 and 3
    - Human immunodeficiency virus (HIV)
    - Coxsackie viruses A and B
    - Varicella
    - Cytomegalovirus (CMV)
    - Epstein–Barr virus
    - Herpes simplex virus
  - Bacterial infections (acute suppurative infections)
    - *Staphylococcal aureus*
    - Streptococcus
- *Abscess of parotid gland:*
  - Tuberculosis (uncommon)
  - Actinomycosis
  - Cat-scratch disease (granuloma, facial swelling, preauricular lymphadenitis)
  - Brucellosis
  - Histoplasmosis
- *Chronic/recurrent sialadenitis:*
  - Benign lymphoepithelial lesion
  - Functional hypersecretion
  - Allergic
  - Drug sensitivity (iodides in drugs or food)
- *Tumors:*
  - Hemangioma (soft, nontender swelling, and bluish hue to the overlying skin)
  - Lymphangioma (diffuse swelling)
  - Mixed tumor (most common, benign tumors, firm, and painless mass)
  - Pleomorphic adenoma
  - Mucoepidermoid tumor
  - Acinic carcinoma and rhabdomyosarcoma (rare)
- *Metabolic and endocrine disorders:*
  - Hypothyroidism
  - Cushing syndrome
  - Diabetes mellitus
  - Anorexia nervosa/bulimia
  - Starvation (parotid hypertrophy)
- *Obstructive enlargement:*
  - Strictures:
    - Congenital
    - Secondary to poor oral hygiene
    - Dental trauma
    - Recurrent infections
    - Calculi
- *Miscellaneous:*
  - Autoimmune disorders:
    - Sjogren syndrome
    - Systemic lupus erythematosus (SLE)
    - Mixed connective tissue disease
    - Sarcoidosis
    - Impaction of Stensen's duct with a food particle.

76. Pica

INTRODUCTION

Pica is a common problem in pediatric office practice. Pica ia defined as compulsive, irresistable, perversion of eating inedible or non nutritive substances. The exact cause of pica is not known, some nutritional and neuropsychiatric causes are considered responsible for it. Various complications can develop following pica and therefore its proper management is important.

- The term "pica" is derived from Latin word magpie, picave, a bird, which is known for its unusual behavior of eating almost anything.
- Pica is defined as persistent or compulsive perversion of appetite with ingestion of inedible or nonnutritive substances over a period of at least 1 month. The mouthing and tasting of objects is considered as normal in infants and toddlers, but certainly inappropriate beyond the age of 2 years.
- Pica can occur throughout life, but occurs most frequently in children. It is also seen in pregnant women, especially in India and Africa.

COMMON TYPES OF PICA

- Eating earth, soil, clay, chalk, etc. (geophagia)
- Consumption of ice (pagophagia)
- Consumption of starch (amylophagia)
- Consumption of hairs and wool (trichophagia)
- Consumption of wood (xylophagia)
- Consumption of excrement (coprophagia)
- Consumption of glass (hyalophagia)
- Other substances such as pebbles, paper, string, ashes, crayons, plastic objects, nails, and screws.

ETIOLOGY

The cause is unknown. Different theories have been proposed.

- *Cultural, ethnic and familial theory:* In some cultures there is custom of eating soil for different illnesses, e.g., morning sickness which leads to perception that nothing is wrong with pica.
- *Nutritional theory:* Iron, calcium, and zinc deficiencies are considered to increase the craving for nonfood substances.
- *Neuropsychiatric causes:*
  - Intellectual disability
  - Developmental disability
  - Child abuse and neglect
  - Family disorganization
  - Schizophrenia
  - Autism
- Genetic disorders like Prader-Willi syndrome.

COMPLICATIONS OF PICA

- Iron deficiency anemia
- Worm infestations
- Lead poisoning
- Life-threatening toxicities
- Intestinal obstruction
- Constipation
- Intestinal ulceration and perforation
- Trichobezoar.

Pollakiuria (Increased Frequency of Micturition)

INTRODUCTION

Pollakiuria or increased frequency of micturition is another very commonly encountered complaint which may or may not be associated with burning micturition.

- Usually older children void six to eight times a day. If the child passes urine more than eight times a day or there is increased frequency compared to usual daily one, it can be considered as pollakiuria (increased frequency of micturition).
- A normal newborn passes urine 10–15 times a day in small quantities which is physiological. A newborn has not matured urinary bladder functions (sympathetic, parasympathetic, and somatic nervous systems). It works as autonomic urinary bladder (involuntary, spontaneous, reflex emptying of the urinary bladder).
- Pollakiuria can be due to certain habits which are not due to underlying disease. It can be due to drinking a large amount of liquids, increased caffeine (tea, coffee) intake, increased citrus fruits intake, beverages, etc. It can also be due to anxiety and change in weather.
- Increased urinary frequency and passing large amount of urine (polyuria) each time may be in a case of diabetes mellitus or diabetes insipidus while increased urinary frequency but passing small quantity of urine each time may be due to incomplete emptying of bladder as in a case of posterior urethral valve. Therefore, it is vital to ascertain the amount of urine passed by the child each time.
- *Red flags:* There are certain red flags indicating some underlying disease which requires prompt attention:
  - Burning or painful micturition
  - Hematuria
  - Loss of bladder control (fullness of bladder, dribbling of urine, incontinence, etc.)
  - Urge incontinence
  - Associated symptoms like fever, pain in abdomen, vomiting, increased thirst, weight loss, and vaginal or penile discharge.
- Look for puffiness of eyelids, pedal edema, and tenderness over abdomen or renal angle. One needs to examine locally for perineal redness, diaper rash in newborns, phimosis in boys, and vaginitis in girls.

COMMON CAUSES OF POLLAKIURIA

- Consumption of large amounts of fluids
- Excessive intake of caffeine-containing liquids (tea, coffee), beverages, citrus fruits, etc.
- Anxiety, stress due to examination, performances in school, sports, etc.
- *Urinary tract infection:*
  - Fever, burning micturition, abdominal or loin pain, and vomiting are common associated symptoms in older children.

- Younger children may present only with fever without focus.
- *Cystitis:* Increased frequency of micturition, lower abdominal pain, urgency, and dysuria suggest cystitis, which is more common in adolescent girls. Usually, fever is not the major symptom in cystitis as it is in acute pyelonephritis.
- *Diabetes mellitus:*
  - Polyuria (especially nocturnal enuresis)
  - Polydipsia
  - Polyphagia
  - Weight loss
  - Generalized weakness
  - Vulvovaginitis (fungal)
- *Diabetes insipidus:*
  - Polyuria (not burning micturition) (recently started secondary nocturnal enuresis)
  - Polydipsia
  - Weight loss
  - Dehydration and dyselectrolytemia
  - May be central (involving neurohypophysis resulting in vasopressin deficiency) or nephrogenic (not responding to vasopressin) in origin
- *Posterior urethral valve:* In this condition, the child may have increased frequency of micturition since he is not able to empty the bladder fully and he passes urine frequently but in small quantity. The urinary bladder may be palpable.
- *Drugs:* Hypervitaminosis D, carbamazepine, antihistaminics, etc., may cause pollakiuria.
- It may be an attention-seeking device by some children.

78. Polydipsia

INTRODUCTION

Polydipsia is an excessive thirst that leads to the consumption of larger than normal volume of fluid. The recommended daily fluid intake varies in neonates, infants, and children, based on age and gender, as follows:

Up to 6 months	150–200 mL/kg/day
7–12 months	600 mL/day
1–3 years	900 mL/day
4–8 years	1,200 mL/day
9–13 years	Boys—1,800 mL/day; girls—1,600 mL/day
14–18 years	Boys—2,600 mL/day; girls—1,800 mL/day

- Polydipsia is a rather uncommon symptom in children. The centers in the ventromedial and anterior hypothalamus integrate signals that decide water ingestion.
- Most common conditions presenting with polydipsia in children are diabetes mellitus and diabetes insipidus. Some drugs may alter thirst and psychological factors also have a profound effect, presenting as polydipsia. Other causes of polydipsia may be neurogenic, endocrinal, metabolic, renal, etc.

COMMON CAUSES OF POLYDIPSIA

- *Metabolic-endocrinal causes:*
  - Diabetes mellitus (polydipsia, polyuria, polyphagia, and weight loss)
  - Diabetes insipidus [antidiuretic hormone (ADH) production is deficit or insensitivity to ADH].
  - Hypercalcemia (anorexia, constipation, failure to thrive (FTT), and renal calculi)
  - Hyperaldosteronism (primary, pseudohyperaldosteronism)
  - Pheochromocytoma
  - Bartter syndrome
  - Neuroblastoma
  - Cystinosis
- *Renal causes:*
  - Sickle cell anemia
  - Renal tubular acidosis (polyuria, polydipsia, FTT, constipation, anorexia, lethargy, and rickets)
  - Nephrogenic diabetes insipidus (X-linked disorder, dehydration, FTT, fever, and no response to vasopressin)
  - Interstitial nephritis
  - Medullary cystic diseases of kidney
- Psychogenic polydipsia (compulsive water drinkers and immature behavior)
- Neurogenic disorder (hypothalamic lesions causing ADH deficiency)
- *Miscellaneous:*
  - Drugs: Diuretics and verapamil
  - Congestive heart failure
  - Hypertension.

Polyphagia

INTRODUCTION

Polyphagia, also called hyperphagia, refers to excessive hunger or increased appetite. There is excessive consumption of food or display of food-seeking behavior.

COMMON CAUSES OF POLYPHAGIA

- Diabetes mellitus (polyphagia, polydipsia, and polyuria)
- Hyperthyroidism (increased metabolic rate, increased appetite, weight loss, diarrhea, tremor)
- Hypoglycemia
- Diabetes insipidus
- Exogenous obesity
- Depression
- Anxiety
- Bulimia
- *Hypothalamic lesions:*
  - Hypothalamic dysfunction
  - Hypothalamic tumors (craniopharyngioma)
  - Tuberculous meningitis
  - Autoimmune disorders
  - Head injury
- *Genetic syndromes:*
  - Prader-Willi syndrome
  - Laurence-Moon-Biedl syndrome
- Cystic fibrosis
- Giardiasis
- Premenstrual syndrome
- *Drugs:*
  - Corticosteroids
  - Cyproheptadine
  - Valproic acid
  - Tricyclic antidepressants
  - Neuroleptics.

Chapter 80: Pruritus

INTRODUCTION

Pruritus is the desire to scratch that is induced by unpleasant skin sensations. It is commonly due to histamine and other endogenous substances.

CAUSES OF PRURITUS

Exogenous Causes

- Contacts (nickel, chemicals, cosmetics, dye, soap, wool, etc.)
- Irritants (soaps, saliva, bubble bath, diaper dermatitis, woolen clothes)
- Allergens (plant dermatitis, colors, cosmetics, etc.)
- *Parasitic infestations and insect bites:*
  - Scabies
  - Papular urticaria (insect bites, scabies)
  - Pediculosis
  - Swimmer's bath
  - Seabath
  - Ancylostoma duodenale
  - Enterobius vermicularis
- Foreign bodies
- *Environmental factors:*
  - Drying of skin (winter season)
  - Excessive bathing
  - High humidity.

Endogenous Causes

- Atopic dermatitis
- Infantile eczema
- Seborrheic dermatitis
- Drug reactions (aspirin, barbiturates, antibiotics, opiates, griseofulvin, etc.)
- Uremia
- Hepatobiliary diseases (cholestasis)
- Hypothyroidism
- Hyperthyroidism
- Diabetes mellitus
- Carcinoid tumors
- Malignancies
- Human immunodeficiency virus (HIV)
- Blood dyscrasias
- Juvenile rheumatoid arthritis
- Systemic lupus erythematosus
- Psychogenic
- Psoriasis
- Urticaria
- Stevens–Johnson syndrome.

81. Ptosis

INTRODUCTION

Ptosis (blepharoptosis) is often an overlooked sign that may serve as a manifestation of other conditions, ranging from a mild and purely cosmetic presentation to a severe and occasionally progressive disorder.

- Ptosis refers to a drooping or inferior displacement of the upper eyelid with associated narrowing of the vertical palpebral fissure. It might be severe in that the pupils are completely covered causing visual disturbances.
- Two separate muscles are involved in the elevation of the upper eyelid, the levator palpebrae superioris which is innervated by the superior branch of the oculomotor (III) cranial nerve and the superior tarsal muscle (Müller's muscle) which is innervated by the cervical sympathetic system and elevates the posterior portion of the eye lid.
- Ptosis may be:
  - Familial or sporadic
  - Acute or chronic
  - Unilateral or bilateral
  - Progressive or nonprogressive
  - Isolated or associated with other ocular anomalies and systemic disorders
  - Congenital (noticed at birth or during the first year of life) or acquired (often associated with neuromuscular disorders)
- *Pseudoptosis:* It resembles ptosis but it occurs because of a different etiology.
  - Pseudoptosis may be related to lack of physical support to the eyelid secondary to a defective ocular globe like anophthalmia and microphthalmia.
  - Dermatochalasis (redundant eye lid skin)
  - Eye infections
  - Corneal abrasions
  - Presence of foreign body in the eye
- *Acute ptosis:*
  - Bell's palsy (facial neve palsy)
  - Botulism (exotoxin produced by *Clostridium botulinum*)
  - Miller Fisher syndrome (variant of Guillain–Barré syndrome)
  - Ophthalmologic migraine
  - Oculomotor (III) nerve palsy (inflammatory, traumatic, and neurotoxic)
- *Chronic ptosis:* It is classified into congenital and acquired varieties.
- *Congenital ptosis:*
  - Isolated congenital ptosis:
    - Muscle fibrosis of levator palpebrae superioris
    - Defective or abnormal muscle innervations
    - May be symmetric or asymmetric and unilateral or bilateral
    - May be familial
    - Hemangioma of eyelid.

- Congenital cranial dysinnervation disorders:
  - A group of disorders resulting from anomalous innervation of the ocular and facial musculature
  - Duane retraction syndrome
  - Blepharophimosis, ptosis, and epicanthus inversus syndrome
  - Congenital fibrosis of the extraocular muscles
  - Marcus Gunn phenomenon
  - Horner syndrome
  - Congenital facial palsy
  - Congenital myasthenic syndromes
  - Turner syndrome
  - Noonan syndrome
  - Rubinstein–Taybi syndrome
- *Acquired ptosis:* It is usually characterized by a progressive and severe course. Several metabolic, neuromuscular, muscular, and traumatic conditions may clinically present with ptosis.
  - Myasthenia gravis
  - Chronic progressive external ophthalmoplegia (mitochondrial disease)
  - Oculopharyngeal muscular dystrophy
  - Myotonic dystrophy.

Pulse Rate—Abnormality

INTRODUCTION

Examination of pulse is routine in clinical medicine. It should be counted for full 1 minute. The pulse rate is a subject of wide fluctuation, especially in newborns and young infants due to crying and excitement. In older children, the pulse rate may be higher after a meal and in afternoon than in the morning. The pulse rate slows as the child grows.

DEFINITION OF PULSE

Pulse is defined as expansion of the vessel wall due to propagation of waves, produced by movement of blood column ejected from the heart during each systolic contraction which is felt by a palpating finger.

Points to Be Noted During Pulse Examination

- Presence/absence
- Rate
- Volume
- Force
- Tension
- Character of pulse
- Radiofemoral/radioradial delay
- Pulse apex deficit
- Condition of the vessel wall
- Other arterial pulsations.

TACHYCARDIA

Cutoff values of resting pulse rate for tachycardia.

Age	Tachycardia
Newborn	>160
<2 years	>120
Older children	>100

- Tachycardia is common in pediatric age group and the cause is often benign.
- Any child with tachycardia requires proper assessment of patient status and cardiac rhythm.

Causes of Tachycardia in Children

- *Life-threatening cardiac conditions:*
  - Supraventricular tachycardia (SVT)
  - Ventricular tachycardia (VT)
  - Atrial fibrillation
  - Atrial flutter
  - Hypertrophic cardiomyopathy (HCM)
  - Cardiomyopathy
  - Myocarditis
  - Pericardial effusion
- *Life-threatening noncardiac conditions:*
  - Hypoxemia
  - Hypovolemia (shock)
  - Hypoglycemia
  - Anaphylaxis
  - Sepsis
  - Toxic response
  - Hyperkalemia
  - Hypocalcemia
  - Hypomagnesemia
  - Pheochromocytoma

- Common conditions:
  - Fever
  - Crying
  - Exercise
  - Pain
  - Anxiety
  - Anemia
  - Drug-induced (caffeine, tobacco, albuterol)
- Other conditions:
  - Kawasaki disease
  - Acute rheumatic fever
  - Hyperthyroidism.

PALPITATIONS

Palpitations describe a noticeable heartbeat that may be concerning to the patient. It refers to a sensation that the heart is beating faster, irregularly, or harder than normal. Palpitations in children are relatively common; many a time, they are completely normal. However, it is important to rule out any serious cause.

Cause of Palpitations

In general, palpitations can be caused by three different mechanisms:
- *High adrenaline state:* It is the most common mechanism in children; a child who is anxious or experiencing an emotion such as fear will be in a high adrenaline state. In this setting, the adrenaline produces a faster and strong heartbeat than normal. Many children with a high adrenaline state experience other symptoms such as chest pain, shortness of breath, dizziness, excessive sweating, or fatigue. These additional symptoms are also due to adrenaline. There is no need of any treatment.
- *Premature cardiac contractions (extra heartbeats):* A premature contracture may come from either atria or the ventricle. They are called premature atrial contractions or premature ventricular contractions. They are atrial fibrillation, atrial flutter, and ventricular tachycardia.
- *Supraventricular tachycardia:* It is due to an abnormal electrical pathway.

Causes of Palpitations in Children

- *Life-threatening cardiac conditions:*
  - Arrhythmias:
    - Wolff-Parkinson-White (WPW) syndrome
    - Prolonged QT syndrome
    - Structural cardiac abnormalities such as Ebstein anomaly, and intracardiac tumor.
  - HCM:
    - Myocarditis
    - Sick sinus syndrome
    - Pacemaker malfunction
- *Life-threatening noncardiac conditions:*
  - Hypoglycemia
  - Toxic exposure
  - Pheochromocytoma
- *Other conditions:*
  - Premature atrial contractions
  - Premature ventricular contractions
  - Fever
  - Anemia
  - Exercise
  - Panic attack
  - Emotional arousal
  - Drug-induced (caffeine, tobacco, antihistaminics)
  - Hyperthyroidism
  - Mitral valve prolapse
  - Acute rheumatic carditis.

BRADYCARDIA

Bradycardia is defined as heart rate below the normal for age, as follows:
- *Newborn:* <100/min

- *<2 years:* <90/min
- *Older children:* <60/min

Conduction system of heart, parasympathetic and sympathetic systems play an important role for bradycardia.

Causes of Bradycardia

- Physiological (athlete, familial)
- Hypothyroidism [decreased basal metabolic rate (BMR)]
- Jaundice [deposition of bile salts and bile pigments at sinoatrial (SA) node]
- Raised intracranial pressure (vagal stimulation)
- Heart block
- Drugs (propranolol, digitalis, clonidine, opiates)
- Structural heart diseases [atrial septal defect (ASD)]
- Long QT syndrome
- Systemic lupus erythematosus (SLE)
- *Surgical trauma:*
  - Closure of ASD
  - Fontan
- The pulse rate increases by 10 for each degree of rise in body temperature. If it is not proportionate, it is called relative bradycardia. Relative bradycardia is seen in enteric fever in older children and adults, brucellosis, Epstein–Barr viral infection, etc.

Pyrexia of Unknown Origin

INTRODUCTION

Pyrexia of unknown origin (PUO) is also called fever of unknown origin (FUO).

- *Definition:* PUO is defined as fever (rectal temperature >38.3°C/100.4°F) documented by a healthcare personnel on several occasions, for which no cause is identifiable after 3 weeks of outpatient evaluation or after 1 week of evaluation as an inpatient that includes detailed history, thorough clinical examination, and initial laboratory assessment.
- *Reasonable working definition of PUO for most clinical purpose is:*
  Fever of >101°F, lasting for >1 week in whom no diagnosis is apparent after initial outpatient or inpatient evaluation which includes detailed history, physical examination, and initial laboratory assessment.
  - Fever without focus (FWF) is defined as fever <7 days' duration where no focus is apparent after detailed history and physical examination.

  FWF and FUO are same where diagnosis is not obvious to the clinician. Those children in whom fever duration falls short of FUO definitions are termed FWF.
- *FUO is differentiated from FWF for the following reasons:*
  - Differential diagnosis (D/D) and most frequent causes are different in each category, infection being the most common cause of FWF while collagen vascular diseases, malignancies, and chronic infections are causes of FUO.
  - Emergency testing and evaluation are needed in case of FWF while children with FUO generally do not need emergency assessment.
  - Empirical antibiotic therapy is not indicated for FUO whereas such therapy is recommended in selected groups of children with FWF after collection of specimens for investigations.

RED FLAG SIGNS IN PYREXIA OF UNKNOWN ORIGIN

- Prolonged appetite loss
- Weight loss
- Sleep disturbances
- Focal complaint
- Organomegaly
- Lymphadenopathy
- Rash
- Clubbing
- Focal signs.

SYSTEMIC APPROACH IN A CASE OF PYREXIA OF UNKNOWN ORIGIN

- Documentation of fever
- Detailed history
- Thorough clinical examination
- Initial laboratory investigations

- Repeated history and daily clinical examination to evaluate development of a new symptom or sign
- Repeat basic laboratory tests
- Additional tests as per clinical evaluation.

HISTORY TAKING

- Fever duration, pattern, and intensity; granulomatous and autoimmune diseases are common in cases of PUO >6 months.
- No response to nonsteroidal anti-inflammatory drugs (NSAIDs) suggests the possibility of noninflammatory causes of fever.
- *History of associated sweating:*
  - Fever, heat intolerance, and sweating: Thyrotoxicosis
  - Fever, heat intolerance, and absence of sweating: Ectodermal dysplasia
- *Associated complaints:*
  - Spontaneously resolved red eyes: Kawasaki disease (KD)
  - Persistent red weeping eyes: Systemic lupus erythematosus (SLE)
  - Persistent nasal discharge and headache: Sinusitis
- *Clues to diagnosis from exposure:*
  - Infected or ill person: Diagnosis of index case, e.g., tuberculosis
  - Cats: Leptospirosis, cat scratch disease, toxocara catis, and tularemia
  - Dogs: Rickettsial disease, leptospirosis, tularemia, and toxocara catis
  - Ticks: Rickettsial disease
  - Unpasteurized milk or raw meat: Brucellosis and toxoplasmosis
  - Pica: Visceral larva migrans and toxoplasmosis
  - Medication: Drug fever
  - Abdominal surgery: Intra-abdominal abscesses
- *Absence of sweating:*
  - Dehydration
- Diabetes insipidus
- Anhidrotic ectodermal dysplasia
- Familial dysautonomia
- Exposure to atropine.

THOROUGH PHYSICAL EXAMINATION

- *Relative bradycardia:*
  - Normally heart rate rises by 10 beats/min per 1°C rise in body temperature for children >2 months old. When the pulse rate remains low in the presence of fever (temperature–pulse dissociation), it is called relative bradycardia. It is commonly associated with:
    - Enteric fever
    - Brucellosis
    - Leptospirosis
    - Drug fever
  - Bradycardia in the presence of fever may be as a result of conduction defect resulting from cardiac involvement with acute rheumatic fever, viral myocarditis, or infective endocarditis.
- *Relative tachycardia:* Pulse rate is elevated disproportionately to temperature and is usually caused by noninfectious diseases or infectious diseases in which a toxin is responsible for clinical manifestations.
- *Eyes:*
  - Bulbar conjunctivitis: KD and leptospirosis
  - Palpebral conjunctivitis: Infectious mononucleosis
  - Phlyctenular conjunctivitis: Tuberculosis
  - Ischemic retinopathy: Polyarteritis nodosa
  - Absent tears and corneal reflex: Familial dysautonomia
  - Choroid tubercle: Miliary tuberculosis, and sarcoidosis

- Roth spot: Bacterial endocarditis
- Uveitis: Sarcoidosis, juvenile idiopathic arthritis (JIA), SLE, KD, and Behcet disease
- Icterus: Hepatitis, leptospirosis, malaria, and typhoid
- Proptosis: Neuroblastoma, thyrotoxicosis, orbital tumor, and Wegener's disease

- *Upper respiratory tract and oral cavity:*
  - Purulent nasal secretions: Sinusitis
  - Pharyngeal hyperemia with exudates: Infectious mononucleosis
  - Pharyngeal hyperemia without exudates: Leptospirosis
  - Hypodontia and conical teeth: Ectodermal dysplasia
  - Smooth tongue with excessive salivation: Familial dysautonomia
  - Oral ulcers: SLE, inflammatory bowel disease, Behcet disease, and PFAPA (periodic fever, aphthous stomatitis, pharyngitis, adenitis) syndrome.
  - Gingival hypertrophy: Leukemia and histiocytosis

- *Musculoskeletal:*
  - Bony tenderness: Malignancy (leukemia), osteomyelitis, and Caffey disease
  - Muscle tenderness: Dermatomyositis, polyarteritis nodosa, leptospirosis, and mycoplasma
  - Arthritis: Collagen vascular disease, brucellosis, tuberculosis, and human immunodeficiency virus (HIV)
  - Hyperactive tendon reflexes: Tuberculous meningitis (TBM), and thyrotoxicosis
  - Hypoactive tendon reflexes: Familial dysautonomia
  - Trapezius tenderness: Subdiaphragmatic abscess

- *Distribution of causes of PUO:*
  - Infectious diseases: 50–60%
  - Rheumatology: 10–20%
  - Hematology/oncology: 5–10%
  - Undiagnosed (self-resolving): 10–20%.

COMMON CAUSES OF PYREXIA OF UNKNOWN ORIGIN

- *Inflammatory:*
  - Infections:
    - Bacterial
    - Viral
    - Protozoal
    - Fungal
  - Collagen vascular diseases:
    - Systemic onset juvenile idiopathic arthritis (SOJIA)
    - SLE
    - KD
    - Wegener's disease
    - Polyarteritis nodosa
    - Behcet disease
  - Malignancies:
    - Leukemia
    - Lymphoma
    - Neuroblastoma
    - Histiocytosis
  - Drug fever:
    - Atropine
    - Antimicrobials
  - Miscellaneous:
    - Inflammatory bowel disease
    - Pulmonary embolus
    - Hematomas
    - Hemophagocytic lymphohistiocytosis (HLH)

- *Noninflammatory causes:*
  - Ectodermal dysplasia
  - Familial dysautonomia
  - Heat hyperpyrexia
  - Diabetes insipidus
  - Thyrotoxicosis
  - Caffey disease.

Common Infectious Causes of Pyrexia of Unknown Origin

- *Bacterial:*
  - Enteric fever
  - Urinary tract infection (UTI)
  - Tuberculosis
  - Bacterial endocarditis
  - Brucellosis
  - Leptospirosis
  - Osteomyelitis
  - Sinusitis
  - Mastoiditis
  - Dental infections
  - Liver abscess
  - Subdiaphragmatic abscess
  - Pelvic abscess
- *Viral:*
  - Epstein–Barr virus (EBV)
  - Cytomegalovirus (CMV)
  - HIV
- *Protozoal:*
  - Malaria
  - Toxoplasmosis
- *Miscellaneous:*
  - Rickettsial disease
  - Chlamydial
  - Fungal.

84 Recurrent Abdominal Pain

INTRODUCTION

Recurrent abdominal pain (RAP) is one of the most common medical problems in children. It is also the condition in which the exact cause of pain cannot be identified in the majority of cases. Most of these patients turn out to have a functional problem. It is seen in almost 10–15% of school-going children. About 10% of children with RAP may be having a serious underlying condition. Hence proper evaluation is very important for diagnosis and management of this problem.

DIAGNOSTIC CRITERIA OF RECURRENT ABDOMINAL PAIN

- At least three episodes of significant abdominal pain occurring over 3 months.
- There should be a clear symptom-free interval between the episodes.
- Severe pain lasts for at least 3 minutes.
- Between 5 and 15 years of age.

Symptoms are maximum between 5 and 7 years and tend to subside around 10 years.

- RAP is a symptom and not a diagnosis, and functional or organic cause or both can coexist.

ETIOLOGY OF RECURRENT ABDOMINAL PAIN

- Nonorganic (functional): 90%
- Organic: 10%.

NORTH AMERICAN SOCIETY OF PEDIATRIC GASTROENTEROLOGY, HEPATOLOGY AND NUTRITION (NASPGHAN) CLASSIFICATION

- Chronic abdominal pain: Long-lasting intermittent or constant abdominal pain that is functional or organic.
- Functional abdominal pain: No anatomic, metabolic, infectious, inflammatory or neoplastic lesions.
- Types of functional abdominal pain:
  - Functional dyspepsia: Upper abdominal pain
  - Irritable bowel syndrome: Functional abdominal pain with alteration in bowel movements
  - Abdominal migraine
  - Functional abdominal pain syndrome.

RED FLAG SIGNS (POINTERS TO ORGANIC PAIN)

- Age <5 years
- Nocturnal pain
- Recurrent vomiting/gastrointestinal (GI) bleed
- Unexplained fever
- Associated symptoms such as headache, pallor, anorexia, and constipation
- Significant weight loss
- Deceleration of linear growth
- Organomegaly
- Joint swelling

- Family history of inflammatory bowel disease.
- Abdominal migraine and abdominal epilepsy are other causes of RAP.

RECURRENT ABDOMINAL PAIN WITH DYSPEPTIC PAIN

- Recurrent pain in the upper abdomen, feeling full earlier than expected when eating
- May be associated with anorexia, nausea, belching, and heart burn
- Endoscopy normal
- Delayed gastric emptying is likely mechanism.
- As per Apley's law, the chance of an organic pathology is high when the pain is away from the umbilicus.
- 25% may be having an underlying pathology like gastroesophageal reflux disease (GERD), peptic ulcer, *Helicobacter pylori*, and gastritis.
- Should be thoroughly evaluated
- 75% functional
- 25% organic like GERD, peptic ulcer, *H. pylori*, giardiasis, pancreatitis, cholecystitis, and appendicitis.

RECURRENT ABDOMINAL PAIN WITH ALTERED BOWEL HABITS

- Functional (75%)
- Organic (25%) like celiac disease, abdomen tuberculosis (TB), human immunodeficiency virus (HIV), Crohn's disease, and food allergies.
- Pain in abdomen, diarrhea, and constipation alone or in an alternating pattern are characteristics.

RECURRENT ABDOMINAL PAIN WITH PAROXYSMAL PERIUMBILICAL PAIN

- Functional >95%
- Organic 5% like abdominal TB, inflammatory bowel disease (IBD), and renal colic.

CLINICAL FEATURES OF FUNCTIONAL RECURRENT ABDOMINAL PAIN

John Apley has aptly summarized the features as follows:
- Slightly underweight
- *Intelligence:* Normal
- *Psyche:* Emotionally disturbed
- *Personality:* Timid and anxious
- *Family history:* Psychological problems
- 5–15 years common age
- More in females.

Characteristics of functional recurrent abdominal pain (FRAP) are as follows:
- Site of pain:
  - The most common site is periumbilical or midepigastric.
  - The pain is away from the umbilicus, the more likely it is of organic pathology.
- Type of pain:
  - Usually transient and intermittent, usually lasts only for a few minutes, rarely for 1–3 hours.
  - Colicky or cramping; sometimes it may be dull and continuous.
- Intensity of pain:
  - May be mild or very severe
  - Child may cry, double over or sit with knees drawn to the chest.
  - He may press the abdominal wall to get relief.
  - No radiation
  - Not related to meals
- Nocturnal pain:
  - Once the child is asleep, he never gets up in the night with pain.
  - If a child gets up in the middle of the night with pain, it is almost always due to an organic cause.
- Role of stress: Role of stress is considered significant in a case of FRAP.

- Associates symptoms:
  - Nausea and vomiting may be present, but the bilious vomiting points to an organic cause.
  - Headache, pallor, anorexia, and constipation are common associated symptoms.

POINTS TO BE ASKED IN HISTORY

- *Duration:* Functional abdominal pain is usually defined as episodic abdominal pain over 3 months or more.
- *Restriction of daily activities:* Restriction of daily activities and absenteeism from school indicates degree of severity in pain.
- *Site of pain:*
  - Functional abdominal pain is usually periumbilical.
  - Pain away from periumbilical region favors organic cause.
- *Any precipitating or aggravating factor:* FRAP is not related to meals, physical activity, defecation, urination, or menstruation.
- *Nocturnal pain:* Nocturnal pain indicates organic pathology.
- *Effect of medicines:* Antacids, H_2 inhibitors, analgesics, and antispasmodics usually are not effective.
- *Condition between the episodes:* Otherwise active and healthy.
- *Bowel habit:* Altered bowel habits such as diarrhea, constipation, or nocturnal bowel movements suggest an organic cause.
- *Appetite:* Appetite remains normal in FRAP.
- *Loss of weight:* Loss of weight indicates an organic disease.
- Family history of migraine and inflammatory bowel disease favor organic etiology.

Following signs should be looked for:
- Anemia (IBD, helminthiasis, and lead poisoning)
- Rash/palpable purpura and arthritis [Henoch-Schönlein purpura (HSP)]
- Iridocyclitis and arthritis (IBD)
- Jaundice (cholelithiasis)
- Right lower quadrant mass (appendicitis)
- Left lower quadrant mass (fecal mass) (constipation)
- Perianal fissure or ulcerations (IBD, constipation)
- Spinal lesions: Neurological signs
- Hepatosplenomegaly (Abdominal TB, HIV).

ORGANIC COMMON CAUSES OF RECURRENT ABDOMINAL PAIN

- *Intestinal causes:*
  - Congenital:
    - Malrotation
    - Strangulated hernia
  - Acquired:
    - Constipation
    - Postoperative adhesions
- *Inflammatory causes:*
  - HSP
  - Crohn disease
  - Peptic ulcer disease
- *Vascular causes:*
  - Abdominal migraine
  - Bowel ischemia
- *Hepatobiliary diseases:*
  - Gall stones
  - Cholecystitis
  - Choledochal cyst
  - Sclerosing cholangitis
- Chronic pancreatitis
- *Renal causes:*
  - Recurrent urinary tract infection (UTI)
  - Urolithiasis
- *Pelvic causes:*
  - Diabetic ketoacidosis
  - Lead poisoning
- *Other causes:*
  - Diabetic ketoacidosis
  - Porphyria
  - Lead poisoning
  - Spinal cord tumors
  - Chronic congetive cardiac failure.

85 Salivation Disorders

INTRODUCTION

Increased salivation (Ptyalism) is a common physiologic sign of teething and irritation. It can also be due to some other reasons which need to be identified.

PHYSIOLOGIC FACTORS

- *Teething:* Irritation of the gums associated with eruption of teeth causes increased salivation and drooling.
- *Reaction to foods:* Ingestion, smell, or sight of certain delicious foods increases salivation. Spicy food is common cause of increased salivation while eating.
- *Nausea:* Any condition causing nausea may result in increased salivation.

PATHOLOGIC CONDITIONS

- *Oropharyngeal lesions:* Oropharyngeal irritation due to infection or chemical can cause increased salivation:
  - Gingivostomatitis
  - Aphthous ulcers
  - Dental caries
  - Tonsillitis
  - Retropharyngeal abscess
  - Foreign bodies
- Gastroesophageal reflux (GER)
- *Drugs:*
  - Iodides
  - Histaminics
  - Pilocarpine
  - Acetylcholine
  - Nicotine acid
  - Sympathomimetic drugs
- *Toxins and poisoning:*
  - *Organophosphorous poisoning:* Increased sweating, salivation, tearing, vomiting, diarrhea, weakness, convulsions, etc., are other features of organophosphorous poisoning.
  - *Acrodynia:* It is caused by mercury poisoning irritability, hypotonia, photophobia, excessive sweating, salivation, painful extremities, and pink rash are characteristics of acrodynia.
  - Other heavy metal poisoning can cause excessive salivation.
  - *Emotional stress:* Excitation, pleasure, and fear like emotional stress can also cause excessive salivation.

DECREASED SALIVATION

Decreased salivation results in dryness of mouth. Therefore, complaint of the patient would be dryness of mouth and not decreased salivation, should be known to the clinician. It is uncommon symptom in children.

Common Causes of Decreased Salivation

- Dehydration (dryness of mucosa-mouth)
- Fever
- Mouth breathing (may be habit, adenoidal hypertrophy)

- Exercise
- *Drugs:*
  - Atropine
  - Antihistaminics
  - Tricyclic antidepressants
  - Opiates
  - Phenothiazines
  - Belladonna
- Salivary glands neoplasms
- *Obstruction of salivary ducts:* Salivary duct obstruction may be due to tumors, inflammation, scarring, or stones.
- Psychiatric disorders (anxiety, depression, hysterical)
- Anhidrotic ectodermal dysplasia
- *Sjogren syndrome:* It is the type of rheumatoid arthritis. Other features are dryness of mouth (xerostomia), dry eyes (keratoconjuctivitis), etc.
- *Salivary gland inflammation:*
  - Mumps
  - Sarocoidosis
- Vitamin A deficiency
- Hypothyroidism
- *Mikulicz syndrome:* There is enlargement of salivary and lacrimal glands due to leukemia infiltration.

DROOLING (SIARLORRHEA)

Drooling (siarlorrhea) is defined as saliva flowing outside the mouth unintentionally. It is very common symptom in daily pediatric practice. Although drooling may occur in healthy children under 2 years of age due to teething, it is commonly observed in neurologically impaired children. Drooling may result from the hypersecretion of saliva, or, more commonly, the impairment of swallowing. It carries a considerable social stigma. In addition to cosmetic and hygienic considerations, psychosocial consequences may arise from this situation.

Common Causes of Drooling

- Developmental
- *Physiological:*
  - Teething
  - Nausea
  - Foods
  - Emotional stimuli
- *Central nervous system (CNS) and muscular disorders:*
  - Cerebral palsy
  - Demyelinating disorders
  - Chorea
  - Encephalitis
  - Pseudobulbar palsy
  - Various myopathies
  - Mental retardation
- Oropharyngeal lesions
- *Retro pharyngeal abscess:*
  - Less than 3-4 years of age
  - Fever, irritability, decreased oral intake
  - Drooling
  - Torticollis
  - Keeping the neck flexed, not able to extend the neck (bolte sign)
- Esophageal obstruction (foreign body)
- Gastroesophageal reflux disease (GERD)
- Drugs and chemicals
- Familial dysautonomia (Riley-Day syndrome).

Chapter 86: Scrotal Swelling

INTRODUCTION

Scrotal swelling is found infrequently in the boys. It may be acute or chronic and painful or painless. Abrupt onset of painful scrotal swelling necessitates prompt evaluation because conditions like testicular torsion and incarcerated inguinal hernia require emergency surgical management.

HISTORY

- *Age at which swelling noted:*
  - New born: Hydrocele, Inguinal hernia, scrotal hematoma, epididymitis, testicular torsion, meconium peritonitis, etc.
  - Older children: Testicular torsion, trauma, inguinal hernia, mumps orchitis, hydrocele, and insect bite.
  - Adolescents: Testicular torsion, varicocele, spermatocele, testicular tumor, and Henoch–Schonlein purpura (HSP)
- *Painful:*
  - Sudden onset of pain and swelling: Torsion of testis
  - Dragging pain: Hernia and hydrocele
  - Inguinal discomfort: Inguinal hernia, epididymitis, etc.
  - Associated flank pain can occur with passage of ureteral calculus.
  - Previous episodes of similar pain may be in a case of intermittent testicular torsion or inguinal hernia.
- Urinary symptoms such as dysuria, urgency, and frequency which indicate urinary tract infection (UTI) can cause associated epididymitis.
- History of (H/o) scrotal trauma may cause hematoma.
- Familial testicular torsion is known.

PHYSICAL EXAMINATION

Physical examination may be difficult with painful scrotum.
- Scrotal wall erythema is common in testicular torsion, epididymitis, incarcerated hernia, and local insect bite.
- Presence of impulse on coughing and reducible swelling indicates inguinal hernia.
- Transillumination test is positive in hydrocele.

COMMON CAUSES OF ACUTE SCROTAL PAIN

- Torsion of testis
- Spermatic cord torsion
- *Epididymitis:*
  - Infectious: UTI, sexually transmitted diseases (STDs), and viral like mumps
  - Noninfectious: Traumatic
- *Scrotal edema or erythema:*
  - Insect bite
  - HSP
- Orchitis: Vasculitis (HSP), viral (mumps), and abscess
- Trauma: Hematocele, scrotal contusion, and testis rupture
- Hernia or hydrocele
- Varicocele
- Testicular tumors
- Spermatocele.

Seizures

INTRODUCTION

Seizure is the most common neurological problem encountered in children. It is a symptom of central nervous system (CNS) dysfunction due to several causes. A proper and detailed seizure history is an important tool for evaluation of a child with seizures. If a clinician had an opportunity to observe the child during an episode or if a video clip of the episode is available, it helps a lot for further evaluation. If the parents have not captured an episode in a video, they should be asked to do so whenever such an event recurs.

DEFINITIONS

Seizures: Seizures is defined as a transient occurrence of signs and/or symptoms resulting from abnormal, paroxysmal, excessive, or synchronous electric neuronal discharge, resulting in motor, sensory, or autonomic disturbances.
- *Convulsions:* Motor manifestations of seizures are called convulsions. Convulsion is a type of seizure, in which there is sudden, violent, irregular movements of the body.
- *Spasms of muscles:* Involuntary muscle contractions are called as muscle spasms. They are found in following conditions:
  - Carpopedal spasm is the characteristic of hypocalcemia and hypomagnesemia (tetany).
  - Painful muscle contractions, particularly of jaw (lock jaw and trismus) and neck muscle in a case of tetanus, a serious disease, caused by bacterial toxin from clostridium tetani.

The goals of the clinical evaluation are confirmation of the paroxysmal event as seizures, defining the semiology, and establishing its etiology. The following questions should be addressed while evaluating a child with seizure:
- Is it a seizure or seizure mimic (e.g., syncope, breath holding spell, benign paroxysmal vertigo, migraine, shuddering attacks, etc.)
- Is it provoked or unprovoked? [Examples of provoked seizures are metabolic, toxic, CNS infections, stroke, trauma, intracranial hemorrhage (ICH), etc.]
- Is it focal or generalized seizures?
- What is the type of seizures? [generalized tonic-clonic (GTC), absence, myoclonic, atonic, etc.]

Generalized tonic-clonic seizure (GTCS): It has two phases: tonic (stiffness) and clonic (twitching/jerking). GTCS starts with opening of eyes, tonic deviation of head and eyes, followed by tonic phase, characterized by sustained contraction of skeletal muscles, forced closure of mouth, tongue biting, epileptic cry, and cyanosis. This is followed by clonic phase with continuous clonic

jerks of facial, trunk, and limb muscles. It is followed by recovery phase, characterized by unresponsiveness bronchial secretions, and urinary and fecal incontinence.
- Are there any comorbidities? (Cerebral palsy, intellectual disability, etc.)
- What is the likely etiology?

POINTS OF EVALUATION IN A CASE OF SEIZURE

- *Age:* The causes of seizures are different at different ages.
  - Common causes of seizures in neonates are metabolic (hypoglycemia and hypocalcemia), hypoxic ischemic encephalopathy (HIE), bacterial meningitis, ICH, inborn error of metabolism (IEM), CNS malformations, etc.
  - Febrile seizures are common in the age group of 6 months to 5 years.
  - Very rarely first episode of febrile seizures develops after the age of 3 years.
- Recurrent seizures are common due to epilepsy, febrile seizures, metabolic disorders, IEM, etc.
- Positive family history for seizures may indicate genetic epilepsy syndromes.
- Presence of an aura (unpleasant feeling or a stereotypical visual or auditory hallucination or abdominal discomfort) and automatism (grimacing, chewing movements, etc.), proceeding an episode of seizure occurs in complex partial seizures (focal seizures with impaired awareness is recent terminology).
- *Type of seizures, focal or generalized:* The focal seizures may be indicating underlying structural lesion which requires neuroimaging for precise diagnosis and management.
- *Duration of an episode:*
  - Duration of typical febrile seizure is <10 minutes.
- Status epilepticus is defined as 5 or more minutes of either continuous seizure activity or repetitive seizures with no intervening recovery or consciousness.
- *Provoked or unprovoked seizures:*
  - Febrile seizures, hypoglycemia, dyselectrolytemia, etc. are examples of provoked seizures.
  - Bacterial meningitis and meningoencephalitis should be differentiated from febrile seizures.
  - Developmental delay, perinatal asphyxia, perinatal or postnatal brain injury are likely to be associated with unprovoked epileptic seizures.
- Look for skin markers like café-au-lait spots, shagreen patch, and port wine stain for neurocutaneous disorders.
- Look for injury marks over forehead and other body parts which may suggest myoclonic jerks.

COMMON CAUSES OF SEIZURES IN NEONATES

- Hypoglycemia
- Hypocalcemia
- Hypomagnesemia
- Hypoxic ischemic encephalopathy
- Bacterial meningitis
- Intracranial hemorrhage
- Central nervous system malformations
- Inborn error of metabolism
- Pyridoxine deficiency (rare).

COMMON CAUSES OF SEIZURES IN CHILDREN

- Febrile seizures
- *Metabolic causes:*
  - Hypoglycemia
  - Hypocalcemia
  - Hypomagnesemia

- Hyponatremia
- Hypernatremia
- Epilepsy
- *Central nervous system infections:*
  - Bacterial meningitis
  - Tuberculous meningitis
  - Viral encephalitis
  - Brain abscess
  - Neurocysticercosis (NCC)
- Encephalopathy (HIE, Reye's syndrome, hepatic uremia, enteric fever, etc.)
- *Raised intracranial pressure (ICP):*
  - Hydrocephalus
  - Space-occupying lesion (SOL) (brain tumor, tuberculoma)
- Intracranial hemorrhage
- *Neurocutaneous syndromes:*
  - Tuberous sclerosis
  - Sturge–Weber syndrome
  - Neurofibromatosis
- Inborn error of metabolism
- Central nervous system malformations.

Short Stature

INTRODUCTION

Short stature is a very common complaint by the parents while the child is brought for any other illness. It is a very common practice to prescribe multivitamins, iron, calcium, zinc, etc. with just assurance to parents or to advice for investigations including for endocrine disorders without any attempt to define the short stature with the help of growth charts and methodological approach, resulting in mishap.

PRINCIPLES OF NORMAL GROWTH

- *Infancy-childhood-puberty (ICP) model:*
  - Infancy component (midgestation to 2-3 years) is mainly determined by nutrition.
  - Childhood component is influenced by growth hormone (GH).
  - Puberty component is superimposed on the decelerating childhood component. It is characterized by gonadal steroids controlling growth, both directly and via enhancement of GH pulse amplitude.
- *Normal growth velocity:*
  - Intrauterine growth: It is the phase of most rapid growth in the life of a human being. The linear growth velocity during this phase is 1.2-1.5 cm/week, peaks at midgestation to 2.5 cm/week and falls to 0.5 cm/week in immediate prenatal period.
  - Average length of the baby at birth is 50 cm. There is increment of 25 cm in the first year of life, 12.5 cm in second year, 6-7 cm each in third and fourth years and thereby 5 cm/year until onset of pubertal growth spurt.
  - The peak growth velocity during adolescence is about 9-11 cm/year for boys and about 7-9 cm/year for girls.
- *Body proportion:*
  - The trunk is relatively larger than the lower segment at birth. The ratio of upper segment (US) (from vertex to symphysis pubis) to lower segment (LS) (symphysis pubis to feet) is being 1.7.
  - US/LS:
    - 3 years → 1.4
    - 5 years → 1.3
    - 8 years → 1.2
    - 10-11 years → 1.1
    - Completion of puberty → 1-1.1
  - LS > US by 5 cm after completion of puberty
  - Arm span is within 5 cm of the height
- *Definition of short stature:*
  - Height is <3rd percentile or <2 standard deviation (SD) of the median height for age and gender according to the population standard.
  - Height is within normal population percentiles, but less than midparental height (MPH) or target height.
  - Height is within normal percentiles for national and parental standards, but growth velocity is <25th percentile over 6-12 months of observation.

Short Stature

- *Pointers toward diagnosis from history:*

Neonatal hypoglycemia, jaundice, and micropenis	Growth hormone deficiency (GHD) and multiple pituitary hormone deficiency (MPHD)
Breech delivery	GHD and MPHD
Small for gestational age	Russell–Silver syndrome and Seckel syndrome
Family history of delayed puberty with short stature with normal final height	Constitutional delay in growth and puberty (CDGP)
Family history of short stature	• Achondroplasia • Hypochondroplasia (autosomal dominant)
Short stature in infancy	• Syndromic short stature • Skeletal dysplasia
Short stature in childhood	• GHD • MPHD • Hypothyroidism • Chronic illness • Turner syndrome
Inadequate dietary intake	Undernutrition
Chronic diarrhea, distention of abdomen, and refractory anemia	Celiac disease
Polyuria and rickets	Renal tubular acidosis
Lethargy, constipation, and weight gain	Hypothyroidism
Headache, vomiting, and visual disturbances	Intracranial tumor like craniopharyngioma
Intracranial tumors, trauma, and surgery	MPHD

- *Pointers toward diagnosis from clinical examination:*

Dysmorphism	Congenital syndromes like Down syndrome, Turner syndrome, mucopolysaccharidosis (MPS), etc.
Pallor	Chronic anemia, celiac disease, malnutrition, chronic renal disease, etc.
Disproportionate short stature	Hypothyroidism, rickets, achondroplasia, MPS, etc.
Hypertension	Chronic renal disease
Frontal bossing, depressed nasal bridge, crowded teeth, and micropenis	Hypopituitarism
Goiter and coarse skin	Hypothyroidism
Central obesity and striae	Cushing syndrome
Increased US/LS	Rickets, achondroplasia, and congenital hypothyroidism
Decreased US/LS	MPS and spondyloepiphyseal dysplasia

- Anthropometry and plotting the data on growth chart is mandatory for evaluation of a case of short stature.

FAMILIAL SHORT STATURE

- One of the most common causes
- Less than 3rd percentile with national standards, but within normal limits with MPH.
- Growth velocity is normal.
- Growth curve follows a line parallel to the 3rd percentile.
- Body proportions are normal.
- Skeletal age is normal.
- Achieves puberty at appropriate age.
- Adult stature is below normal.

CONSTITUTIONAL DELAY IN GROWTH AND PUBERTY

- Another common cause of short stature
- More common in boys
- Born with normal weight and length, grow normally in first year.
- Growth then decelerates during second and third years, <3rd percentile for height, continue to grow parallel to 3rd percentile with normal growth velocity throughout childhood.
- The onset of puberty and adolescent growth spurt is delayed.
- Due to delayed skeletal age, lineal height gain continues beyond the time when their peers have stopped growing.
- History of (H/o) delayed puberty in either parents is often present, but not always.
- Body proportions may range from normal to eunuchoid, the latter probably caused by inadequate spine growth due to lack of gonadal steroids at appropriate time.
- Skeletal age less than chronological age (2 years), but equivalent to height age.
- Cause of constitutional delay in growth and puberty (CDGP) is not clear, transient GH deficiency is likely.
- CDGP and familial short stature (FSS) often coexist leading to height shorter than normal.

UNDERNUTRITION

- Most important cause of short stature in India.
- Features of undernutrition including vitamin and mineral deficiency signs are common.
- Weight is less for height.
- Delayed puberty
- Weight for height or BMI are better clinical pointers to undernutrition as the cause of short stature.
- Iron, calcium, vitamin D, and zinc deficiency can cause short stature.

INTRAUTERINE GROWTH RESTRICTION (IUGR)

- Birth length (sometimes BW) <10th percentile for gestational age
- In contrast to appropriate for gestational age (AGA) or preterm babies, small-for-dates (SFD) babies often do not show catch-up growth; 30% do not achieve their genetic potential. Those who are destined to achieve a normal height percentile will have usually shown good catch-up by 2 years of age.

GROWTH HORMONE DEFICIENCY

- Usually, normal weight and length at birth
- Neonatal hypoglycemia, jaundice, micro penis, etc.
- They grow normally in the first year of life as growth in this phase is influenced by nutrition and is mediated by insulin and related growth factors.
- Growth falters in early childhood leading to severe stunting.
- Immature facies, doll-like face, prominent cheeks, child-like voice, small hands and feet, frontal and parietal bossing, and depressed nasal bridge
- Body proportions are preserved
- Low growth velocity
- Retarded bone age.

HYPOTHYROIDISM

- Short stature
- Puffy face with coarse features
- Bradycardia
- Delayed relaxation of ankle jerk.

CUSHING SYNDROME

- May be due to exogenous steroid administration or adrenal tumors
- Short and obese
- Purplish striae
- Muscular weakness—myopathy
- Buffalo hump
- Hypertension.

TURNER SYNDROME

- Short and female
- Webbing of neck
- Low posterior hairline
- Wide carrying angle
- Short 4th/5th metacarpals or metatarsals
- Delayed puberty and infertility
- Autoimmune thyroid disorder
- Celiac disease
- Horseshoe kidney
- Coarctation of aorta.

COMMON CAUSES OF SHORT STATURE

- *Physiological short stature:*
  - FSS
  - CDGP
- *Pathological short stature:*
  - Malnutrition and rickets
  - Malabsorption:
    - Celiac disease
    - Human immunodeficiency virus (HIV)
  - Chronic illness:
    - Chronic anemia
    - Chronic renal diseases
    - Renal tubular acidosis
    - Chronic liver disease
    - Chronic lung diseases
    - Giardiasis
    - Thalassemia
  - Endocrine disorders:
    - Growth hormone deficiency
    - Hypothyroidism
    - Cushing syndrome
  - Syndromic disorders:
    - Turner syndrome
    - Noonan syndrome
    - Down syndrome
    - Edward syndrome
    - Patau syndrome
    - Russell–Silver syndrome
  - Skeletal dysplasia:
    - Achondroplasia
    - Hypochondroplasia
    - Osteogenesis imperfect
  - Medications:
    - Prolonged steroid intake
    - Methylphenidate.

CHAPTER 89: Splenomegaly

INTRODUCTION

The spleen is the largest lymphoid organ in the body, in the left upper quadrant of the abdomen. It is an intraperitoneal organ. It weighs about 10 g at birth, 130 g at puberty, and 250 g in the adults. The size and shape of the spleen is roughly like a clinched fist.

The spleen must enlarge at least twice the normal size to become clinically palpable. However, in newborns and infants up to the age of 3 months, a just palpable spleen can be normal. The enlarging spleen traverses from the left hypochondrium to midline and right iliac fossa. It is also described in centimeters below the left costal margin as follows:
- *Mild enlargement:* 1-2 cm below the left costal margin
- *Moderate enlargement:* 3-7 cm below the left costal margin
- *Massive enlargement:* >7 cm below the left costal margin

A wandering spleen, the result of elongated mesenteric connections, may appear and disappear in sitting and lying down positions. A wandering spleen may appear in unusual places and may be mistaken for another organ or mass.

FUNCTIONS OF SPLEEN

- *Reservoir function:*
  - Sequestration crisis in sickle cell anemia
  - Enlargement of spleen in a case of portal hypertension due to congestion; splenic size decreases following massive gastrointestinal (GI) bleed (hematemesis) in a case of portal hypertension.
- *Hemopoiesis:*
  - Fetal spleen
  - Hemolytic anemias (thalassemia)
  - Osteopetrosis
  - Myelofibrosis
  - Chronic iron deficiency anemia
- *Culling:* Removal of damaged or abnormal cells; excessive culling activity may result in hypersplenism.
- *Immune functions:*
  - Production of immunoglobulin M (IgM)
  - Opsonophagocytosis.

SPLENOMEGALY AND CONSISTENCY

- *Soft splenomegaly:* Epstein–Barr virus (EBV), enteric fever
- *Firm splenomegaly:* Malaria, tuberculosis, lymphoma, leukemia, storage disorders
- *Tender splenomegaly:* Splenic abscess, splenic infarct.

Causes of Splenomegaly

- *Normal variants:*
  - 15-30% of neonates
  - 10% of healthy, thin children
  - Wandering spleen

- *Infections:*
  - EBV
  - Cytomegalovirus (CMV)
  - Human immunodeficiency virus (HIV)
  - Hepatitis A, B, and C
  - Malaria
  - Kala-azar
  - Enteric fever
  - Bacterial endocarditis
  - Septicemia
  - Brucellosis
  - Rickettsial infections
  - Leptospirosis
  - Toxoplasmosis
  - Syphilis
  - Splenic abscess
- *Hematological disorders:*
  - Hemolytic anemia:
    - Thalassemia
    - Sick cell anemia
    - Spherocytosis
    - Rhesus (Rh) and ABO incompatibility
    - Autoimmune hemolytic anemia
  - Extramedullary hematopoiesis:
    - Osteopetrosis
    - Pyknodysostosis
    - Myelofibrosis
    - Iron deficiency anemia (in 10–15% of chronic iron deficiency anemia)
  - Neoplasms:
    - Hemangioma
    - Leukemia
    - Lymphoma
    - Histiocytosis
    - Metastatic
- *Storage disorders:*
  - Gaucher disease
  - Niemann–Pick disease
  - Mucopolysaccharidosis
  - Gangliosidosis
  - Wolman disease
  - Glycogen storage disease
- *Vascular congestion:*
  - Portal hypertension with congestive splenomegaly:
    - Cirrhosis of liver
    - Wilson disease
    - Galactosemia
    - Tyrosinosis
    - Cystinosis
    - Chronic hepatitis
    - Cystic fibrosis
    - Hemosiderosis
  - Extrahepatic lesions:
    - Splenic vein thrombosis
    - Chronic congestive heart failure
    - Constrictive pericarditis
    - Splenic trauma
- *Collagen disorders:*
  - Juvenile idiopathic arthritis (Still's disease)
  - Systemic lupus erythematosus
- *Miscellaneous:*
  - Sarcoidosis
  - Congenital cyst
  - Hydatid cyst.

Cause of Splenic Abscesses

- Brucellosis
- Bacterial endocarditis
- Salmonellosis (enteric fever)
- Sickle cell disease
- Falciparum malaria following infarct
- Plague.

Strabismus

INTRODUCTION

The word strabismus is derived from the Greek word meaning, a squinting. It refers to misalignment of the eyes. Strabismus has been estimated in about 5% of children younger than 5 years of age. It is important to detect and treat strabismus at the earliest because 30–40% of children with strabismus will develop secondary amblyopia (loss of vision). The infants are rarely born with aligned eyes and it may be difficult to assess the alignment till 3 months of age.

TYPES OF STRABISMUS

- The types are named according to direction of the abnormal eye movement.
  - Esotropia (turning in)
  - Exotropia (turning out)
  - Hypertropia (turning upward)
  - Hypotropia (turning downward)
- Strabismus is also classified as nonparalytic (concomitant) and paralytic (nonconcomitant). The nonparalytic strabismus is common in children, while paralytic in adults.

COMMON CAUSES OF STRABISMUS

About 50% of cases of strabismus in children are hereditary. The causes of strabismus can be divided into congenital, acquired, and associated with syndromes. The causes of strabismus in children are not apparent; it should be evaluated by a pediatric ophthalmologist.

Congenital Strabismus

- *Pseudo strabismus:* In young infants and children, a broad, flat nasal bridge, and prominent epicanthal folds may create a false impression of strabismus.
- *True congenital strabismus:* Nonparalytic esotropia (turning in) or exotropia (turning out) may be seen up to age of 6 months. Esotropia is more common than exotropia. The nonparalytic (concomitant) strabismus accounts for a large number of cases in childhood. The cause of this problem is not known.
- *Central nervous system (CNS) insults:* Hypoxic, infective, vascular, and hemorrhagic insults to the developing CNS may result in strabismus and other conditions like microcephaly and cerebral palsy
- *Congenital oculomotor nerve (III nerve) paralysis:* It is usually unilateral and may be observed to occur in families. Ptosis, hypotropia, and exotropia are the manifestations.
- *Congenital fourth (IV nerve) palsy:* It creates weakness of superior oblique extraocular muscle and torticollis may result as the child tries to correct the vision.
- *Congenital familial external ophthalmoplegia:* It is autosomal dominant condition. It causes bilateral ptosis with partial or

complete paralysis of external ocular muscles. The affected children keep the chin held up.
- *Mobius syndrome:* This is an uncommon syndrome and there is hypoplasia or agenesis of several cranial nerve nuclei. The face is mask-like because of facial paralysis with several other deformities.
- Double elevation palsy: There is congenital weakness of both superior rectus and inferior oblique muscles. The eye cannot be rotated upward.
- Infant born to drug-dependent mothers are known to develop strabismus in almost 25% cases.

Acquired Strabismus
- *Child exotropia:* This is most common divergent strabismus in children. One eye will shift outward when the child is fixating at a distance. The onset is found commonly between infancy and 5 years of age.
- *Interference with foveal vision:* Refractive error and cataract-like disorders may prevent fusion of sight on fovea, resulting in strabismus.
- *Tumors:* Tumors involving the orbit, either primary or metastatic as well as primary eye tumors like retinoblastoma may cause strabismus. Exophthalmos and hemorrhages of retina, conjunctivae, and lids are other manifestations of eye tumors. A white pupillary reflex is a sign of retinoblastoma. Intracranial tumors manifest with signs of raised intracranial pressure, involvement of cranial nerves, and strabismus.
- *Increased intracranial pressure:* Any cause of raised intracranial pressure may involve cranial nerves, especially sixth nerve, resulting in strabismus. Many children with hydrocephalus have sixth nerve palsies and strabismus.
- *Orbital injury and head trauma:* Fracture of orbital bones may cause entrapment of eye muscles, resulting in strabismus.
- *Myasthenia gravis:* Ptosis, ophthalmoplegia, facial muscles weakness, and strabismus are manifestations of myasthenia gravis.
- Benign sixth nerve palsy may develop 1-3 weeks after an upper respiratory infection and improves within 4-6 weeks.
- Guillain-Barré syndrome
- Miller Fisher syndrome (ophthalmoplegia, ataxia, and hyporeflexia)
- Ocular myopathy
- Vascular disorders
- Ophthalmoplegia migraine
- Infections (meningitis, encephalitis, tuberculous meningitis (TBM), polio, orbital cellulitis, etc.)
- Drugs and toxins (lead and other heavy metal poisoning and botulism)
- Thyrotoxicosis
- Diabetes mellitus.

Syndromes with Dysmorphism and Strabismus
- Down syndrome
- Edward syndrome
- Turner syndrome
- Noonan syndrome
- Cri du chat syndrome
- Marfan syndrome
- Laurence-Moon-Biedl syndrome
- Prader-Willi syndrome
- William syndrome
- Osteopetrosis
- Rubinstein-Taybi syndrome
- Apert syndrome.

91 Stridor

INTRODUCTION

- Stridor is a harsh, high-pitched, vibrator noisy sound caused by partial obstruction on laryngeal area or trachea.
- It can be almost always heard without stethoscope.
- Stridor is usually heard during inspiration, but sometimes may be biphasic.
- Inspiratory stridor is produced when a child breaths against a closed glottis.
- Expiratory stridor results due to semi-approximated vocal cords causing resistance to exhalation.
- Biphasic stridor may result due to subglottic or glottic anomaly or a severe obstruction of the extrathoracic airway.
- Stridor must be differentiated from stertor. Stertor is a noisy breathing sound like snoring, caused by partial obstruction of the upper airway at the level of pharynx and nasopharynx.

STRIDOR IN NEONATES

- Laryngomalacia is the most common cause (90%) of laryngeal stridor in neonates and infants.
  - Manifestations occur usually after the first week or two of birth. If it is immediate after birth, think of birth trauma or congenital malformation.
  - It is intermittent. It disappears or decreases during sleep and rest and gets aggravated during crying or excitement. It is much less in prone position, but increases in supine position.
  - The voice, cry, feeding, and general health remain unaffected.
  - Dyspnea with chest retractions occur during inspiration.
  - The manifestations begin to decrease after 7-9 months and disappear by the age of 18-24 months.
- When stridor manifesting at birth, always consider the possibility of birth trauma (injury to recurrent laryngeal nerve resulting in vocal cord paralysis).
- Prolonged intubation can cause inflammation or stenosis of larynx, resulting in stridor.
- In infants, if the stridor is worsening, there is strong possibility of an anatomical obstruction or vocal cord paralysis.
- If the stridor is accompanied by severe respiratory distress, laryngeal or tracheal atresia is a strong possibility which is a serious condition.
- Lymphangioma or goiter-like mediastinal or neck tumors may cause compression and produce stridor.

STRIDOR IN LATER INFANCY AND CHILDHOOD

- *Acute laryngotracheobronchitis (ALTB):*
  - Most common cause of acute and inspiratory stridor in children

- It is also called as croup.
- *Haemophilus influenzae* and parainfluenza are most common viruses as etiological agents.
- Barking cough, respiratory distress, and lower chest retractions are characteristics. Severe ALTB may cause cyanosis and respiratory failure.
- *Acute epiglottitis:*
  - Caused by *H. influenzae* type B (HIB), pneumococcus, or staphylococcus
  - Inspiratory stridor, dyspnea, muffling of voice, dysphagia, and drooling are characteristics.
- *Diphtheria:*
  - Laryngeal diphtheria is known to present with stridor.
  - Hoarseness of voice, aphonia or dysphonia, barking cough, dyspnea, and restlessness are other features of laryngeal diphtheria. "Bull neck" appearance due to lymphadenitis is the characteristic.
- *Laryngeal foreign body:* Sudden development of inspiratory stridor in a child who is otherwise normal, particularly if he is left to eat unattended is a classical story of a foreign body impacted in the larynx.
- *Retropharyngeal abscess:*
  - A retropharyngeal abscess manifests with respiratory stridor only when it causes compression on the larynx.
  - Abrupt onset of high fever, dysphagia, throat pain, refusal of feeding, keeping neck flexed, and drooling of saliva in younger than 3-4 years child should raise the strong suspicious of retropharyngeal abscess.
- *Laryngospasm:* Laryngospasm due to tetany may manifest with stridor.
- *Trauma:* Any trauma resulting from instrumentation, corrosive agents, or inhalation of smoke may be responsible for laryngeal edema and acute stridor.

COMMON CAUSE OF STRIDOR

Acute Stridor

- Laryngotracheobronchitis
- Epiglottitis
- Diphtheria
- Bacterial tracheitis
- Laryngeal foreign body
- Retropharyngeal abscess
- Allergic laryngeal spasm
- Vocal cord palsy
- Prolonged intubation.

Chronic Stridor

- Laryngomalacia
- Congenital or acquired subglottic stenosis
- Laryngeal webs
- Tracheomalacia
- Vascular ring
- *Compression from masses:*
  - Laryngeal cyst
  - Lymphangioma
  - Goiter
  - Hemangioma
  - Polyp
- Posterior laryngeal cleft.

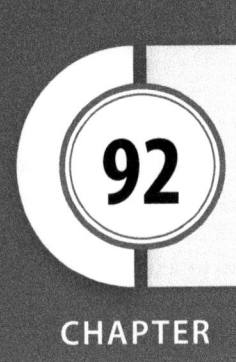

Syncope

INTRODUCTION

Syncope is defined as a sudden and transient loss of consciousness with inability to maintain postural tone. Syncope is more common in older children and adolescents. The incidence peaks around the age of 15–19 years and appears to be a female predominance. The syncope is uncommon before the age of 6 years.

TYPES OF SYNCOPE

There are three types:
1. Neurocardiogenic syncope (vasovagal/vasodepressor)
2. Cardiovascular-mediated syncope
3. Noncardiovascular syncope.

Neurocardiogenic Syncope (Vasovagal)

- The most common cause of syncope in the normal children is neurocardiogenic syncope. It is also called as vasovagal, vasodepressor, or fainting syncope.
- It is classically associated with a prodrome that includes diaphoresis, warmth, pallor, or feeling lightheaded and is often triggered by a specific event or situation such as pain, medical procedures (needle phobia, seeing blood, etc.), or emotional distress (anger, pain, etc.). Postural changes like prolonged standing or sitting are other triggers.
- It is characterized by hypotension and bradycardia.
- Most patients with a vasovagal syncope episode will have prodromal features followed by loss of motor tone. Once the person is in horizontal position, he regains consciousness rapidly within few minutes. Some patients may have tonic-clonic motor activities for few seconds, which should not be confused with a seizures.
- Vasovagal syncope has an excellent prognosis.
- Vertigo, ataxia, and seizures should be differentiated from syncope.

Cardiovascular-mediated Syncope

- Cardiovascular-mediated syncope is less common in children than in adults.
- It has a high mortality and incidence of sudden death.
- A detailed cardiac history and important red flags suggest a need for an urgent pediatric cardiology referral. Several cardiac disorders are known to present as cardiovascular syncope in children.
- *Cardiac red flags in history of syncope:*
  - Syncope during exercise or exertion
  - Family history of sudden cardiac death
  - History of hyperpnea or cyanosis
  - History of chest pain and palpitation
  - History of (H/o) cardiac murmur
  - Medications known to cause long QT syndrome or arrhythmias

- A detailed history, thorough clinical examination, and electrocardiogram (ECG) have a diagnostic yield of 50%. All patients with risk factors for cardiac disease should be evaluated by performing echocardiography and Holter or event monitor.
- EEG and neuroimaging are not indicated unless it is suggestive of seizures or seizures-associated syncope.
- *General measures:*
  - Reassurance to parents and the patient
  - Encourage to maintain adequate hydration (1.5–2 liters of water per day)
  - Enhance dietary salt intake (2.5 g/day)
  - Learn to avoid triggers
  - Isometric counter pressure maneuvers such as leg crossing, buttock tensing, and squatting may help in appropriate situations.

DIFFERENTIATING FEATURES OF SYNCOPE AND SEIZURES

Features	Syncope	Seizure
Relation to posture	Common	No
Precipitating factors	• Prolonged standing • Pain, fever • Heat • Dehydration • Emotion	• Sleep deprivation • Withdrawal of drug
Skin color	Pallor	Cyanosis/normal
Diaphoresis	Common	Rare
Convulsions	Rare, brief	Common
Abnormal movements	Minor twitching	Rhythmic, jerks
Injury	Rare	Common
Urinary incontinence	Rare	Common
Tongue biting	No	Can occur
Postictal confusion	No	Common
Focal neurologic signs	No	May be

CAUSES OF NEUROCARDIOGENIC SYNCOPE

- *Reflex vasodepressor:*
  - Vasovagal
  - Pain (needle prick)
  - Emotion (seeing blood)
- *Systemic illness:*
  - Hypoglycemia
  - Anemia
  - Dehydration, hypovolemia
  - Infection
  - Adrenal insufficiency
- *Drugs:*
  - Vasodilators
  - β-blockers
  - Sedatives
  - Drugs causing prolonged QT internal
  - Antihistaminics
- *Miscellaneous:*
  - Sneezing
  - Defecation
  - Micturition
  - Panic attack
  - Anxiety.

CAUSES OF CARDIOVASCULAR-MEDIATED SYNCOPE

- Cardiac arrhythmias
- Long QT syndrome (congenital/drug induced)
- Wolf–Parkinson–White (WPW) syndrome
- Aortic stenosis
- Hypertrophic obstructive cardiomyopathy
- Coronary artery anomalies [anomalous left coronary artery from the pulmonary artery (ALCAPA)]
- Mitral valve prolapse
- Cardiac tumors (atrial myxoma).

Tall Stature

INTRODUCTION

Tall stature is an uncommon condition in pediatric practice. Methodological evaluation of a child with all stature guides for further investigations and management.

DEFINITION

Tall stature is defined as height of the child is >2 standard deviation (SD) above the population mean for age and sex, using growth charts based on local reference standards.

If there is significant discrepancy between the midparental centile and child's height, detailed assessment is indicated.

HISTORY

- A detailed history of early growth including birth weight and length should be obtained.
- Birth weight and length are usually above 2 SD in children with primary growth disorders such as Sotos, Beckwith-Wiedemann, and Marfan syndromes. They continue to show accelerated growth velocity in infancy and early childhood.
- Children with constitutional tall stature are within normal range for birth weight and length and demonstrate accelerated growth velocity in early childhood.
- Neonatal hypoglycemia can be a feature of Beckwith-Wiedemann syndrome.
- An underlying endocrine disorder is suspected when growth initially follows a low centile and then crosses up growth chart centiles.
- History of eating habits, weight gain, and pubertal changes should be taken in all cases.
- Simple obesity can lead to tall stature and advanced skeletal age.
- Symptoms such as palpitation, muscle weakness, diarrhea, weight loss, and heat intolerance suggest hyperthyroidism.
- History of ophthalmic problems such as lens subluxation, glaucoma, and retinal detachment suggests Marfan syndrome or homocystinuria.
- Pituitary tumor and secreting growth hormone (GH) may present with impairment of vision.
- Developmental delay and learning difficulties are associated with Klinefelter syndrome, homocystinuria, Sotos syndrome, etc.

PHYSICAL EXAMINATION

- Serial measurement of height, weight, head circumference, upper segment/lower segment (US/LS) ratio, span, and BMI (body mass index) and plotting them on standard growth chart is an important step for the evaluation.
- Measuring the height of each biological parent, sibling, and other family members is necessary. It is essential to calculate midparental height centile range for final adult height.

- A significant discrepancy between the height of the child and midparental centile indicates a growth disorder than constitutional tall stature.
- Measuring sitting height and arm span is essential.
- Marfan and Klinefelter syndromes are associated with disproportionate tall stature.
- Arm span is more than height in Marfan and Sotos syndromes.
- Head circumference is more than 2 SD in most patients with Sotos syndrome.
- Precocious puberty is associated with an early pubertal growth spurt, but results in a shorter than expected final height due to the premature closure of the epiphyses.
- Tachycardia, tremors, diarrhea, hair loss, exophthalmos, and goiter are signs of hyperthyroidism.
- GH-secreting pituitary adenoma may present with bitemporal hemianopia.
- Sotos syndrome is characterized by dysmorphic features such as prominent forehead, hypertelorism, large ears, and high-arched palate.
- Looks for other dysmorphic and syndromic features.
- Macroglossia and earlobe creases are features of Beckwith–Wiedemann syndrome.

Constitutional (Familial) Tall Stature
- Birth weight and length are normal
- Parents are tall.
- Predicted adult height with midparental target range and normal height velocity.
- Tall stature becomes apparent from 3 to 4 years of age
- Clinical examination is normal.
- Onset of puberty within normal range.

Obesity
- Exogenous obesity is becoming a global epidemic.
- May be associated with tall stature and advanced skeletal age.
- May mimic Cushing syndrome.
- Associated with elevated levels of insulin.

Klinefelter Syndrome
- 47, XXY (other variants—47, XXX, 48 XXXY, 48 XX YY, and 49 XX XX Y)
- Tall stature with eunuchoid body proportions (increased arm span to height ratio)
- Hypogonadism (small testes)
- Pubertal failure or arrest
- Gynecomastia
- Behavioral problems and learning difficulties.

Marfan Syndrome
- Autosomal dominant
- *Skeletal features:*
  - Long arms (arm span >5 cm than height)
  - US/LS ratio reduced
  - Arachnodactyly
  - Joint laxity
  - Wrist and thumb sign
  - Scoliosis and chest deformities
  - High-arched palate
  - Flat feet
- *Cardiovascular anomalies:*
  - Mitral and aortic valve incompetence
  - Pulmonary stenosis
  - Aortic root dilatation and dissection
- *Eyes abnormalities:*
  - Myopia
  - Dislocation of lens
  - Hypoplastic iris
- Hernias.

Homocystinuria
- Autosomal recessive inborn error of metabolism

- Disproportionate tall stature
- Dislocation of eye lens
- Severe myopenia
- Thromboembolic and cardiovascular complications.

Sotos Syndrome (Cerebral Gigantism)
- Autosomal dominant
- Excessive prenatal and postnatal growth
- Increased birth weight
- Tall forehead
- Large head
- High-arched palate
- Down slanting palpebral fissures
- Flushed cheeks
- Large chin
- Large hands and feet
- Scoliosis
- They are tall during childhood but attain normal adult height due to an advanced skeletal age.

Beckwith–Wiedemann Syndrome
- Autosomal dominant
- Neonatal hypoglycemia.
- Macrosomia
- Macroglossia
- Hemi hypertrophy
- Transverse ear crease
- Organomegaly
- Omphalocele
- Wilms' tumor, hepatoblastoma, and germ cell tumors are common.

Growth Hormone Excess (Acromegaly)
- Excessive GH production prior to fusion of epiphyses.
- GH-producing pituitary adenoma or growth hormone-releasing hormone (GHRH) excess from hypothalamic tumors
- McCune–Albright syndrome can present as excessive GH secretion and tall stature.
- Multiple endocrine neoplasia is another cause.
- Prominent soft tissues, prognathism, frontal bossing, large hands and feet, etc. are other features.
- May be signs and symptoms of compression of optic chiasma due to pituitary tumor.

ALGORITHMIC APPROACH TO A CHILD WITH TALL STATURE

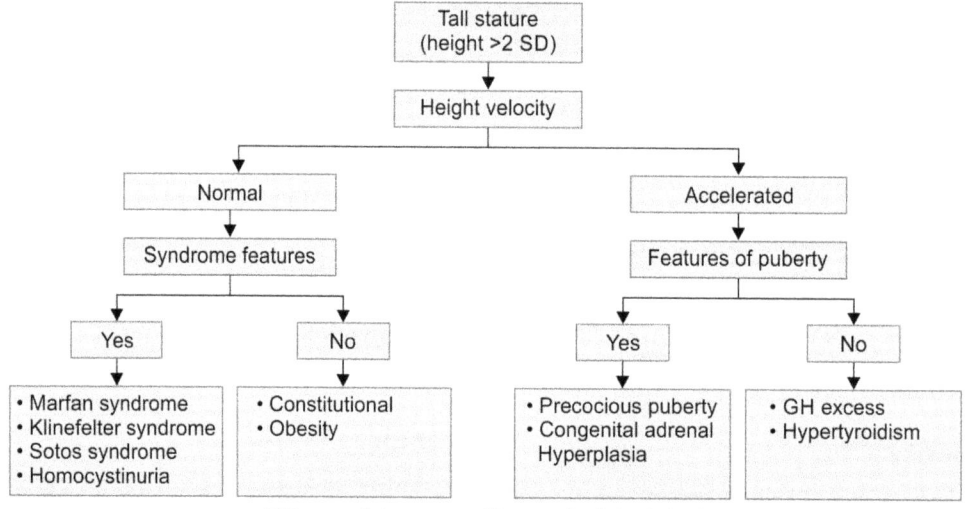

(GH: growth hormone; SD: standard deviation)

Teething and Disorders of Teeth

INTRODUCTION

The human dentition is categorized as primary (deciduous), transitional (mixed), and secondary (permanent).

PRE-DENTITION PERIOD

This is from birth to 6 months. Occasionally, there may be a neonatal tooth present at birth, and mandibular central incisors are common. It is a supernumerary tooth and is often lost soon after birth.

DECIDUOUS DENTITION

The deciduous teeth start to erupt at the age of 6 months and it is completed by the age of approximately 2 years. The pattern of eruption of deciduous dentition is as follows:

Tooth	Maxillary	Mandibular
Central incisors	8–12	6–10
Lateral incisors	9–13	10–16
First molar	13–19	14–18
Canine	16–22	17–23
Second molar	25–33	23–31

PERMANENT DENTITION

The permanent dentition is composed of 32 teeth. The permanent teeth begin to erupt and replace the primary teeth at 6 years of age. The permanent teeth complete eruption by approximately 13 years, with the exception of 3rd molar (wisdom tooth) which usually erupts at the age of 21 years.

	Maxillary	Mandibular
First molar	6–7	6–7
Central incisors	7–8	6–7
Lateral incisors	8–9	7–8
Canine	11–12	10–12
First premolar	10–11	10–12
Second premolar	10–12	10–12
Second molar	12–13	11–13
Third molar	17–21	17–21

MIXED DENTITION

Permanent teeth start to erupt at the age of 6 years and deciduous teeth gradually wobble and fall out as the child grows. All deciduous teeth will be replaced by permanent teeth by the age of 12–13 years. This transition period is called as "mixed dentition stage".

DELAYED DENTITION

The first tooth usually begins to erupt by the age of 6 months, although the exact age can vary from one baby to another. In some cases delayed tooth eruption is a trait that runs in the family and can be inherited from either parent. If there are no other associated medical or developmental issues, then there is no need to be concerned for delayed teething. The baby will catch up with no issues. The appearance of the first tooth may be delayed until after first birth day in some children.

Common Causes of Delayed Dentition

- Most common cause is normal variation or familial
- *Nutritional:*
  - Rickets
  - Malnutrition
- *Endocrinal causes:*
  - Vitamin D deficiency and nondeficiency rickets
  - Hypothyroidism
  - Hypopituitarism
  - Hypoparathyroidism
  - Pseudohypoparathyroidism
- *Chromosomal disorders:*
  - Down syndrome
  - Apert syndrome
  - Angelman syndrome
  - Cockayne syndrome
- *Inherited disorders:*
  - Achondroplasia
  - Ectodermal dysplasia
  - Cleidocranial dysostosis
  - Osteopetrosis
  - Pycnodysostosis
  - Ellis-van Creveld syndrome
  - Osteogenesis imperfecta
  - Mucopolysaccharidosis
  - Progeria
- *Congenital infections:*
  - Congenital syphilis
  - Congenital rubella
- *Other causes:*
  - Serious systemic illness
  - Phenytoin therapy.

Discoloration of Teeth

- Poor orodental hygiene
- Certain foods and beverages
- Dental caries
- Oral iron therapy (black colored)
- Tetracycline therapy
- Chlorhexidine containing mouth rinses
- Trauma
- Fluorosis
- Porphyria
- Lead poisoning.

95 Toeing In

INTRODUCTION

In the evaluation of the relatively common parental concern about toeing in, examination of the child should begin at the toes and move up to the hip. The main stay of treatment is parental reassurance. In the majority of children, the problem resolves spontaneously by 8 years of age.

The causes are grouped by the anatomic location of the underlying problem.

FOOT PROBLEMS

- *Metatarsus adductus:* This deformity of the forefoot is most likely a result of forefoot position in utero. The medial deviation of the forefoot is apparent at birth. The forefoot can be abducted and is not fixed. The adduction may be compounded by the sleeping position, lying in prone with the feet turned in. Metatarsus adductus is the most common cause of toeing in infants, gets corrected spontaneously.
- *Metatarsus varus:* This is congenital subluxation of the tarsometatarsal joint, with adduction of the metatarsals. It is due to compression of the forefoot in adduction, in utero. A deep vertical crease is seen on the medial side of the foot at the tarsometatarsal joint. Unlike adductus, it is not corrected by abducting. It requires serial casting as early as possible after the birth.
- *Talipes equinovarus:* In mild clubfoot, the forefoot adduction may be more severe than the eversion and equine deformities.
- *Flatfeet (pronated feet):* The child with pes planus tends to stand with the feet in a valgus position, with the heel everted and the forefoot turned out. As this position is not the most stable for walking or running, the child will toe in to shift the center of gravity toward the center of the foot.

LEG PROBLEMS

- *Internal tibial torsion:* Internal tibial torsion is a common cause of in toeing. It is the most likely result of intrauterine positioning and is accentuated by infants sleeping prone. The simplest clinical examination of tibial torsion is comparison of the relative positions of the medial and lateral malleoli while the child sits with legs extended and the patellae pointing straight ahead. Normally, the medial malleolus sits anterior to the lateral malleolus in the transmalleolar axis. Fortunately, it gets corrected with due course of time. Splints are not required.
- *Knock knees:* The children with knock-knees develop toe in to maintain body's center of gravity centrally.
- *Tibia vara:* Bilateral tibia vara results in toeing in.
- *Bow legs:* The children with bow legs develop toeing in when they walk.

HIP PROBLEMS

- *Femoral anteversion:* In this situation, the head of femur assumes a more anteriorly directed angle as it sits in the acetabulum. Toeing in is the result of an effort to make hips more stable while walking. On examination, with the legs extended and the pelvis flat, there is excessive internal rotation (>80) and limited external rotation (<30) of the hips. Femoral anteversion may be associated with developmental dysplasia of hip, Perthes disease, congenital talipes equinovarus, etc. This entity is more common in girls with toeing in after the age of 3 years.
- *Paralytic conditions (muscle force imbalance):* Cerebral palsy, sequelae following poliomyelitis, and myelomeningocele are conditions associated with toeing in.
- Spasticity of internal rotation of the hip is common in children with cerebral palsy.
- Maldirection of the acetabulum in which acetabulum is directed anteriorly, the child develops toeing in and swings the femoral head back into the hip joint for stability.

96 Toeing Out

INTRODUCTION

Toeing out is a less common problem than toeing in. In most children, toeing out is a result of intrauterine position. Hardly, there is a pathological condition associated with toeing out, and therefore requires no therapy.

FOOT PROBLEMS

- *Talipes calcaneovalgus:* In this deformity, the foot is extremely dorsiflexed and elevated, but it is flexible. There is rapid correction with passive exercise in infancy.
- *Everted flatfeet:* The children with hypermobile, pronated feet may stand in toeing out position, when they walk they tend to toe in to improve the center of gravity.
- *Triceps surae muscle contracture:* Children with cerebral palsy have toeing out because of spasticity affecting the triceps surae muscles (gastrocnemius and soleus). The foot is held in an equines position.
- *Vertical talus (rocker-bottom foot):* The forefoot is abducted and dorsiflexed. They have congenital vertical talus and flatfoot.

LEG PROBLEMS

- *External tibial torsion:* It may be congenital or acquired. The medial malleolus lies much more anterior to the lateral malleolus (more than normal 5-15). External tibial torsion may be a consequence of femoral anteversion, in which external rotation of hip is restricted, or of contracture of the iliotibial band in which the internal rotation of the hip is limited.
- *Congenital absence or hypoplasia of fibula:* It is uncommon congenital condition. There is shortening of the peroneal and triceps surae muscles resulting in bowing of tibia and equinovalgus of the foot. The lateral malleolus is absent.

HIP PROBLEMS

- *Femoral retroversion:* It is very rare. The retroverted position of the femoral head results in limited internal rotation and excessive external rotation of the hip.
- Flaccid paralysis of the internal rotators of the hip
- *Physiological rotation in newborns:* Newborns, whose intrauterine position was cross-legged, have a relative external rotation contracture of the hips. When the legs are extended, the toes will point out. It improves rapidly with age.
- *Maldirection of the acetabulum:* The acetabulum may face posteriorly, resulting in outward turning of the leg.
- *Slipped capital femoral epiphysis (SCFE):* It is most common in obese adolescent boys. There is unilateral toeing out with painful hip.

97 Umbilicus—Abnormalities

INTRODUCTION

Normally, umbilicus is located at the midpoint of the line joining the tip of xiphoid process and symphysis pubis. It is retracted and inverted. Everted umbilicus may be due to gross distention of abdomen like ascites or organomegaly. It may be grossly inverted in obesity. Transverse umbilicus (smiling umbilicus) is a sign of ascites. In neonates, look for umbilical sepsis, umbilical granuloma, or any fistulae.

UMBILICAL HERNIA (FIG. 1)

Umbilical hernia is a common pediatric condition. The majority of umbilical hernias spontaneously resolve by 2 years of age. Very few children with umbilical hernia may require surgery if it persists or gets obstructed.

Causes of umbilical hernia:
- Normal variant
- Diastasis recti abdominis (rectus muscles separated laterally) (very common)
- Hypothyroidism
- Mucopolysaccharidosis (MPS)
- Down syndrome
- Beckwith-Wiedemann syndrome.

Umbilical hernia should be differentiated from following conditions as they require different modes of management.

- *Supraumbilical and infraumbilical hernia (Fig. 2)*: Supraumbilical hernia is a hernia just above the umbilicus, specific type of epigastric hernia rather than a type of umbilical hernia. Supraumbilical hernia is very unlikely to resolve spontaneously at any age and surgical correction is usually

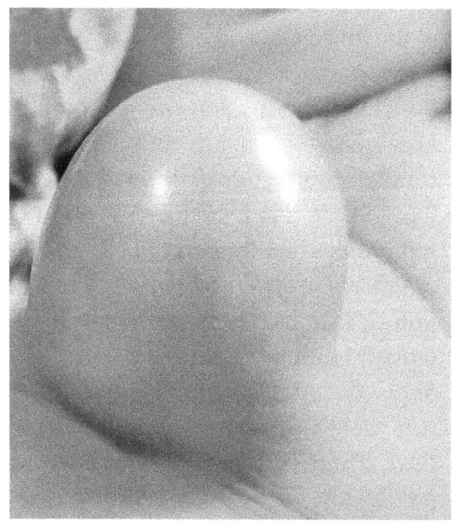

Fig. 1: Umbilical hernia.

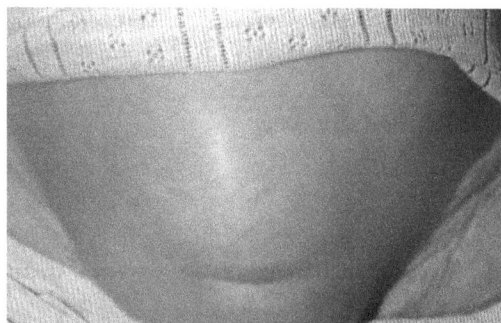

Fig. 2: Supraumbilical hernia.

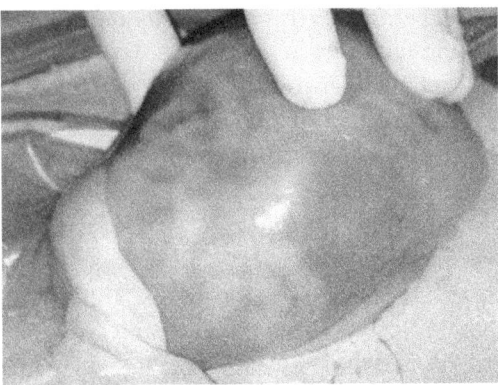

Fig. 3: Omphalocele.

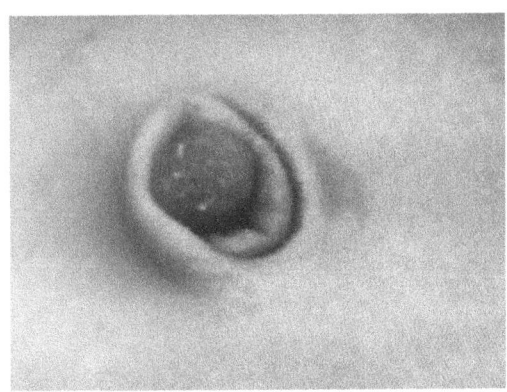

Fig. 5: Umbilical granuloma.

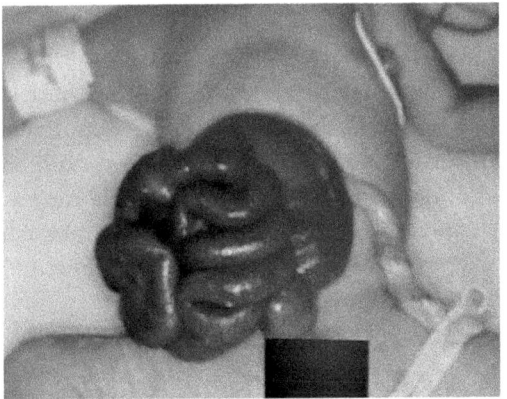

Fig. 4: Gastroschisis.

recommended. Similarly, infraumbilical hernia can also occur.
- *Omphalocele* (**Fig. 3**): Omphalocele, also known as exomphalos, is a birth defect of the abdominal wall. The intestines, liver, or other organs stick outside the abdomen through the umbilicus. The organs are covered in a thin, nearly transparent sac that hardly ever is open or broken. There is herniation of abdominal contents into umbilical cord, covered by peritoneum not by skin. It is often associated with genetic syndromes. It requires surgery.
- *Gastroschisis* (**Fig. 4**): The umbilical cord is intact in gastroschisis. There is evisceration of bowel through a defect in the abdominal wall, usually found on the right side of the cord without any overlying membrane. It needs surgery.
- *Umbilical granuloma* (**Fig. 5**): The umbilical cord usually dries and separates within 6-8 days after birth. The raw surface becomes covered by a thin layer of skin, scar tissue forms, and then it is usually healed within 10-14 days. Mild infection or incomplete epithelization may result in a moist granulating area at the base of the cord with a mucoid or mucopurulent discharge. Good results are usually obtained by cleansing with alcohol several times a day. The granuloma may be cauterized with silver nitrate, repeated at interval of several days until the base is dry. Some Indian pediatricians have experience of application of common salt crystals with good results.
- *Umbilical polyp* (**Fig. 6**): Umbilical granuloma must be differentiated from umbilical polyp, a rare anomaly resulting from persistence of all or part of the omphalomesenteric duct or the urachus. The tissue of the polyp is firm, bright red, and a mucoid secretion. The polyp is communicating with ileum or

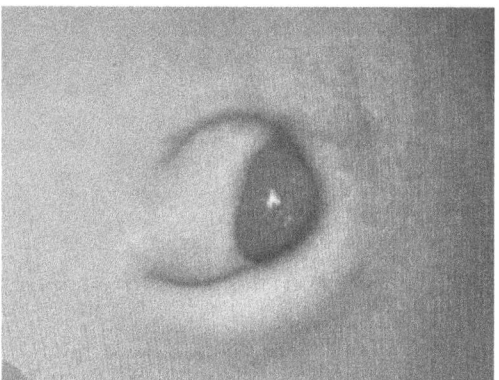

Fig. 6: Umbilical polyp.

bladder. Histologically, the polyp consists of intestinal or urinary tract mucosa. Treatment is surgical excision of the omphalomesenteric or urachal remnant.
- *Hemorrhage from umbilical cord:* Hemorrhage from umbilical cord may be the result of trauma, loose ligation of the cord, or failure of normal thrombus formation. It may also indicate hemorrhagic disease of the newborn, factor XIII deficiency, or local infection. Patients with factor XIII deficiency usually present with prolonged umbilical stump bleeding. Delayed fall of umbilical cord is known to occur in factor XIII deficiency.

DELAYED SEPARATION OF UMBILICAL CORD

Umbilical cord separation usually occurs between 7 and 14 days of life. Separation of umbilical cord occurring after 3 weeks of life is considered as abnormal, delayed separation.

Causes of delayed separation of umbilical cord:
- Prematurity
- Neonatal sepsis
- Excess use of antiseptic to clean the umbilical cord, probably it prevents normal colonization of umbilicus and delays its separation.
- *Immunodeficiencies:*
  - Leukocyte adhesion defect (LAD)
  - Defective gamma interferon
- Histiocytosis X
- Factor XIII deficiency.

SINGLE UMBILICAL ARTERY

A normal umbilical cord consists of one umbilical vein, which later becomes ligamentum teres, and two umbilical arteries, which become the lateral umbilical ligaments. One-third of infants with single umbilical artery have associated congenital anomalies. It is recommended that number of umbilical arteries should be examined and documented in each baby at the time of birth.

Associated malformations with single umbilical artery:
- *Genitourinary (33%):* Renal agenesis, dysgenesis, hypoplasia, ambiguous genitalia
- *Musculoskeletal (37%):* Club foot, vertebral anomalies
- *Cardiovascular (30%):* Patent ductus arteriosus (PDA), ventricular septal defect (VSD), dextrocardia
- *Gastrointestinal (28%):* Imperforate anus, tracheoesophageal fistula
- *Respiratory (9%):* Pulmonary hypoplasia
- Trisomy 18.

98. Unequal Pupils

INTRODUCTION

Unequal pupils (anisocoria) may be physiologic or due to underlying disease of the eye or central nervous system (CNS). It may be difficult at times to decide which eye is abnormal, the larger or the smaller. The associated symptoms and signs are important clues to decide it. For complete evaluation, help of a pediatric ophthalmologist is essential. About 20% of the people, who may have some degree of anisocoria, should be kept in mind before extensive evaluation for ophthalmic or CNS disorder.

COMMON CAUSES OF UNEQUAL PUPILS (ANISOCORIA)

- Unequal pupil size is found in about 20% of population.
- *Familial trait:* Some varieties of anisocoria may be inherited as an autosomal dominant trait. Other family members should be examined for the same.
- *Sporadic occurrence:* Some degree of anisocoria is common and no pathologic importance.
- *Ocular causes:*
  - Anisometropia: When acuity of vision is different in both the eyes, the more myopic eye may have a large pupil.
  - Amblyopia: When binocular fusion fails, there is suppression of visual image from one eye and the pupils may be unequal.
  - Blindness: Unequal papillary size is common with blindness.
  - Ocular trauma: The pupil may be mydriatic following injury.
  - Corneal abrasion
  - Keratitis: Herpes simplex is a common cause.
  - Cataract
  - Iritis
  - Glaucoma
- *CNS disorders:*
  - Horner syndrome:
    - Miosis, ptosis, and decreased facial sweating on affected side are the common manifestations.
    - Birth injury affecting brachial plexus is the most common cause.
    - Trauma, cervical rib, enlarged cervical lymph nodes, mediastinal lesions, and thyroid disorders are other causes of Horner syndrome.
  - Hutchinson pupil: The dilated pupil results from third nerve compression, commonly due to supratentorial tumor or hematoma.
  - Adie pupil (tonic pupil): The pupil reacts slowly or not at all the light. The accommodation reflex is also slow. The most common causes are varicella, herpes zoster and familial dysautonomia involving ciliary ganglia.
  - Encephalitis and meningitis
  - Migraine: may be due to III nerve involvement.

- Epilepsy
- Multiple sclerosis (rare in children)
- *Parinaud syndrome:* The pupil does not react to light, but accommodation reflex is present. The associated signs may be paresis of upward gaze, nystagmus and eyelid retraction. Parinaud syndrome indicates involvement of mid brain and common cause are hydrocephalus and pineal tumor.

- *Drugs and toxins:*
  - Miotic or mydriatic and cycloplegic drugs
  - Atropine aerosolized in treatment of bronchial asthma
  - Scopolamine in patches used to reduce vomiting children who are on chemotherapy. The children may touch it and then rub into the eyes.
  - Organophosphates.

Upper Gastrointestinal Bleeding

CHAPTER 99

INTRODUCTION

Gastrointestinal (GI) bleeding is quite alarming and a frightening condition. It is an emergency which requires urgent attention and prompt action.

Gastrointestinal bleeding can be classified into two, depending on the site of pathology:
1. *Upper GI bleeding:* Proximal to the ligament of Treitz (duodenojejunal junction)
2. *Lower GI bleeding:* Distal to the ligament of Treitz.

MANIFESTATIONS OF UPPER GASTROINTESTINAL BLEED

- Hematemesis (vomiting of fresh blood)
- Melenemesis (vomiting of altered blood)
- Melena (passage of black, tarry, sticky, and offensive loose stools).

Hematemesis

Presence of blood in the vomiting is called hematemesis. It should not be confused with hemoptysis (blood in sputum).

Differences between Hemoptysis and Hematemesis

	Hemoptysis	Hematemesis
Appearance of blood	Bright red and frothy	Coffee ground mixed with food
Preceding symptom	Cough	Vomiting
Associated symptoms	• Cough with expectoration • Fever	• Abdominal pain • Vomiting
Following day	Rusty sputum	Black, tarry, sticky, and offensive stools (melena)

Melena

- Passage of black, tarry, sticky, and offensive stool is termed melena. Black stool due to oral iron therapy should be differentiated from melena. Black stool due to oral iron is nonsticky, well-formed stool, and may be associated with constipation.
- With bleeding from upper GI tract, hydrochloric acid in the stomach converts hemoglobin to acid hematin. Blood should enter the colon slowly so that the colonic bacteria can convert the hematin into hemochromogens, which are black.
- Massive bleeding from upper GI tract; hardly passed blood may be fresh looking and not melena.
- It takes about 14 hours for blood to be broken down within the intestinal lumen. Therefore, if transit time is >14 hours, the patient will have melena.
- Melena can persist for 4–7 days after treating the source of bleeding.

- Blood in the intestine for longer periods of time leads to elevated blood urea levels.
- The minimum quantity of blood required to produce melena is 50 mL.
- The melena can be confirmed by stool examination for occult blood for 3 consecutive days.
- Other causes of black stool: Oral iron therapy, lead, spinach, beets, blueberries, etc.

Examination of Stool for Occult Blood

- Stop iron for 5-7 days prior to test, if the child is on oral iron therapy.
- Stop nonsteroidal anti-inflammatory drugs (NSAIDs) and aspirin before the test.
- Meat should not be consumed for 2-3 days before the test.
- Liquid stool is desirable for the test.
- If the test for occult blood is positive with only outer layer of stool, site of bleeding is likely to be lower GI tract and if it is positive with only core of stool, it indicates upper GI bleeding.
- Test should be performed for 3 consecutive days.
- Vitamin C can give false-negative test.

COMMON CAUSES OF UPPER GASTROINTESTINAL BLEEDING

- Swallowed maternal blood in newborns
- Hemorrhagic disease of newborn
- Gastritis, peptic ulcer (drug induced, inflammation)
- Drug induced: NSAIDs, aspirin, steroids, and anticoagulants
- Esophageal varices (portal hypertension)
- Chronic liver disease (coagulopathy)
- Generalized bleeding tendency
- Cow's milk protein allergy
- Stress ulcer (Curling's ulcer): Septicemia, burns
- Vascular malformation in esophagus
- Malrotation
- Mallory-Weiss syndrome.

CHAPTER 100: Urticaria (Hives)

INTRODUCTION

Urticaria is divided into two categories—acute and chronic. Acute urticaria lasts <6 weeks, while chronic urticaria is present or recurs for >6 weeks. Urticaria is characterized by the presence of wheals that come and go and are pruritic. Individual lesions usually last <4 hours, although they may persist for 24–48 hours. Longer lasting urticarial lesions suggest vasculitis or hereditary angioedema. The wheals vary in size, ranging from a few millimeters to many centimeters. There may be even giant urticaria covering large areas. At times, the central area of lesions may take on a dusky hue, suggesting target-like lesions, which should not be mistaken for erythema multiforme. There may or may not be other associated signs and symptoms associated with urticaria. Immunogenic and nonimmunogenic mechanisms may be involved.

COMMON CAUSES OF URTICARIA

- *Drugs:* Drug reactions are the most common causes of urticaria. Almost any drug is potential offender. Penicillins, nonsteroidal anti-inflammatory drugs, aspirin sulfas, analgesics, chloroquine, hormones, and diuretics are common to cause urticaria. Aspirin may be responsible for the exacerbation of chronic urticaria. The effects of aspirin may last for few weeks.
- *Foods:* Foods are another common cause of acute urticaria. The causative factor may be food protein, color, or an added preservative. The common foods are nuts, milk, fish, tomatoes, strawberries, yeasts, naturally occurring salicylates, citric acid, dyes, benzoic acid, etc. Often more than one food may be responsible for it.
- *Infections and infestations:*
  - Streptococcal infection
  - Viral hepatitis
  - Infectious mononucleosis
  - Adenovirus
  - Coxsackievirus
  - Mycoplasma
  - Giardia
  - Hookworm
  - Roundworm
  - Malaria
  - Giardiasis
  - Scabies
  - Insect bites
  - Mosquito bites
  - Scorpion bites
- Physical factors (dermatographia, cholinergic factors)
- Cold
- Pressure
- Solar
- Allergic rhinitis
- Bronchial asthma
- Systemic diseases (lymphoma, malignancies, autoimmune thyroiditis, hyperthyroidism, etc.)
- Psychogenic urticaria
- Angioedema
- Anaphylaxis.

Vomiting

INTRODUCTION

Vomiting is defined as forceful expulsion of stomach contents, usually associated with contraction of abdominal muscles.

VOMITING REFLEX

Vomiting is a highly coordinated reflex. Usually, it is preceded by increased salvation and begins with involuntary retching. Violent descent of the diaphragm and contraction of the abdominal muscles with relaxation of the gastric cardia actively force gastric contents into the esophagus. This process is coordinated by the vomiting center in the medulla, which is influenced by the afferent innervation and indirectly by the chemoreceptor trigger zone (CTZ) and higher central nervous system (CNS) centers.

REGURGITATION

Vomiting should be differentiated from regurgitation. Regurgitation is passive expulsion of stomach contents. It is a normal phenomenon in infants due to poor lower esophageal sphincter tone. As the tone improves with the age, regurgitation decreases and gradually disappears. It may be due to aerophagia, ingestion of air while feeding, especially with bottle feeding. The child does not develop dehydration, gains weight, and remains playful inspite of regurgitation. It does not require any investigation or medicine. Parents should be explained for proper feeding technique and burping. Reassurance to the parents is important.

VOMITING AND RED FLAGS

- *Persistent/severe vomiting:* It may be a manifestation of preicteric/anicteric hepatitis. Persistent and severe vomiting in a diagnosed case of hepatitis is considered as one of the danger signs for hepatic failure.
- *Suspected surgical abdomen* (intestinal obstruction, appendicitis, pancreatitis): It requires urgent surgical evaluation.
- Bilious vomiting should be considered as red flag sign.
- *Cushing triad* (Bradycardia, hypertension, and irregular respiration), along with vomiting, highly suggests raised intracranial pressure (ICP). It is an emergency for proper diagnosis and management.
- *Failure to thrive (FTT):* FTT warrants urgent Ixs for renal tubular disorders, chronic renal failure (CRF), inborn errors of metabolism (IEM), adrenal gland disorders, etc.

EVALUATION

Age

- Vomiting in neonates may be due to faulty feeding technique, gastroesophageal reflux disease (GERD), sepsis, urinary

tract infection (UTI), IEM, and surgical conditions like necrotizing enterocolitis (NEC), intestinal obstruction, and GI tract malformations.
- In case of nonbilious, projectile vomiting in a 3–4-week-old infant, hypertrophic pyloric stenosis should be suspected. Appearance of swelling in left hypogastric area after giving the feed, which disappears after vomiting, is a classic story of hypertrophic pyloric stenosis. After the vomiting, the baby is hungry and wants to feed again. Persistent vomiting may cause hypochloremic metabolic alkalosis. It may present as FTT.
- In infants and young children gastroenteritis, UTI, acute otitis media (AOM), pneumonia, GERD, IEM, raised ICP, and surgical conditions are common.

Contents of Vomiting
- Vomitus containing food particles and nonbilious vomiting indicate pathology before the second part of duodenum. Common conditions are gastritis, hypertrophic pyloric stenosis, GERD, etc.
- Bilious vomiting: It suggests obstruction distal to ampulla of Vater. Duodenal atresia, annular pancreas, and intestinal obstruction are common causes.
- Bilious vomiting is always abnormal in neonates, suggesting serious conditions like intestinal malformation, intestinal obstruction, NEC, and sepsis. In older children, occasionally, bilious vomiting may be following multiple episodes off severe vomiting due to retrograde entry of intestinal contents into the stomach due to duodenogastric reflux.
- Presence of blood in vomitus indicates hematemesis.

Type of Vomiting
- It can be projectile or nonprojectile. Projectile vomiting is forceful where vomitus falls away. Projectile vomiting can be seen in obstructive conditions like pyrolic stenosis, annular pancreas, and malrotation. Projectile vomiting without nausea or hypersalivation is suggestive of raised ICP.
- Recurrent vomiting is seen in migraine, cyclical vomiting, motion sickness, abdominal epilepsy, psychogenic, etc.

Post-tussive Vomiting
It is common in children with pertussis and bronchial asthma.

Associated Symptoms
- Loose stool (acute gastroenteritis)
- Severe anorexia, pain in right hypochondrium, and dark colored urine (hepatitis)
- Headache, irritability, and convulsions [CNS infections like acute bacterial meningitis (ABM), tuberculous meningitis (TBM), and encephalitis]
- Fever without focus in young children and fever with urinary symptoms in older children (UTI)
- Abdominal pain (renal calculus, cholecystitis, pancreatitis, etc.)
- Constipation (intestinal obstruction)
- Polyuria, weight loss, pain in abdomen, and acidotic breathing [diabetic ketoacidosis (DKA)]

COMMON CAUSES OF VOMITING

Medical Conditions
- Faulty feeding (in infants)
- Gastroenteritis
- GERD

- Drug induced
- Hepatitis
- UTI
- Raised ICP
- DKA
- IEM
- Uremia
- Psychogenic.

Surgical Conditions

- Hypertrophic pyloric stenosis (3–4 weeks)
- Duodenal atresia, annular pancreas (bilious vomiting and scaphoid abdomen)
- Intestinal malrotation, obstruction
- Appendicitis
- Intussusceptions
- Renal colic
- Peritonitis.

Chapter 102: Weight Loss

INTRODUCTION

Significant weight loss in children is defined as loss of weight >5% of maximum weight noted in the last 3 months or failure to gain weight in past 3 months despite adequate nutrition. Transient weight loss in the course of an acute illness may not be worrisome, but weight loss >5% in the last 3 months requires careful evaluation.

Certain terminologies related to weight loss should be understood distinctly to clarify their exact meaning and related disorders.

- *Underweight:* The person whose weight is considered as too low to be healthy is considered as underweight. Dieting, frequent physical activity, high body metabolic rate, family tendency, or some illness are common causes for underweight.
- *Wasting:* It means low weight for height. It is the type of malnutrition in young children (<5 years). It suggests acute malnutrition, the result of more recent food deficit or an illness.
- *Emaciation:* It is defined as a state of extreme thinness from absence of fat and muscle mass. It is marasmus-like manifestations in older children and adults.
- *Cachexia:* It is extreme weight loss and muscle wasting with almost no fat. The person with only skin and bones is called cachexia. It is commonly associated with human immunodeficiency virus (HIV), tuberculosis, malignancy, severe hyperthyroidism, and chronic severe disease like end-stage renal disease.

Cachexia is associated with elevated cytokines—interleukin-1 (IL-1), IL-6, tumor necrosis factor (TNF), interferon V, etc.

WEIGHT LOSS IN NEONATES

A full-term, exclusively breastfed, healthy newborn loses 7–10% of the birth weight, but regains back to birth weight within 10 days to 2 weeks time. Later on, most newborns gain weight at a rate of 30 g/day in the first month.

Common Causes of Weight Loss in Neonates

- Feeding problem
- Dehydration (common in hot months in tropical countries)
- Acute infection
- Malnutrition
- Failure to thrive (FTT)
- Gastroesophageal reflux disease (GERD)
- Pyloric stenosis
- Milk protein allergy
- Child neglect
- Congenital adrenal hyperplasia
- Congenital heart disease
- Inborn errors of metabolism (IEM)
- Congenital infections [cytomegalovirus (CMV), rubella, herpes simplex virus (HSV), syphilis, tuberculosis (TB), etc.]

COMMON CAUSES OF WEIGHT LOSS IN CHILDREN

- *Physiological causes:*
  - Dieting (adolescent girls)
  - Increased physical activity
- *Gastrointestinal disorders:*
  - Gastroesophageal reflux disease
  - Chronic diarrhea
  - Inflammatory bowel disease
  - Hepatitis
  - Pancreatitis
  - Constipation
- *Malabsorption disorders:*
  - Celiac disease
  - Cystic fibrosis
  - Worm infestations (giardiasis, round worms, hook worm, etc.)
- *Metabolic causes:*
  - Diabetes mellitus
  - Diabetes insipidus
  - Hyperthyroidism
  - Addison disease
  - Hypopituitarism
  - Hypercalcemia
  - Inborn errors of metabolism
- *Cardiovascular causes:*
  - Chronic congestive cardiac failure (CCF)
  - Constrictive pericarditis
  - Infective endocarditis
- *Nutritional disorders:*
  - Protein–energy malnutrition (PEM)
  - Iron deficiency
  - Zinc deficiency
- *Neurological causes:*
  - Diencephalic syndrome
  - Chronic increased intracranial pressure
  - Hydrocephalus
  - Chronic subdural hematoma
- *Malignancy:*
  - Acute lymphocytic leukemia (ALL)
  - Lymphoma
  - Neuroblastoma
  - Wilms tumor
  - Hepatoblastoma
- *Emotional disorders:*
  - Depression
  - Anorexia nervosa
  - Bulimia
  - Rumination
- *Miscellaneous:*
  - Chronic infections
  - Tuberculosis
  - Chronic inflammatory diseases
  - Sarcoidosis
  - Chronic renal failure
  - Drugs.

Index

Page numbers followed by *f* refer to figure and *t* refer to table

A

Abdomen
  distention of 59
  generalized distention of 59
Abetalipoproteinemia 15
Abscess 69, 222
  deep neck 190
  mastoid 214
  retropharyngeal 70, 242, 256
Accessory muscles, use of 67
Acetabulum, maldirection of 267
Achalasia 66
Achondroplasia 183, 208
Acrodynia 241
Acromegaloid facies 89, 90*f*
Acromegaly 208
Active rickets, sign of 208
Adenoid facies 89, 90*f*
Adenoma sebaceum 211, 211*f*
Afibrinogenemia 26
Agarwal and Khadilkar growth charts 132
Alae nasi, flaring of 67
Alagille syndrome 91, 91*f*
Alexander disease 183
Allopurinol 181
Altered sensorium 6, 67
  causes of 8
Androgen deficiency 144
Anemia 41, 97, 159, 208, 215, 216
  acute 216
  causes of 216
  chronic 5, 208, 216
  diagnosis of 215
  grades of 215
  hemolytic 159, 216
Angiomas 70
Angularis oris muscle 86*f*
Anhidrosis, causes of 81
Anisocoria, causes of 271
Ankle jerk, delayed relaxation of 250
Anthropometry 131
Anus 64
Anxiety 224
Aorta, coarctation of 163, 250
Aortic thrombosis 163

Apert syndrome 83, 206, 254
Aqueductal stenosis 183
Arginine vasopressin, hyposecretion of 77
Arnold–Chiari malformation 16, 65, 183
Ascites 12, 73, 160
  causes of 13
  etiology of 12
  high-gradient 13
  low-gradient 13
Ash leaf 211, 211*f*
Astrocytoma 16
Ataxia 14-16, 189
  causes of 16
  telangiectasia 15, 16, 210
  toxic causes of 15
Athetosis 188
Atopic facies 90
Autoimmune disorders 26
AVPU pediatric response scale 6, 7
Axillary temperature 17

B

Bacteremia 119
Barotrauma 69
Beckwith–Wiedemann syndrome 207, 260, 262
Bed wetting 76
Behcet's disease 204
Bell's palsy 85
Bematuria, asymptomatic 152
Bernard–Soulier syndrome 26
Biliary atresia 176*f*
  partial 212
Biliary obstruction 158
Biliary tract, involvement of 157
Birth defects 61
Black measles 106
Bleeding 24, 217
  abnormal 23
  disorder 23, 25, 26
  manifestations 23, 218
  site of 178
  skin lesions 24, 24*f*
  tendency 3

Blindness
  causes of 170
  congenital 170
  hysterical 171
  impairment of 170
Blood
  loss 216
  pressure, measurement of 163
Bloody diarrhea 3, 57
Bloom syndrome 210
Blue sclera 208, 208*f*
  causes of 208
Body mass index 94, 197
  chart 198*f*, 199*f*
  calculation of 197
Body temperature, measurement of 17
Bone
  diseases 83
  marrow failure 26
Boston criteria 121*t*
Bow legs 27, 265
  causes of 28
  symptoms of 28
Bowel habit 240
Bowel sounds 29, 30
  absence of 29
Brachycephaly 4
Bradycardia 232, 250
  causes of 233
Bradykinesia 188
Brain
  abscess 214
  stem, tumors of 196
  tumors 15
Brainstem 6
Branchial cleft cyst 180, 190, 191*f*
Breastfeeding
  faulty technique of 99
  problems 100
Breath
  holding spell 215
  shortness of 215
Breathing
  abnormal 68
  apneustic 68
  types of 67

Bristol stool chart 43f
Bronchiectasis 146
Brucellosis 181
Buffalo hump 250
Bulging flanks 12
Bullous myringitis 69
Burning micturition 31

C

Cachexia 3, 279
Café-au-lait
    lesions 210, 210f
    spots 210
Caffey disease 83
Canavan disease 183
Candidiasis 66
Captopril 181
Caput succedaneum 4
Carbamazepine 181
Cardiac failure, congestive 16, 219
Cardiovascular disorders 80
Cardiovascular mediated
    syncope 257
    causes of 259
Caries 212
Carotenemia 174
Carotid cavernous sinus fistula 83
Cat's eye 209, 209f
    causes of 209
Cataract 32, 209
    causes of 33
Cavernous sinus thrombosis 83
Celiac disease 250
Cells, proliferation of 157
Cellulitis 69, 190
Central nervous system 51, 52, 97, 242, 253
    infections 246
    malformations 245, 246
Cephalohematoma 4
Cephalosporins 181
Cerebellar
    ataxia, acute 14
    vermis, agenesis of 16
Cerebral
    cortex, quick evaluation of 6
    gigantism 262
    palsy 54, 65
Cerebrospinal fluid 122
Cerumen 214
Cervical rib 180
Chediak-Higashi syndrome 210
Cherry-red spot 213, 213f
    causes of 213

Chest
    abnormal shapes of 37
    emphysematous 38
    kyphoscoliotic 37f
    normal shapes of 37
    pain 35
        causes of 35, 36
    retractions 67
    shape of 37
    sounds, abnormal 67
Chiari malformation 16
Chickenpox 106
Chikungunya 110
Childhood obesity 197
    causes of 200
    risk factors of 200
Chlamydia trachomatis 84
Cholesteatoma 214
Chorea 187, 188
Choroid 171
Chromosomal disorders 34
Ciliary body 171
Circumcision 24
Cleidocranial dysostosis 208
Clubbing 40, 41
    causes of 40
    grades of 40
    mechanism of 40
Coagulation disorders 25, 26, 79
Coarse facies 87
Cognition 6
Collagen disorders 160, 252
Collagen vascular diseases 164
Colonic obstruction 30
Coma 7
Complete blood count 102, 122
    interpretation of 102
Conductive deafness 151
Congenital anomalies 15, 45
    classification of 61
Congenital hearing loss 150
    causes of 150
Congestion, vascular 252
Conjunctivitis 84
    allergic 84
    bacterial 84
    viral 84
Connective tissue disorders 97
Consciousness 7
    quick evaluation of level of 7
Constipation 42, 43
    acute 42
    causes of 45
    chronic 42
    functional 45

Convulsions 244
Corrosives 66
Cough 46, 47
    duration of 46
    etiological principles of 46
    evaluation of 46
    mechanism of 46
    pattern of 46, 47f
    reflex 46
    severe 212
Cranial meningocele 5
Cranial nerve palsy 65
Craniostenosis 5
Craniosynostosis 83
Craniotabes 207, 208f
    causes of 208
C-reactive protein 122
Cretinism 212
Cricopharyngeal incoordination 65
Cri-du-chat syndrome 206, 207, 209, 254
Crohn disease 66
Crouzon syndrome 83, 208
Cry, types of 49
Crying child 10, 48
Cushing syndrome 250
Cushingoid face 88
Cyanosis 50, 67
    causes of 51
    mechanism of 50
    peripheral 50
    types of 50
Cystic hygroma 180, 191f
Cystitis 225
Cytomegalovirus 180

D

Dacryocystitis 84f
Dandy-Walker
    malformation 16
    syndrome 5, 16, 183
Dapsone poisoning 213
Deafness 150
    sensorineural 151
Deciduous dentition 263
Deep tendon reflex 16
Degenerative diseases 15
Delayed dentition 263
    causes of 264
Dengue fever 110
Dental problems 70
Depressed nasal bridge 211, 211f
    causes of 212

Depressor anguli oris muscle,
    hypoplasia of 86
Dermatomyositis 66
    juvenile 116
Dermoid cyst 190, 191f
Development
    delayed 52
    domains of 53
    principles of 52
Diabetes
    insipidus 77, 81, 96, 225
    mellitus 77, 96, 225, 254
        gestational 197
Diamond-Blackfan syndrome 208
Diarrhea 56
    causes of 57
    chronic 57, 58
    disease
        acute 49, 57
        clinical types of 57
    persistent 57
    starvation 56
DiGeorge syndrome 206, 207
Digital clubbing 40
Digital thermometer 17
Diphtheria 146, 256
    tetanus, and pertussis
        vaccination 49
Disease-specific growth
    charts 132
Disruption 61
Disseminated intravascular
    coagulation 219
Distal phalangeal diameter 40, 41f
Diurnal enuresis, causes of 77
Dolichocephaly 4
Doll's eye phenomenon 7, 8
Double quotidian fever 22
Down syndrome 33, 205-207, 210,
    212, 254
Drooling 242
    causes of 242
Drowsy 7
Drug 26, 33, 45, 81, 118, 204, 210
    ingestion 217
    rash, with eosinophilia and
        systemic symptoms
        syndrome 118
    reaction 181
    therapy 24
Dysautonomia, familial 81
Dysentery 57
Dyskinesia 188
    drug-induced 194
Dysmorphism 61, 254

Dysphagia 65
    causes of 65
Dysplasia 62
Dyspnea 67, 95
Dystonia 188
    drug-induced 194

E

Ear 64
    discharge 214
    external 69
    trauma 69
Earache 69
Ecchymosis 25
Eccrine sweat glands 80
Ectodermal dysplasia 81, 207, 208
Ectopic ureter 77
Eczema 214
    chronic 69
Edema 12, 71, 215
    angioneurotic 73f
    generalized 72
    localized 72
    morning 73
    nonpitting 71, 71f
    pitting 71
    scrotal 243
Edward syndrome 33, 207,
    209, 254
Ehlers-Danlos syndrome 206, 208
Electrocardiogram 35
Elfin facies 88, 88f
Emaciation 279
Emotional disorders 280
Empyema 183
Encephalitis 210
Encephalocele 16, 83
Encephalomyelitis, acute
    disseminated 16
Encephalopathy 246
    hypoxic ischemic 245
Encopresis 74
    causes of 75
    classification of 74
    nonretentive 74
    primary 74
    retentive 74
    secondary 74, 75
Endocrine disorders 34, 176, 222
Enterobius vermicularis 31
Enterocolitis, necrotizing 60
Enuresis 76
    primary 76
    secondary 76

Eosinophils 102
Epicanthal fold 206, 206f
    causes of 206
Epididymitis 243
Epigastrium 2
Epiglottitis, acute 256
Epilepsy 246
Episode, duration of 245
Epistaxis 78
    causes of 79
    recurrent 78
Epstein-Barr virus 108, 203
Erythema 243
    infectiosum 109
    nodosum 118
        causes of 118
Escherichia coli 120
Esophageal duplication 65
Esophageal spasm 66
Esophageal web 66
Esophagus
    candidiasis of 201
    disorders affecting 65
Estrogen
    exogenous sources of 144
    secreting tumors 144
Eustachian tube
    dysfunction 70
    obstruction 69
Everted flatfeet 267
Exercise intolerance 215
Exophthalmos 82
Exotropia, child 254
External tibial torsion 267
Eyes 64, 218, 235
    discharge 84
    ophthalmic examination
        of 220
    slanting of 207
    upward slanting of 207f

F

Fabry disease 33, 81
Face 63
Facial measurements 63
Facial nerve paralysis
    acquired 85
    congenital 86
Facial paralysis 85
Facies 87, 218
Failure to thrive 36, 57, 92
Fanconi disease 210
Farber's disease 213
Fatigability 95, 215

Fatigue 97
  causes of 97
Fecal incontinence, categories
    of 74
Feeding
  difficulty 100
  disorders, classification of 99
  issues 99
  problems, complications
    of 100
Femoral anteversion 266
Femoral retroversion 267
Fetal alcohol syndrome 206, 209
Fever 3, 17, 19, 22, 101, 159, 160
  basics of 17
  biphasic 21, 21f
  continuous 19, 19f
  enteric 246
  factitious 22
  hectic 21
  intermittent 20f, 21
  mechanism of 18
  of short duration 101
    causes of 103
  of unknown origin 22
  pattern 22
  periodic 22
  persistent 19
  prolonged 3, 22
  recurrent 22
  relapsing 21
  remittent 19, 20f
  scarlet 111
  short duration of 102
  types of 19
  with rash 105
  without focus 119, 121, 123
Fibula, hypoplasia of 267
Flat chest 37f
Flatfeet 265
Floppy infant 124
  central causes of 126
  peripheral causes of 126
Fluid-thrill 12
Fluorosis 212
Foot problems 265, 267
Foveal vision 254
Fractures 172
Fragile X syndrome 207
Friedrich ataxia 16
Functional constipation 45
  pathogenesis of 44
Functional recurrent abdominal
    pain, clinical features
    of 239

Fungal infections 181
Funnel chest 37, 37f, 38f
Furuncle 69

G

Gait
  abnormality in 128
  antalgic 128
  ataxic 128
  circumduction 128
  disorders 127
  duck 129
  equinus 129
  festinate 129
  hemiplegic 128
  high stepping 129
  limping 128
  reeling 128
  scissoring 129
  short limb 129
  stamping 129
  tandem 128
  waddling 129
Galactosemia 32
Gangliosidosis 213
Gastrocolic reflex 56
Gastroenteritis, acute 30
Gastroesophageal reflux 241
  disease 48, 66, 70, 96, 201
Gastrointestinal bleeding 24, 273
Gastrointestinal diseases 204
Gastrointestinal disorders 98, 280
Gastrointestinal system,
    microanatomy of 56
Gastroschisis 269, 269f
Gaucher disease 210, 213
  infantile 210
Genetic microcephaly 186
Genitals 64
Genu
  valgum 28
  varum 27
Geographic tongue 202, 202f
German measles 108
Gigantism, pituitary 183
Glanzmann thrombasthenia 26
Glasgow coma scale 6, 7
Glaucoma 170
Global developmental delay,
    causes of 55
Glomerular hematuria 153
Glomerulonephritis, acute 72
Glycogen storage disease 96
Glycoprotein 26

Goiter 180
Goldberg's syndrome 213
Gonorrhea 84
Granulomatous, chronic 181
Gray matter disorders 183
Gray platelet syndrome 26
Gross hematuria 152
Group A streptococcal
    pharyngitis 118
Growth 249
  charts 131-133, 185
    interpretation of 141
  hormone 96, 262
    deficiency 249
    excess 262
  patterns, abnormal 141
  retardation 215
Guillain-Barré syndrome 16, 65,
    66, 172
Gynecomastia 143
  neonatal 143
  pathological causes of 144
  physiologic 143

H

Haemophilus influenzae 84, 120,
    256
Halitosis 145
  causes of 146
Hand-foot-and-mouth disease
    109
Harrison's sulcus 38, 38f
Head
  bobbing 67
  circumference 185, 186
  trauma 254
Headache 147, 148
  causes of 148
  types of 148
Head-to-toe assessment 63
Hearing loss 150
  acquired 151
  congenital 150
Heart
  disease, congenital 96
  failure, congestive 72, 100, 215
Heat
  loss 19
    defective 19
  production 19
Helicobacter pylori 239
Heliotrope rash 117
Hematemesis 3, 154, 273

Hematocrit 219
Hematological diseases 160
Hematological disorders 159, 160, 252
Hematoma 25
  subdural 5
Hematopoiesis, extramedullary 208
Hematuria 152
  causes of 153
  extraglomerular 153
  microscopic 152
  persistent 152
  symptomatic 152
Hemiballismus 188
Hemoglobin 219
Hemolytic facies 87, 88f
Hemophilia 83
  A 26
  B 26
Hemopoiesis 251
Hemoptysis 154, 273
  causes of 154
  true 154
  types of 154
Hemorrhage 83, 270
  intracranial 183, 245, 246
  subconjunctival 212, 212f
  vitreous 209
Hemostasis, systemic disorder of 23
Henoch–Schönlein purpura 116
Hepatic mass 3
Hepatitis
  autoimmune 212
  neonatal 176
Hepatocyte involvement, features of 156
Hepatomegaly 156, 157
  causes of 157
  classification of 156
Hepatosplenomegaly 159, 160, 218
Hernia 243
  infraumbilical 268
  supraumbilical 268, 268f
Herpangina 203
Herpes simplex 69
  virus 120
Herpes zoster 69, 70, 107
Hip problems 266, 267
Hippocratic facies 90
Histiocytic disorders 181
Histoplasmosis 118, 181
Holoprosencephaly 206
Homocystinuria 261

Horn cell, anterior 126, 173
Horse-shoe
  dullness 12
  kidney 250
Human immunodeficiency virus 96, 181
Hurler syndrome 208, 212, 213
Hydralazine 181
Hydrocele 243
Hydrocephalus 5, 16, 208, 209
  causes of 183
  congenital 83, 183
Hyperbilirubinemia
  conjugated 175
  unconjugated 175
Hyperhidrosis 80
  familial 80
Hypertelorism 205, 205f
  causes of 205
Hypertension 3, 72, 163, 250
  causes of 163
  drug-induced 164
  essential 164
  idiopathic intracranial 11
  malignant 221
  portal 157
Hyperthermia 22
Hypertrophic pyloric stenosis 30
Hypervitaminosis A 208
Hypocalcemia 245
Hypogastirum 2
Hypoglycemia 33, 245
Hypogonadism, secondary 144
Hypohidrosis 81
  causes of 81
Hypomagnesemia 245
Hypopituitarism 210
Hypoplasia 86, 86f, 209, 267
Hypotelorism 206
  causes of 206
Hypothermia 169
  causes of 169
Hypothyroidism 87f, 215, 250
  congenital 205, 212
Hypotonia 126
  assessment of 125f
  types of 124
Hypoxemia, chronic 97

I

Icterus 160
Immune thrombocytopenia purpura 212

Incontinence
  primary 75
  true 74
Indian Academy of Pediatrics 42
Infancy-childhood-puberty model 247
Infections 9, 80, 82, 97, 118, 146, 159, 160, 176, 193, 203, 222, 252
  bacterial 101, 102, 222
  congenital 32, 150
  viral 101, 181, 222
Infectious disorders 85
Infectious mononucleosis 108, 146
Inflammation 157, 171
Inflammatory bowel disease 118
Infrared radiation emission detectors 18
Infrared thermometer 17
Inner canthal distance 205, 205f
Internal tibial torsion 265
Interphalangeal diameter 40, 41f
Interstitial lung disease 97
Intestinal obstruction 29
Intestinal pseudo-obstruction 30
Intracranial aneurysm 170
Intracranial pathology 48
Intracranial pressure 9, 15, 254
Intrauterine growth restriction 94, 96, 142, 197, 249
Intrauterine infections 157
Iris, inflammation of 171
Iron deficiency 280
  anemia 208
  chronic 208
Ischemia, intestinal 29

J

Jaundice 3, 159, 174
  causes of 176
  cholestatic 175
  mistaken for 174
  neonatal 175
  recognition of 175
  uniocular 175
Jaw, tumors of 210
Jobber syndrome 16
Joints 64
Jugular venous pressure 12
Juvenile idiopathic arthritis 181
  systemic onset 114

K

Kala-azar 181
Kawasaki disease 112
Kayser–Fleischer ring 212, 212f
   causes of 212
Kernicterus 209
Kidney
   disease, chronic 26
   injury, acute 163
Klinefelter syndrome 206, 210, 261
Knock knees 28, 265
Kupffer cells 157
Kwashiorkor 12
Kyphoscoliosis 39
Kyphosis 39

L

Labyrinthitis 196
   acute 15
Lacunar skull 208
Laron dwarfism 209
Larsen syndrome 206
Laryngeal foreign body 256
Laryngeal muscles, weakness of 162
Laryngitis 162
Laryngospasm 256
Laryngotracheobronchitis, acute 255
Larynx 162
Lassitude 215
Laurence–Moon–Biedl syndrome 254
Lead poisoning 212
Leg problems 265, 267
Leonine facies 90
Leopard syndrome 83, 206
Leukemia 181, 212
   acute lymphocytic 181
Leukodystrophy, metachromatic 183, 213
Limbs
   lower 173
   upper 173
Lipomas 65
Liver 156
   cryptogenic cirrhosis of 212
   disorders 26
   span of 156
Lock jaw 209
Long philtrum 206f, 207
Lordosis 39
Low set ears 207, 207f
Lowe syndrome 33
Lower gastrointestinal bleeding 178
   causes of 179
Lump, abdominal 1
Lung abscess 146
Lycopenemia 174
Lymph node 160, 180
   characteristics of 180
Lymphadenopathy 160, 180, 190, 218
   generalized 181
   location of 181
   postauricular 70
Lymphangioma 83
Lymphocytes 102
Lymphomas 181

M

Macrocephaly 5, 182
   causes of 183
Macroglossia 184
   causes of 184
Malabsorption
   disorders 280
   syndrome 57, 58, 96f
Malformation 61
   congenital 61
Malignancy 26, 104, 159, 160, 280
   esophageal 201
Malignant disorders 158
Malnutrition 57, 97
Mandible 64
   hypoplasia of 209
Marfan syndrome 208, 254, 261
Mask-like face 90
Mass
   abdominal 1, 3
   location of 2
   lymph node 180
Mastoiditis 69
Maxilla 64
McCune–Albright syndrome 210
Measles 106
   atypical 106
   hemorrhagic 106
Mechanical injury 212
Mechanical intestinal obstruction 30
Medulloblastoma 16
Megalencephaly, causes of 183
Melena 273
Meningitis, bacterial 119, 150, 183, 214, 245
Meningococcemia 114
Mercury clinical thermometer 17
Metabolic diseases 160
Metabolic disorders 15, 32, 34, 158, 222
Metabolism, inborn error of 96, 245, 246
Metatarsus
   adductus 265
   varus 265
Methemoglobinemia 50, 51
Metoclopramide 210
Microcephaly 5, 185
   acquired 186
   causes of 186
   primary 186
   secondary 186
Micrognathia 209, 209f
   causes of 209
Micropenis 210
Micturition 76
   increased frequency of 224
Migraine 171
Mikulicz syndrome 242
Miller–Fisher syndrome 16
Mitochondrial disorders 15
Mobius syndrome 86, 254
Mongolian spots 211, 211f
Mongoloid facies 87, 87f
Monkey facies 88, 88f
Moon face 88, 88f
Mouth, disorders affecting 65
Movement disorders 187-189
   causes of 187
   evaluation of 187
   lesion of 188
Mucopolysaccharidosis 5, 33, 59, 87f, 183, 212
Multisystem genetic disorders 34
Mumps 70
Muscles 126, 173
   force imbalance 266
   spasms of 244
Muscular disorders 126, 242
Myasthenia gravis 65, 83, 254
Myelodysplastic syndrome 219
Myoclonus 188, 189
Myringitis 214

N

Nail changes 218
Nasal
   diphtheria 79
   examination 78

foreign body 79
picking 79
snuffle 67
Nausea 241
Neck masses 190
 causes of 190
Necrotizing fasciitis 113
Neoplasia 82, 85
Neoplasms 194
Nephrotic syndrome 12, 215
Nerves, peripheral 126, 173
Neuroblastoma 15, 16
Neurocardiogenic syncope 257
 causes of 258
Neurocutaneous syndromes 246
Neurodegenerative disorders 170
Neurofibroma 180, 183
Neurofibromatosis 210
Neurologic disorders 80, 196
Neuromas 65
Neurometabolic disorders 170
Neuromuscular disorders 65
Neuromuscular junction 126, 173
Niemann-Pick disease 33, 213
Nonsteroidal anti-inflammatory
 drugs 24, 79, 274
Nonsyndromic hereditary
 congenital deafness 150
Noonan syndrome 33, 205, 207,
 210, 254
Normal growth
 principles of 247
 velocity 247
North American Society
 of Pediatric
 Gastroenterology,
 Hepatology and
 Nutrition
 classification 238
Nose 64
Nuchal rigidity 193
 causes of 193
Nutritional disorders 280
Nystagmus 195
 acquired 196
 causes of 195
 congenital 195

O

Obesity 97, 164, 197, 261
 childhood 197
 constitutional 200
 primary 200
 secondary 200

Obstruction 160
Ocular anomalies 34
Ocular myopathy 254
Oculocephalic reflex 7, 8
Oculocerebrorenal syndrome 33
Oculodentodigital syndrome 206
Oculomotor nerve, congenital 253
Odynophagia 201
 causes of 201
Omphalocele 269, 269f
Ophthalmoplegia
 congenital familial external 253
 migraine 254
Opsoclonus 196
Optic
 atrophy, congenital 170
 neuritis 171, 220
 neuropathy 221
Oral cavity 236
Oral iron therapy 212
Oral ulcers 202
Orbit, osteomyelitis of 82
Orbital cellulitis 82
Orbital fossa, fracture of 83
Orbital hypertelorism 205
Orbital injury 254
Orbital tumors, primary 82
Orchitis 243
Organophosphorus
 poisoning 241
Orofacial dyskinesia 188
Oropharyngeal lesions 241
Osteogenesis imperfecta 208
Osteomyelitis, acute 172
Osteopetrosis 83, 85, 254
Otalgia 69
 primary 69
 secondary 70
Otitis externa 69, 214
Otitis media 69
 acute 69, 214
 chronic suppurative 214
Otorrhea 214
 causes of 214
Ototoxic medications 150
Outer canthal distance 205, 205f
Overflow incontinence 74
Oxycephaly 4

P

Pain
 colicky abdominal 3
 dyspeptic 239
 intensity of 239

nocturnal 239
site of 35, 239
types of 239
Palatal paralysis 65
Pallor 3, 159, 215
 causes of 215
Palmar pallor 218
Palpable lymph nodes 180
Palpebral fissure length 205
Palpitations 232
 causes of 232
Papilledema 220
 causes of 220
 signs of 220f
Papillomas 65
Paralytic ileus 29
Paresis 173
Parinaud syndrome 209
Parkinson's gait 129
Parotid gland
 abscess of 222
 swelling 222
Paroxysmal periumbilical
 pain 239
Patau syndrome 33, 207, 209
Pectus
 carinatum 37, 38f
 excavatum 37, 38f
Pedal edema, demonstration
 of 71f
Pemphigus vulgaris 204
Perichondritis 69
Peritonitis 29, 30
Pertussis 212
Petechiae 24
Pharyngitis, acute 70
Pharynx, disorders affecting 65
Phenothiazines 210
Phenylketonuria 206
Phenytoin 118, 181
Philadelphia protocol 121t
Pica 223
 complications of 223
 types of 223
Pierre-Robin syndrome 209
Pigeon chest 37, 37f, 38f
Pittsburg guidelines 121t
Plagiocephaly 4
Plague 181
Plasmodium malariae 21
Platelet 102
 disorders 25
Poisoning 241
Poliomyelitis 65, 172

Pollakiuria 224
  causes of 224
Polydipsia 226
  causes of 226
Polymorphs 102
Polyphagia 227
  causes of 227
Poor orodental hygiene 145, 212
Porphyria 212
Portal venous circulation,
    disorder of 157
Posterior fossa
  congenital anomalies of 15
  tumors 16
Potter facies 89, 89f
Potter syndrome 207
Prader-Willi syndrome 207,
    210, 254
Prematurity, retinopathy of
    170, 209
Primary enuresis 76
  causes of 77
Progeria 83, 209
Progeroid face 90, 90f
Pronated feet 265
Proptosis 82, 83
  causes of 82
Protein energy malnutrition
    59, 280
Pruritus 174, 228
  causes of 228
Pseudo-hemoptysis 154
Pseudohypertelorism 206
Pseudoparalysis 172
Pseudoptosis 229
Pseudo-strabismus 253
Pseudotumor cerebri 221
  causes of 11
Ptosis 229
  acquired 230
  acute 229
  chronic 229
  congenital 229
Puberty 249
  gynecomastia 143
Puddle sign 12
Puffy face 12, 250
Pulse 231
  examination 231
  rate 231
Purpura 24
Pycnodysostosis 83, 208
Pyrexia of unknown origin 234
  causes of 236, 237
Pyridoxine deficiency 245

Pyrogens 18
  endogenous 18
  exogenous 18

Q

Qualitative platelet function
    disorders 26

R

Rachitic rosary 38, 39f
Racial 205, 212
Radiation 33
Raised intracranial pressure 10,
    220, 246
  benign 221
Ramsay Hunt syndrome 70
Rapid breathing 68
Rash, appearance of 105
Rattling sounds 67
Readiness criteria 77
Rectal temperature 18
Recurrent abdominal pain
    238-240
  diagnostic criteria of 238
  etiology of 238
Red blood cells production 216
Red flag signs 234, 238
Reference growth charts 132
Reflex
  immaturity of 209
  vasodepressor 258
Regurgitation 276
Renal artery
  stenosis 163
  thrombosis 163
Renal failure, chronic 96
Renal malformations,
    congenital 163
Renal tubular acidosis 96
Respiratory signs 68
Respiratory tract infection,
    lower 103
Retentive postures 44, 44f
Retinal detachment 209
Retinal hemorrhage 221
Retinitis pigmentosa 170
Retinoblastoma 209, 209f
Retraction chest, unilateral 37f
Reye's syndrome 158, 246
Rhabdomyosarcoma 70, 210
Rhinitis
  allergic 79
  chronic 145

Rickets 5, 83, 208
Rickettsial diseases 113
Risus sardonicus 89, 89f
Rochester criteria 121t
Rocker-bottom foot 267
Romberg sign 14
Rubella 108
  syndrome, congenital 86, 108
Rubinstein-Taybi syndrome 206,
    207, 254

S

Salivary ducts, obstruction of 242
Salivation 241
  Salivation disorders 241
Sandhoff disease 213
Sarcoidosis 83, 97, 118, 181
Scalp hair 63
Scaphocephaly 4
Scleroderma 66
Scorbutic rosary 38
Scrotal pain, acute 243
Scurvy 83, 172
Secondary enuresis 76
  causes of 77
Seizures 9, 244, 245, 258
  causes of 245
  provoked 245
  types of 245
  unprovoked 245
Sepsis, neonatal 120
Septic arthritis 172
Septo-optic dysplasia 170
Setting sun sign 209, 209f
Shagreen patch 210, 210f
Shield-like chest 39, 39f
Shock 215
Short philtrum 207
Short stature 247, 250
  causes of 250
  familial 249
  pathological 250
Sialadenitis
  chronic 222
  recurrent 222
Siarlorrhea 242
Sick appearance 3
Sickle cell arthropathy 173
Single isolated fever spike 22
Single umbilical artery 270
Sinus, infected 180
Sinusitis 70
Sjögren syndrome 66, 81, 242
Sjögren-Larsson syndrome 206

Skeletal disease 170
Skeleton 64
   muscular disorders 194
Skin 64
   changes 218
   rashes, types of 105
Skull 63
   abnormal shapes of 4, 4f
   bossing of 208
   normal shapes of 4f
   towering of 4
Slipped capital femoral epiphysis 267
Small bowel obstruction, acquired 30
Snoring 67
Soft splenomegaly 251
Soto's syndrome 183, 206, 262
Sounds, abnormal 67
Space-occupying lesions 183
Spasmus nutans 196
Speech delay 54
Spermatic cord torsion 243
Spermatocele 243
Spinal cord, upper 196
Spleen, functions of 251
Splenic abscesses, causes of 252
Splenomegaly 3, 12, 251
   causes of 251
Spranger's disease 213
Sputum 47
Standard growth charts 132
Staphylococcus aureus 84, 120
Stereotype 189
Sternocleidomastoid muscle 67
Steroid face 88, 88f
Stiff neck 193
Stool
   examination of 274
   patterns 42
Strabismus 253, 254
   acquired 254
   causes of 253
   congenital 253
   true congenital 253
   types of 253
Straight leg raising test 2
Streptococcus pneumoniae 120
Stress
   emotional 241
   role of 239
Stridor 67, 255
   acute 256
   causes of 256
   chronic 256
Stroke, posterior circulation 16

Strychnine poisoning 210
Stupor 7
Sturge–Weber syndrome 82
Sulfhemoglobinemia 50
Sulfonamides 118, 181
Sunflower cataract 33
Suppurative infections, acute 222
Sweat glands 80
Sweating 80
   absence of 235
   excessive 80
Swelling
   abdominal 1
   scrotal 243
Syncope 257, 258
   neurocardiogenic 257
   types of 257
   vasovagal 215
Syndromic hereditary congenital deafness 150
Syphilis 181, 204
   congenital 172, 208, 212
Systemic diseases 9
Systemic disorders 153
Systemic lupus erythematosus 72, 115, 173, 181

T

Tachycardia 231
   causes of 231
   relative 235
Tachypnea 67
Talipes
   calcaneovalgus 267
   equinovarus 265
Tall stature 260
   constitutional 261
Tay-Sachs disease 183, 213
Teeth
   discoloration of 212, 264
   disorders of 263
Teething 241, 263
Telecanthus 206, 206f
   causes of 206
Temporal artery thermometer 18
Temporal bone
   anomaly 150
   neoplasma 70
Temporomandibular joint
   arthritis 209
   dysfunction 70
Testicular tumors 243
Testis, torsion of 243

Tetanus 209, 214
Tetracycline therapy 212
Thalassemia major 5, 206, 208, 212
Thrombocytopenia 25, 79
   causes of 26
   purpura 24
Thrombotic microangiopathy 26
Thyroglossal cyst 180, 190, 190f
Thyroid
   abscess 180
   swelling 180
Thyroiditis 180
Thyrotoxicosis 254
Tibia vara 265
Tiredness 215
Toe walking 129
Toilet training 76
Tonic-clonic seizure, generalized 244
Tonsillitis 70, 146
Tourette syndrome 189
Toxins 33, 81, 241
Tracheoesophageal fistula 65
Transient hematuria 152
Trauma 9, 33, 79, 83, 162, 171, 196, 201, 210, 212, 243, 256
Traumatic oral ulcers 203
Treacher–Collins syndrome 207, 209
Tremor 188, 189
Trendelenburg gait 129
Triangular face 89
Triceps surae muscle contracture 267
Trigonocephaly 4, 206
Trisomy 33, 205-207, 209
Tuberculosis 96, 118, 204, 219
   orbital 82
Tuberculous meningitis 183, 214
Tuberous sclerosis 183, 210
Tumors 70, 85, 183, 222, 254
   esophageal 65
   mediastinal 65
   metastatic 82
   secondary 82
   vascular 82
Turner syndrome 33, 83, 205-207, 250, 254
Tympanic membrane perforation 214
Tympanic thermometer 18
Tympanostomy tube drainage 214

U

Ulcers
　acute 202
　chronic 202
　recurrent 203
Umbilical cord 270
　delayed separation of 270
Umbilical granuloma 269, 269f
Umbilical hernia 268, 268f
　causes of 268
Umbilical polyp 269, 270f
Umbilicus, abnormalities 268
Unconsciousness 7
Undernutrition 249
Underweight 279
Unequal pupils, causes of 271
Upper gastrointestinal
　　　bleeding 273
　causes of 274
　manifestations of 273
Upper respiratory tract 236
　infection 49, 103
Uremia, hepatic 246
Urethral valve, posterior
　　　circulation 225
Urinary bladder outlet
　　　obstruction 77
Urinary symptoms 3, 243
Urinary tract infection 22, 44, 77,
　　　95, 103, 119, 224

Urticaria 275
　causes of 275
Uveitis 171

V

Varicella 106
　neonatal 107
　syndrome, congenital 107
Varicocele 243
Vascular disorders 82, 254
Vascular malformations 191
Vasoconstriction, peripheral 215
Vertical talus 267
Vertigo, benign paroxysmal 196
Vestibular system, disorders
　　　affecting 196
Vincent's angina 146
Vision
　impairment of 170
　loss of 170, 221
　sudden loss of 171
Vitamin K deficiency 26
Voice
　hoarseness of 161
　mechanism 161
　organs 161
　overusing of 162
Vomiting 276
　causes of 277
　contents of 277
　post-tussive 277

　reflex 276
　types of 277
von Willebrand disease 26

W

Waardenburg syndrome 206
Watery diarrheal disease 57
Weight loss 279
　causes of 279, 280
Werdnig-Hoffman disease 65
Wheezing 67, 68
White blood cell 122
White matter disorders 183
WHO growth charts 132
Whooping cough 212
Williams syndrome 205, 206, 254
Wilson disease 159, 212
Wolff-Parkinson-White
　　　syndrome 36
Wolman disease 213

Y

Yellow sclera 174

Z

Zinc deficiency 280

EU GSPR Authorised Reprsentative
Logos Europe, 9 rue Nicolas Poussin
1700, La Rochelle, France
Phone: +33 (0) 6 67 93 73 78
E-mail: contact@logoseurope.eu

www.ingramcontent.com/pod-product-compliance
Ingram Content Group UK Ltd.
Pitfield, Milton Keynes, MK11 3LW, UK
UKHW050456150426
5217IPUK00025B/1715